Partnerships for women's health

Partnerships for women's health

Striving for best practice within the UN Global Compact

EDITED BY MARTINA TIMMERMANN
AND MONIKA KRUESMANN

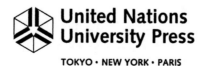

United Nations University Press

TOKYO · NEW YORK · PARIS

The views expressed in this publication are those of the authors and do not necessarily reflect the views of the United Nations University.

United Nations University Press
United Nations University, 53-70, Jingumae 5-chome, Shibuya-ku, Tokyo 150-8925, Japan
Tel: +81-3-5467-1212   Fax: +81-3-3406-7345
E-mail: sales@unu.edu   general enquiries: press@unu.edu
http://www.unu.edu

United Nations University Office at the United Nations, New York
2 United Nations Plaza, Room DC2-2062, New York, NY 10017, USA
Tel: +1-212-963-6387   Fax: +1-212-371-9454
E-mail: unuony@unu.edu

United Nations University Press is the publishing division of the United Nations University.

Cover design by Curtis Christophersen

Printed in the United States of America

ISBN 978-92-808-1185-8

Library of Congress Cataloging-in-Publication Data

Partnerships for women's health : striving for best practice within the UN Global Compact / edited by Martina Timmermann and Monika Kruesmann.
    p. ;   cm.
  Includes bibliographical references and index.
  ISBN 978-9280811858 (pbk.)
  1. Women—Health and hygiene. 2. Women—Health and hygiene—India. 3. Global Compact. I. Timmermann, Martina. II. Kruesmann, Monika.
  [DNLM: 1. Global Compact. 2. Women's Health. 3. Developing Countries. 4. International Cooperation. WA 309 P273 2009]
  RA564.85.P367   2009
  362.1082—dc22   2009041596

CONTENTS

FIGURES

TABLES

BOXES

CONTRIBUTORS

Moazzam Ali, a physician by training, is currently assistant professor at the Department of Global Health Policy, Institute of International Health at the Graduate School of Medicine, University of Tokyo, from where he also received his doctorate in public health. Prof. Ali has also earned master's degrees in public health and in business administration.

Rama V. Baru, Centre of Social Medicine and Community Health, Jawaharlal Nehru University, New Delhi, is an expert on health policy, international health, privatisation of health services and inequalities in health. Prof. Baru is the author of *Private Health Care in India: Social Characteristics and Trends* (Sage), the regional editor of *South Asia for Global Social Policy* (Sage), and an acclaimed advisor to the Government of India, the WHO, and the Indian Council for Medical Research.

Kai Bethke has been UNIDO's regional director for Mexico, Central America and the Caribbean since November 2007. He joined UNIDO in 2000 as head of both the public private partnership and corporate social responsibility (CSR) Programmes, which support small and medium-sized enterprises (SMEs) in developing countries through fostering cooperation with large buyers from the economic sector.

Manuela Bösendorfer is working as a consultant at UNIDO in Vienna, Austria.

Judith Bueno de Mesquita is currently a part-time teacher in the School of Law at Essex University. From 2001–2008 she was a senior research officer in the Human Rights Centre, in support of the mandate of the UN Special Rapporteur on *the right to the highest attainable standard of health*, Paul Hunt.

Anu Chopra holds Masters degrees in Business Administration and Sociology. She worked with GTZ for nearly two decades. Currently Ms. Chopra is a business developer and M&E specialist with expert experience in financial management, project management, monitoring & evaluation, and public private partnerships (PPP) in the context of development cooperation.

Iris J. Driessle studied business administration at the Ludwig Maximilian University in Munich. After postgraduate studies on the commonwealth, she continued her academic career as a research assistant at the Institute for Social and Health Economics, Munich. Her current research focuses on rural development and the paradigm shift in the pharmaceutical industry.

Nirmal Kumar Ganguly is the Boston University 2008 Distinguished Visiting Scholar in Global Health. Prior to that, he served as director-general at the Indian Council of Medical Research, New Delhi. Among many eminent positions in the Indian scientific community, Prof. Ganguly serves as senior advisor to the Health Minister and advisor to the Secretary of the Department of Biotechnology of the Government of India.

Arabinda Ghosh is the joint director of the Administrative Training Institute, Government of West Bengal, India. Dr. Ghosh has a PhD in Economics and a Masters in Development Management from the Asian Institute of Management, Manila, Philippines. An acclaimed master trainer, he published *Training of Trainers Manual on Human Development* which was a Planning Commission-UNDP sponsored project.

Christina Gradl is a doctoral candidate at the Department for Business and Ethics, Martin Luther University Halle-Wittenberg, Germany. She was awarded the first Kofi Annan Fellowship in Global Governance during which she worked and studied at KARL STORZ GmbH & Co. KG, the UNGC office in New York and Harvard University.

Jörg Hartmann heads GTZ's Centre for Cooperation with the Private Sector. The centre initiates partnerships with business in developing countries. It is the focal point of the German Global Compact Network and works on behalf of the German Ministry of Economic Cooperation and Development.

Paul Hunt served as UN Special Rapporteur on *the right to the highest attainable standard of health* (2002–2008) and Rapporteur of the UN Committee on Economic, Social and Cultural Rights (1999–2002). A professor at the University of Essex (UK) and an adjunct professor at the University of Waikato (New Zealand), Prof. Hunt was one of the authors of OHCHR's *Principles and Guidelines for a Human Rights Approach to Poverty Reduction Strategies*.

A. Kurian Joseph is director of the Joseph Nursing Home in Chennai, India. Among his many professional activities, Prof. Joseph serves as deputy secretary-general of the Asia and Oceania Federation of Obstetrics and Gynaecology (AOFOG) (2007–2009), as co-chair of the Indian Association of Gynaecological Endoscopists (2009) and as board member of the International Society of Gynecological Endoscopy (2007–2011).

Diana Kraft is the project manager of the GTZ Strengthening partnerships and networks for sustainable and renewable energy project. From 2006 to 2007 she managed development partnerships (PPP) in India, the Philippines and Mongolia for GTZ. From 2004 to 2005 she was a research fellow and project manager at the Department for Economic Ethics, Martin Luther University Halle-Wittenberg.

Alka Kriplani is unit head in the Department of Obstetrics & Gynaecology at AIIMS, New Delhi, India. As of 2009, Prof. Kriplani is vice-president of FOGSI (Federation of Obstetricians and Gynaecological Societies of India) and editor of the *Asian Journal of Obst & Gynae Practice* (AJOG).

Monika Kruesmann is a PhD student in the Department of International Relations, London School of Economics and Political Science, and was formerly Assistant Director in the Australian Government Department of Education. She holds a Master of Arts (International Relations) from the Australian National University, and has worked and studied in India, the Pacific region, London and Tokyo.

Peter Laser has been Director of International Business Development at KARL STORZ GmbH & Co. KG in Tuttlingen, Germany since 2006. He is the CSR Manager and responsible for all activities related to KARL STORZ's membership in the United Nations Global Compact. From 1998 to 2005 he served as country director of KARL STORZ Endoscopy India Pvt. Ltd. in India.

Klaus M. Leisinger is the president and chief executive officer of the Novartis Foundation for Sustainable Development. From 2005 to 2006 he served as special advisor to the United Nations secretary-general for the UN Global Compact. His advice is sought by numerous institutions such as the World Bank, UNDP, ADB, MIT and Harvard University.

Arvind Mathur works as national professional officer for Health Systems and Community Health at the WHO. He is a medical graduate from Meerut Medical College and holds an MD in Social and Preventive Medicine, Diploma of the National Board in Community Medicine and a Diploma in Hospital Administration. He is currently pursuing a Master of Business Administration degree (HRD) with the Indira Gandhi National Open University.

Suneeta Mittal is heading the Department of Obstetrics & Gynecology and is director-in-charge, WHO-CCR in Human Reproduction at the All India Institute of Medical Sciences (AIIMS), New Delhi. Due to her pioneering professional contributions, Prof. Mittal is an internationally acclaimed WHO expert on emergency contraception and medical abortion and the regional editor of the *WHO Reproductive Health Library*.

Günter Neubauer is the director of the Institute of Health Economics (IfG) and professor (emeritus) of health economics at the Bundeswehr University Munich, Germany. From 1990 to 1998 he served as a member of the Advisory Council for the Concerted Action in Health Care. Prof. Neubauer is currently an expert member on numerous scientific boards.

Madhurima Nundy is a research scholar at the Centre of Social Medicine and Community Health, Jawaharlal Nehru University. Her doctoral study looks at the transformation of the non-profit hospitals in Delhi. She has worked as a technical consultant with the National Commission on Macroeconomics and Health on issues relating to health financing, public private partnerships and gender and health.

Mary Robinson is the president of Realizing Rights: The Ethical Globalization Initiative. Prior to that, she served as United Nations High Commissioner for Human Rights (1997–2002) and President of Ireland (1990–1997). Prof. Robinson was the chair of the Business Leaders Initiative on Human Rights (BLIHR) until 2009 and is a founding member of the Council of Women World Leaders.

Malabika Roy serves at the Indian Council of Medical Research (ICMR) which she joined in 1984. She is an expert on maternal and child health including fertility regulation. Dr. Roy has published in international and national journals and serves on expert committees of the Government of India and international organizations such as the WHO and the Population Council.

Sybill Storz has been serving as CEO of KARL STORZ GmbH & Co. KG since 1996. Dr. h.c. mult. Storz has received numerous international honours for her outstanding business leadership. In 2005, amongst other awards, she received the *Chevalier de la Légion d'honneur* (Knight of the Legion of Honour) by decree of then French President Jacques Chirac.

Martina Timmermann served as director of studies on Human Rights and Ethics in the Peace and Governance Programme at the United Nations University headquarters in Tokyo and Bonn (2004–2007). In 2008 she joined the TIMA GmbH (Transition and Integration Management Agency, established in 1996) as vice-president and managing director of international projects.

Nicolaus von der Goltz is the private secretary to the minister of the Federal Ministry for Economic Cooperation and Development since 2006. Prior to that, he served as desk officer at the Federal Ministry for Economic Cooperation and Development, Division for Cooperation with the Business Sector, based in Bonn.

FOREWORD

Mary Robinson

President, Realizing Rights: The Ethical Globalization Initiative;
Former Chair of the Business Leader Initiative on Human Rights (BLIHR);
Former UN High Commissioner for Human Rights

The year 2010 celebrates the 15th anniversary of the Beijing Platform for Action. This milestone document for women's human rights was launched at the Fourth World Conference on Women in Beijing in 1995 and complements another key document, whose sixtieth anniversary was celebrated in 2008 – the Universal Declaration of Human Rights. Both of these anniversaries are times to celebrate our successes in improving the lives of people around the world, and also a time to reflect on our failures and shortcomings. Perhaps most importantly, it is a time when we can reflect that, despite the vast changes that have occurred since 1948, and the vast changes that continue to be wrought by forces connected to globalisation, the essential truth of universal human rights, belonging to all people everywhere, endures and remains inalienable.

Indeed, in an era of complex interdependence and competition, human rights are more relevant now than they have ever been. This fact is recognised in the proliferation of international legal documents concerned with human rights protection; in the many government and non-government reports and projects on human rights issues; in the normative power of human rights arguments in decision-making bodies; and most of all in the daily lives of all the world's peoples, many of whom continue to suffer human rights violations on a daily basis.

Women suffer most from human rights violations. The extent to which women continue to be disadvantaged and discriminated against is alarming, and remains a cause of great concern. As well as reaffirming the international community's commitment to human rights, the Millennium Declaration of 2000 explicitly recognises that gender equality and the empowerment of women must be promoted to alleviate poverty and stimulate genuinely sustainable development. This commitment goes to the heart of a vital understanding about the nature of human rights: they are part of a web of interconnected issues including security, development, poverty and governance. No one of these can be secured without the others, and each must be treated in a coordinated, mutually reflective way. Only then is long-term improvement in people's lives possible.

Despite such formal understandings of the cross-cutting nature of human rights work, not all rights do in reality receive equal attention. A vital precondition for achieving the goals outlined in the Millennium Declaration, for instance, is good health and equal access to the best attainable health care.

Poor people suffer the highest burden of disease. Illness in turn makes people poorer. The extent to which ill health is holding back human and economic development was very clearly demonstrated in the work of Jeffrey Sachs and his colleagues in the Commission on Macroeconomics on Health. Access to health for all will be achieved only if greater attention is paid to the links between health and the realisation of fundamental human rights. Implementing the right to the highest attainable standard of health should therefore be the ultimate objective of action in the field of public health.

Further, whereas many are increasingly aware of the relationship between health and poverty, fewer seem to realise the crucial links between health, human rights and gender equality. Being born a boy or a girl has a significant impact on health and access to health care, with women continuing to suffer a greater disease and mortality burden – for social as well as biological reasons. Every day, an estimated 1,600 women – overwhelmingly in the developing world, starting with Liberia, followed by Afghanistan, Pakistan and India – die of preventable complications during pregnancy and childbirth. Such statistics point to tragic failures at all levels of government, in both the developing and the more developed world. In many countries, stigma and discrimination continue to prevent women from accessing the health care they need and are entitled to have.

These statistics also point, however, to a great opportunity. We are all increasingly familiar with debates and discussions about the relative authority and power of both the public and private sectors to shape the context in which human rights are protected and provided for. States are still the primary actors in the provision of public goods; but we know that the private sector is playing an increasingly important role, too – not only through provision of material resources, but through active collaboration with public sector agencies and with individuals and communities. This is particularly the case in developing countries, where the poorest and most vulnerable people live; as globalisation facilitates increased transnational trade and business links, opportunities for public private partnerships aiming at complying with the UN human rights framework and shared ethical standards also increase. The way these opportunities are being grasped and brought to fruition is evident in the activities of many companies and organisations that have signed on to the United Nations Global Compact. The distinction of the Global Compact lies in its recognition of the fact that securing and protecting human rights is not a matter of charity. Rather, it is a matter of deeply embedding rights within governance and policy-making.

The development and implementation of the Women's Health Initiative (WHI), as described in this volume, provides salient suggestions and insights for other public private partnerships. Many of the authors point out that partnerships are most effective and sustainable where they recognise the legitimate interests of all the partners, and develop ways to further every party's objective. They also point to the need for ongoing review and adaptation to ensure projects can meet their objectives in response to changing circumstances on the ground.

The emphasis on innovation and transfer in the Women's Health Initiative further shows that public private partnerships for human rights are part of an ongoing process of necessary experimentation. Rights work is long-term work; there are no easy fixes or simple solutions, and prolonged dedication to clear goals is necessary to ensure that where projects are successful they may be sustained, and where not they can be reviewed.

The chapters in this volume show that it is possible to embrace the strengths of existing knowledge and practice in public private partnerships, while also pioneering new methods and principles. They do also show, however, some of the challenges that must be addressed if public private partnerships that aim at the advancement of the poor, women, health and human rights are to meet their potential.

In particular, the experience of the WHI shows the vital importance of developing *sustainable* participatory projects, which can be maintained and become self-supporting after initial project start-up phases have passed. To be truly sustainable, health care projects must be aligned and integrated with existing national health systems with the involvement of the governments and civil societies concerned. It is here that the principles of the Paris Declaration are very useful to guide the practice of any initiatives in health at the country level.

In this respect, the WHI in India offers useful lessons learnt and abundant sources for reference and further learning. The experiences of this initiative, although it was conducted on a comparatively small scale, underline the relevance of our earlier findings on Global Health Partnerships. Beyond that, it may help encourage small and medium-size actors at the local, national and regional levels to dare to come on board with this pertinent but challenging undertaking.

In order to succeed, public private partnerships must have clear, shared understandings of the project's objectives and priorities; these must be reviewed and all partners must be equally kept accountable. Business and public agency imperatives are valid, but there is a careful line to tread in making sure none of these take over.

Despite, or perhaps more accurately because of, these challenges, I am particularly encouraged by the decision to open the project to external review, which has resulted in this volume. By allowing independent, systematic assessment and analysis, the Women's Health Initiative not only embraces a higher standard for legitimacy, but opens up a resource of information and guidance for other projects and partners. It provides a valuable and needed approach for transparent and balanced assessment of business projects that are committed to be undertaken in compliance with the principles of the UN Global Compact.

This points to one other, vital, aspect of work that seeks to improve human rights: collaboration, cooperation and transparency in information-sharing are the most effective bases on which to develop and implement interventions.

I am very happy to share in the story of the Women's Health Initiative. I would like to thank all the authors, the project leaders and partners for their contributions; and I would like to express particular thanks to the doctors and patients who, by making this idea part of their lives, demonstrated that improving women's health and human rights can be not only a possibility but a daily reality.

ACKNOWLEDGEMENTS

This book project has come to life thanks to the invaluable assistance and support of various people and institutions.

First, we wish to thank the Deutsche Gesellschaft für Technische Zusammenarbeit (GTZ) and the Asian Women's Fund for their financial support of this project. We are also grateful to Dr. hc. mult. Sybill Storz from KARL STORZ GmbH & Co. KG and Dr. Achim Deja from TIMA GmbH for their continuous professional cooperation.

We extend our appreciation to the former United Nations University rector, Prof. Dr. Hans van Ginkel, who agreed to this "new in style and approach" United Nations University academic endeavour. We equally extend our deep gratitude to the current rector, Prof. Dr. Konrad Osterwalder, who provided us with his unflinching support so that we could finalise this project successfully. We thank the United Nations University, and particularly Max Bond, for continuously supporting this project over the years. Within this context, we also deeply appreciate the logistical and administrative assistance provided by Yoshie Sawada at the Peace and Governance Programme of the United Nations University. We thank Millie Carlson for her patient editorial support during the first stages of language editing. And we deeply appreciate the United Nations University Press, especially Naomi Cowan, for her meticulous work and patient attention during the publication process, as well as Liz Paton for doing a marvellous job copy-editing this volume.

In the long process of making this book, there have been many more supporters whom to name here would be impossible because of the sheer number. However, some do need to be mentioned because of their selfless support in organising the two project-related workshops. In this regard we would like to express our gratitude and appreciation to Jasja van der Zijde who – actually invited as a guest to the workshop in Bonn – generously gave her professional support during the final stages of the workshop organisation and during the conference itself. Vilma Liaukonyte, Sharon Kirabo-Steffens, Francesca Burchi and Pit Pruessner, all from UNU-EHS, made a formidable team and decisively contributed to the success of our workshop in Bonn in 2006.

Memorable support was also given to us during our first workshop in Chennai in 2005. We are particularly grateful to Prof. Gundapuneni Koteswara Prasad and his students from Madras University who were there for us with their steadfast support during the course of preparing and running the workshop. We highly appreciate the work of Timothy Webster, then intern at UNU Tokyo, who meticulously typed the transcripts of the workshop discussions. Our gratitude also extends to the KARL STORZ ground staff in India who gave us a helping hand when organising the logistics for the 2005 workshop in Chennai and during the UNU field mission in April 2007. A particular "thank you" also goes to UNDP India which gave us additional and much appreciated logistical support in organising that mission. Staying at the HABITAT compound was a new and very pleasant experience.

We finally thank all our contributors as well as interview partners and workshop participants for sharing their knowledgeable insights and for showing continuous patience in this challenging and exciting process of a book production. Each person has an indispensible share in the overall result and successful outcome of this volume.

Martina Timmermann and Monika Kruesmann
September 2009

Introduction

Women's health through PPP within the UN Global Compact – At the nexus of business, ethics and human rights

MARTINA TIMMERMANN

Improving the health of people in low- and middle-income countries will be a major international concern for the next few decades. The necessity of improving individual health as well as health care systems has found its most fundamental reflection in several of the UN Millennium Development Goals (MDGs),[1] which were articulated in the *Millennium Declaration* as a common vision for the new century by the UN member states at the historic summit in New York in 2000.[2] In the economic and social sphere, especially, this vision is linked to specific, measurable targets for the first 15 years of the century. Collectively, the MDGs constitute the single most important normative mandate for the United Nations in its development operations.[3]

By the end of 2008, however, it seemed that this vision would not match reality. The World Bank's *Global Monitoring Report 2008* warns that most countries will fall short of the Millennium Development Goals.[4] Among the eight MDGs, the prospects are worst for

Partnerships for women's health: Striving for best practice within the UN Global Compact,
Timmermann and Kruesmann (eds),
United Nations University Press, 2009, ISBN 978-92-808-1185-8

the health-related targets, especially MDG5, with its ambitious goal of achieving a reduction of 75 per cent in the maternal mortality rate between 1990 and 2015. In an even more recent report by UNICEF, such warnings are further underlined.[5] Ann Venneman, Director of UNICEF, in her announcement of the UNICEF report commented: "As the 2015 deadline for the Millennium Development Goals draws closer, the challenge for improving maternal and newborn health goes beyond meeting the goals ... Success will be measured in terms of lives saved and lives improved."[6]

About 90 per cent of maternal deaths occur in sub-Saharan Africa and Asia (see Chapter 1 in this volume). The rate of maternal mortality in developing countries is more than 100 times higher than in industrialised countries, making it the health statistic that shows the greatest disparity between developing and industrialised countries. In October 2007, the United Nations Population Fund (UNFPA), the World Health Organization (WHO), the United Nations Children's Fund (UNICEF) and the World Bank released the first new international (estimated) data in five years, which revealed that women continue to die of pregnancy-related causes at a rate of about one a minute.[7]

> The total number of women dying in pregnancy or childbirth has ... shown a modest decrease between 1990 and 2005. In 2005, 536,000 women died of maternal causes, compared to 576,000 in 1990.... Although maternal mortality ratios (the number of maternal deaths per 100,000 live births) are declining globally, and in all regions, the decline is too slow to meet the target of Millennium Development Goal 5.... Meeting that goal would have required an annual drop of 5.5 per cent, whereas the recorded declines have been less than 1 per cent.[8]

With regard to the Asia-Pacific region, most countries are not on track to achieve MDG5, which makes any contribution to the improvement of women's health in those countries a highly important endeavour. Among them, India – with a current population of more than 1 billion people, an impressive 24 per cent ratio of young adolescents, a very low contraceptive prevalence rate, an increasing rate of sex-selective abortions, and an estimated 136,000 maternal deaths per annum – is a focus of grave international concern (see Chapter 7 in this volume).

In India, roughly 30 million women experience pregnancy each year, and 27 million give live birth.[9] The maternal mortality rate is estimated to be 407 deaths per 100,000 live births, which makes India one of the countries with the worst maternal death records. Such numbers indicate a pressing priority for the Indian government, as well as the international community, which is equally obliged by international human rights treaties and the Millennium Declaration, to tackle maternal and child mortality and to develop policies for the improvement of maternal health.

India itself, a signatory to the Millennium Declaration, has made those eight goals the guidelines in setting its political priorities. This is reflected in its several national health and population policy plans, such as the National Health Policy 2002 (NHP-2002), the Tenth Five Year Plan (2002–2007) and the current Eleventh Five Year Plan (2007–2012) as well as Vision 2020 India (see Chapters 8 and 9 in this volume). These plans contain, as major government goals, the achievement of population stabilisation, the promotion of reproductive health and the reduction of infant and maternal mortality. Because of the strong urban–rural and inter-state disparity in terms of access to public health services, it is "a principal objective of NHP-2002 to evolve a policy structure which reduces these inequities and allows the disadvantaged sections of society a fairer access to public health services".[10] Paying tribute to the strong role of the private sector, the government, the corporate sector and the voluntary and non-voluntary sectors are expected to work towards this goal in partnership.

Still, to reach this complex array of goals there are several hurdles to overcome, especially with regard to India's health care system and politics (see Chapters 7, 8 and 9 in this volume). Until 2002, health care was not a priority for the political agenda.[11] This was reflected by the very low level of national expenditure on health care as a share of gross national product (GNP). There was also an obvious neglect of rural areas in terms of providing health services. And, finally, there was a lack of effective measures to tackle the persistent problems of poor people's difficulties in getting access to health facilities and of low investment in human resources and organisation capabilities for the public health sector. In 2005, K. Srinath Reddy, the convenor of the core Advisory Group on Public Health and Human Rights of the National Human Rights Commission of India, brought the Indian government's inadequate response to the growing health challenge to public attention in his stock-taking of India's health policies. In detail, he criticised the government's poor allocation of money spent on health and the inefficient utilisation of allocated resources.[12]

Within this context, public private partnerships (PPPs) have become key instruments of governmental health care policies (on PPPs in general see Chapter 4 in this volume; on PPPs in India, see Chapter 9 in this volume). However, the issues of whether such PPPs can help the government to fulfil its obligations, reach its political goals and contribute to good governance while solving the issue of accountability are central in the ongoing debate between the government, health care and development specialists, human rights activists and non-governmental organisations.

The case of India thus vividly illustrates the urgent need and paramount relevance of finding convincing answers to the question of how to achieve the health-related MDGs, and especially MDG5, by the target date of 2015.

Heading towards MDG5 with a comprehensive approach of integration

Any measures for reducing maternal mortality and for strengthening women's human rights to the best attainable physical and mental health need a comprehensive approach, starting with political determination and considering the particular social and cultural environment. It is crucial to keep in mind that reproductive health status depends heavily on income and gender, so gender-sensitive health policies are vitally necessary. Further, policies must recognise that achieving women's health goals under MDG5 involves issues of social justice, ethics and equity; diverse and comprehensive approaches must therefore be integrated within a broader framework. These are central understandings of the Women's Health Initiative, our case study, which recognises that integration is necessary at all levels, beginning with the international conceptions of human rights, through the specific health care needs of women and girls, to the public and private institutions and governance structures under which policies and programmes are implemented.

Integrating a human rights approach

The United Nations High Commissioner for Human Rights stressed in 2007 that the human rights approach is absolutely crucial to prevention, and emphasised the need for "addressing the political, social and economic inequalities behind mortality and the disease burden".[13]

The human rights approach to development is encapsulated in international human rights law. It is fundamentally based on the understanding that human rights are *not* about charity or the *goodness* on governments' or anyone else's part in providing some favour to the poor; rather, human rights contain certain obligations and entitlements. Human rights are underpinned by universally recognised moral values, which in the form of international human rights law create three major obligations for states:

1. the obligation to respect people's rights;
2. the obligation to protect those rights (that is, to prevent others from violating such rights); and
3. the obligation to create conditions that make human rights possible.

Within this rights-based approach, individuals are considered to be "rights holders", whereas (mainly) governments are recognised as "duty bearers". Among their duties is the establishment of equitable laws and systems that enable individuals to exercise and enjoy their rights and to seek judicial recourse for violations under the rule of law. As rights holders, people can claim their legitimate entitlements. This approach is genuinely democratic because it specifically emphasises the participation of individuals and communities in political decision-making processes that directly affect them. States accept those obligations through ratifying international human rights treaties, which are binding under international law. If states fail to give effect to such rights, there are a number of different accountability mechanisms,[14] including tribunals, parliamentary processes, a health ombudsperson, international human rights treaty monitoring bodies, and so on, which can take action. With regard to the perceived notion of the "punishment" in those mechanisms, however, and because of the complexity of the challenge of providing adequate health care, it seems more promising to use non-judicial procedures and strengthen self-commitment.

Integrating women's health rights and needs

The judicial implications derived from the rights-based approach as well as the right to health have not been central to the debates on women's reproductive and maternal health. One reason for this lack of interest may be that, in contrast to other rights, "the right to health has not yet gained the same human rights currency as more established rights".[15] (See also Chapter 2 in this volume.)

The right to health, enshrined in Article 12 of the International Covenant on Economic, Social and Cultural Rights (ICESCR), stipulates that everyone has the right to the highest attainable standard of physical and mental health. This does not mean that a person has a "right to be healthy", but refers to freedoms and entitlements. In terms of freedoms, it includes the right to control one's health and body, as well as the right to be free from interference (such as torture). In terms of entitlements, the right to health refers to the possibility of having access to the best attainable health care, as well as to the enjoyment of the broad range of conditions that make good health possible. The right to health and the approach to health based on human rights are fundamentally built on this dynamic of freedoms and entitlements.

Integrating women's and girls' specific health (care) needs

The right to health creates an obligation for governments to provide the best attainable health care for both women and men. Nevertheless, there are gender-related differences in terms of their health care needs, which are noted in various documents.

With specific regard to women's health, the ICESCR and the Convention on the Elimination of All Forms of Discrimination against Women (CEDAW) are of particular relevance. State signatories have to take steps to improve women's reproductive and maternal health, and thereby live up to the values and obligations manifested in several human rights provisions, such as the right to the best attainable health care (the Convention on the Rights of the Child (CRC), Article 24; CEDAW, Article 12); the right to life, survival and development (CRC, Article 6); the right to an adequate standard of living (CRC, Article 27); the right to be free from harmful traditional practices (CRC, Article 24.3); the right to non-discrimination (CRC, Article 2; CEDAW, Articles 1, 2); the duty of the state to undertake legislative, administrative and other measures for the implementation of rights (CRC, Article 4; CEDAW, Articles 3, 4); and the right to international cooperation (CRC, Article 24.4).

In particular, CEDAW (Article 12) notes:

1. States Parties shall take all appropriate measures to eliminate discrimination against women in the field of health care in order to ensure, on a basis of equality of men and women, access to health care services, including those related to family planning.

2. Notwithstanding the provisions of paragraph I of this article, States Parties shall ensure to women appropriate services in connection with pregnancy, confinement and the post-natal period, granting

free services where necessary, as well as adequate nutrition during pregnancy and lactation.[16]

Another important document pointing out the gender differences in access to health care is the Beijing Platform for Action (1995), which states that:

> Women have different and unequal access to and use of basic health resources, including primary health services for the prevention and treatment of childhood diseases, malnutrition, anaemia, diarrhoeal diseases, communicable diseases, malaria and other tropical diseases and tuberculosis, among others ... Women's health is also affected by gender bias in the health system and by the provision of inadequate and inappropriate health services to women.[17]

Women's health needs differ from those of men not only as a result of biological distinctions but also because of gender differentials. Women face higher exposure to some risk factors. They are biologically more vulnerable than men to a number of reproductive health problems, including reproductive tract infections and sexually transmitted diseases. And, unlike men, women need health services when they are not ill, for example to carry pregnancies to term, to deliver safely or to avoid unwanted pregnancies.

Women's complex reproductive and maternal health care needs cut across all sectors of society, and require that any measure for the improvement of women's maternal and reproductive health and health care has to be addressed at multiple levels and in multiple sectors of society. Thus, it is essential to provide and improve access to reproductive health programmes that respond effectively to social, cultural, economic and gender factors.[18]

As a first step in improving the gravely unsatisfactory provision of women's reproductive and maternal health care, suggestions have been made to routinely address women's reproductive health issues within the context of primary health care provision. This, however, requires a strong public health system.

In addition, it has been noted that the indicators for achieving the ambitious goal of reducing maternal mortality by 75 per cent by 2015 are outdated. Consequently, there has been a growing demand for the use of supplementary information sources, such as UNICEF's 1997 *Guidelines for Monitoring the Availability and Use of Obstetric Services.*[19]

In acknowledgment of such differences, governments need to develop gender-specific responses in their health care services and politics. To develop adequate services, it is obviously also necessary to take a closer look at women's specific health and health care needs.

Yet the development and maintenance of viable public health and monitoring systems go beyond the issue of women's reproductive health and reach to the core of ongoing worldwide debates on how best to set up and maintain quality health care provisions.[20]

Integrating health care politics

In Kofi Annan's MDG roadmap (2001), as in most of the following discussions on measures against maternal mortality, strong emphasis has been put on strengthening the health care sector.

> The ["Making Pregnancy Safer"] initiative is based on the premise that achieving substantial and sustained reductions in maternal and neonatal mortality is critically dependent on the availability, accessibility and quality of maternal health care services, and therefore efforts must necessarily be focused on strengthening health-care systems.[21]

For several reasons, this demand poses serious challenges not only to national and local governments in South Asia and sub-Saharan Africa but also to the international community (see Chapter 1 in this volume). All of them are struggling with two very pertinent questions: How can we finance viable health care systems? How can we implement human rights and women's rights and pay adequate tribute to women's health needs?

Integrating the private sector

In addition to the obligation of the state to provide the best attainable health care – as rightfully demanded by human rights protagonists – such questions put enormous pressure on governments in developed countries, and even more so in developing countries. Designing, building and maintaining viable health care systems has thus become one of the most central issues for governments worldwide. Within this process, awareness has been rising that new models need to be developed – models that combine governmental obligations with complementary support activities by the private sector. As another consequence, there is also increasing recognition of the crucial role and the responsibilities of the private sector in the promotion and protection of human rights (see Chapters 2 and 3 in this volume).

This has even been reflected in international human rights law. Originally, international human rights law imposed obligations on states but not on non-state actors. In more recent times, however, the increasing role played by non-state actors in the economic and social spheres has been taken more into consideration. This was highlighted in a resolution adopted by the UN Sub-Commission on the Promotion and Protection of Human Rights, which states that, even though states have the primary responsibility towards human rights, "transnational corporations and other business enterprises, as organs of society, are also responsible for promoting and securing the human rights set forth in the Universal Declaration of Human Rights".[22]

In response to this general development, the question has been raised of how international human rights law can be applied to non-state actors. One suggested way is to apply it *indirectly*, by the duty of the state to protect. The alternative would be the *direct* application of human rights norms to business (see Chapter 2 in this volume).

The second option seems to be flourishing more strongly, as reflected, for instance, in documents such as the International Labour Organization (ILO) *Tripartite Declaration of Principles Concerning Multinational Enterprises and Social Policy* (2000), the Organisation for Economic Co-operation and Development (OECD) *OECD Guide-*

lines for Multinational Enterprises (2008), and the UN "Norms on the Responsibilities of Transnational Corporations and Other Business Enterprises with Regard to Human Rights" (2003).[23] An example has been *A Guide for Integrating Human Rights into Business Management*, which was developed by the Business Leaders Initiative on Human Rights, the UN Global Compact and the Office of the High Commissioner on Human Rights in 2006.[24]

Still, even if business and human rights norms are brought together from a legal point of view, another major (and more political) question is how best to *involve* corporate business in public policies? What are, or should be, the common binding ethics? And, most importantly, who will finally be held accountable to whom?[25]

Integrating the concept of public private partnership

The state is increasingly losing ground as a provider of the public good "health" but is still obliged to fulfil its responsibility towards its citizens by providing equal access to the best attainable health services. In order to meet the increasing financial and organisational challenges associated with this obligation, one solution has been sought in the development of public private partnerships (PPPs). PPPs are understood as a "cooperative venture between the public and private sectors, built on the expertise of each partner, that best meets clearly defined public needs through the appropriate allocation of resources, risks and rewards"[26] (for details see Chapter 4 in this volume).

There are a great number of different PPPs that, on varying levels, engage the expertise or capital of the private sector. There are examples not only of straight contracting-out but also of traditionally delivered public services. Other forms may include simpler partnerships that are publicly administered but within a framework that still allows for private finance, design, operation and (possibly) temporary ownership of an asset.

On a positive note, PPPs in general – but especially in the health sector – are contributing to fund-raising and tackling the financial challenges facing governments.[27] They help in developing stronger planning strategies and setting standards for future practice, and they contribute to improving access to products and the delivery of services. On a more critical note, there have been complaints about the exclusion of important stakeholders in the planning and implementation process, the lack of a clear definition of the roles and responsibilities of partners, the lack of information on national policies (or the disregard of such information) and, as a consequence, the wasting of resources.

A major issue in the debate on PPPs in the health care sector is the question of who is accountable to whom. Since traditionally the state is responsible for providing the public good "health", the question that arises is: Who actually sits in the driver's seat and controls or manages the provision of health care when the private sector is involved via PPPs? The generally accepted answer is that PPPs may contribute to improving the delivery of health care services but should be excluded from the political process of defining public priorities.

Concerns regarding business interference in government affairs are being countered by PPP defenders with the argument that, in the case of a successful PPP, not only does the private sector benefit from the partnership, but so too do the other partners and the target public as well. The important issue of binding ethics, norms and procedures is to be solved by recognising that, in successful public private partnerships, the public and private competitors automatically serve as each other's watchdogs. An ideal PPP, therefore, should represent a win–win situation for all partners and the target public. But what will happen in international PPPs that operate in foreign settings? What happens when there are different legal and ethical settings? What will happen to the request for transparency? In short, how do partners make sure that their partners comply with what they have promised to deliver and that they are accountable?

Integrating the UN Global Compact

Perhaps the most prominent international forum for this debate has been the UN Global Compact (GC) Initiative, which was started by UN Secretary-General Kofi Annan at the World Economic Forum in Davos in 2000. The Global Compact, first consisting of nine and then of ten ethical principles,[28] provides a framework for engaging the private sector on voluntary terms. By joining the GC, companies commit themselves to comply with the Ten Principles and to provide an annual report, the so-called Communication on Progress (CoP). Such a voluntary, self-commitment approach seems to be attractive: 5,209 business participants and 1,598 non-business participants were registered by the end of 2008.[29]

Why do companies join the GC and commit themselves to such principles? Just for branding or marketing purposes? This was probably a major incentive at the beginning. Meanwhile, however, studies by Goldman Sachs in 2006 and on a smaller scale by TIMA (Transition Integration Management Agency) in 2004, have indicated that adhering to such principles pays off for the following reasons:[30]

1. When joining the GC, companies decide to invest in their personnel by adhering to the ILO labour standards and human rights standards. This approach strengthens positive dispositions and leads to stronger commitment and loyalty from the employees. A positive effect of this increased loyalty is greater sustainability of business activities.

2. The GC is a crucial tool for strengthening good corporate governance, which, again, leads to a reduction in financial, economic and social risks; this is rewarded by the financial investment world.

3. The GC provides important foundations for process responsibility and leadership, which leads to higher value creation and an increase in corporate business value. Companies that decide to take over process responsibility also choose more competitive and cost-effective structures, which help them survive in this new global era of a genuinely changing international socio-economic environment.

4. Taking over process responsibility in a credible way necessarily contributes to gaining and keeping the trust of clients and customers in this new global market structure.

Figure 0.1 The Ten UN GC principles

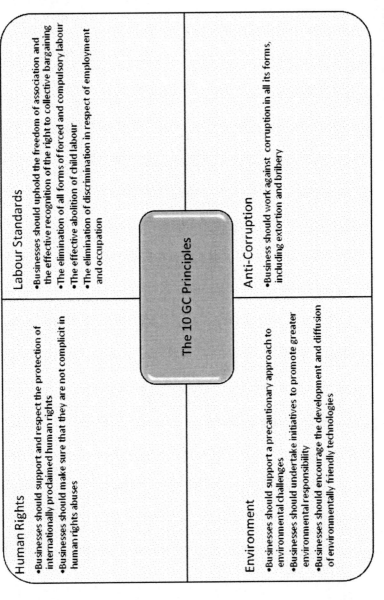

Human Rights
- Businesses should support and respect the protection of internationally proclaimed human rights
- Businesses should make sure that they are not complicit in human rights abuses

Labour Standards
- Businesses should uphold the freedom of association and the effective recognition of the right to collective bargaining
- The elimination of all forms of forced and compulsory labour
- The effective abolition of child labour
- The elimination of discrimination in respect of employment and occupation

The 10 GC Principles

Environment
- Businesses should support a precautionary approach to environmental challenges
- Businesses should undertake initiatives to promote greater environmental responsibility
- Businesses should encourage the development and diffusion of environmentally friendly technologies

Anti-Corruption
- Business should work against corruption in all its forms, including extortion and bribery

Source: the author based on information retrieved from <http://www.unglobalcompact.org/AboutTheGC/TheTenPrinciples/index.html>

5. And, finally, through its universal principles the GC provides an overarching ethical framework, or ethical bridge, to all members of the world market(s), irrespective of their faith, race or sex. It is therefore a UN platform in the finest sense, where the world can meet and work while building mutual trust, reliability and stability in all sectors through business activities framed and accepted by the Global Compact.

Human rights implementation in business practice poses one of the strongest challenges. To human rights defenders, such a voluntary approach seems clearly insufficient. They insist on stronger forms of review and auditing. The search for compliance mechanisms and approaches for identifying good or best practices that live up to the promises and declarations of the GC has thus become a major focus of interest.

Paul Hunt, in his 2006 report to the Human Rights Council, noted that with particular regard to the human right to the best attainable health care and the role of business:

> there is a new maturity about the health and human rights movement. "Naming and shaming", test cases and slogans all have a vital role to play in the promotion and protection of the right to health, but so do indicators, benchmarks, impact assessments, budgetary analysis, and the ability to take tough policy choices in a manner that is respectful of international human rights law and practice.[31]

In spite of this development, the alarming results of the 2009 UNICEF report, the Millennium Development Report 2008, and the 2007 study by UNFPA, UNDP and the World Bank emphasise only too vividly that there is an urgent need to go beyond declarations, debates and reporting issues if we want to keep some chance at least of meeting MDG5 by 2015.[32]

This raises another important question. How can international public private partnerships that are embedded in the UN Global Compact be designed in order to be successful? What can be learned from other experiences?

Integrating lessons learnt from former health PPPs

Kent Buse from the Overseas Development Institute, London, found in his analysis of 22 global health PPPs largely focused on products and communicable diseases that such PPPs could demonstrate not only seven achievements but also seven challenges, which he provocatively called the "seven deadly sins".[33] As positive achievements of global health partnerships (GHPs), Buse considered the opportunities of PPPs (1) to be rapidly established with many partners (3–300+), (2) to raise profiles and funds for certain issues, (3) to stimulate research and development, (4) to improve access to products, (5) to enhance service delivery capacity, (6) to strengthen policy and planning processes, and (7) to establish norms and standards.

In contrast, however, Buse also found seven particular challenges, the "seven deadly sins", which, if unmet, will hamper effectiveness, efficiency and overall success for a PPP.

As the first challenge, Buse found that in many of his analysed PPPs there was a lack of respect for the primacy of national planning. This meant the failure of the ideas of the Paris Agenda of 2006, which aims at aid alignment, the use of government channels and national governmental budget support.[34] Even in the conceptual phase, PPPs may avoid adequate consideration of the national health sector, including evidence-based processes for national priority-setting and planning. The resources provided for national health policy already reflect shifting agendas linked to Medium-Term Expenditure Framework[35] and Poverty Reduction Strategy Papers.[36] It may therefore happen that existing parallel, pooled and sector budget support is not made use of to limit transaction costs. Issue-specific GHPs in particular find it difficult to accept the Paris Agenda, which may lead to an (unwanted) shift of resources from high-priority activities to this issue-specific area, including a lack of synchronicity with planning/budget cycles and high transaction costs as well as non-consideration of recurrent costs in light of budget constraints. Still, Buse also found some positive developments when looking at global health PPPs, most notably increased policy dialogue at the national level and respect for national priorities.

As a second major challenge, Buse found in his sample of 22 GHPs that not all stakeholders had an equal voice in decision-making. He particularly noted an imbalance between civil society, the private sector and the public. For effectiveness, buy-in and commitment, however, stakeholder involvement is necessary. Any PPP should therefore aim at ensuring seats for all stakeholders and improving its constituency management.

Buse's third finding was that there was a particular feeling of denial of, or even contempt for, the public sector in the 1990s. According to his analysis, there was a dominant perception that the market is good and the public sector is bad. Scandals at the WHO as well as controversial debates on the efficiency and effectiveness of PPPs and research and development versus service delivery added to this negative image. Consequently, programmes shifted from the WHO to GHPs and caused fragmentation.

The fourth challenge according to Buse is a mix of idleness, complacency and irresponsibility. Buse is referring not to the core group of partners that actually make cooperation possible, but to his analysis of evaluations of GHPs that comment on a lack of specificity of objectives, roles and responsibilities, which may then lead to inadequate work performance, misunderstandings, mistrust, a lack of commitment, a lack of mutual accountability and problematic performance monitoring. Buse criticises the fact that, despite developing norms and standards, few partnerships screen for corporate social responsibility. As a solution he recommends more business-like approaches to consolidated partnership-wide planning. He also notices insufficient oversight in global health PPPs, including a lack of screening criteria when looking for corporate partners. Buse suggests designing individual policies and guidelines in order to manage conflicts of interest, and stresses the need to communicate transparently by developing and sharing strategic and operational plans; by organising board meeting agendas, backgrounders and decisions; by making governance arrangements; by developing arrangements for managing constituencies and by writing performance reports against objectives.

As a fifth challenge, Buse states that miserliness in giving or meeting funding needs prevents "permanent reward". As a consequence, he concludes that there are serious GHP financing challenges. He found a particular gap (an average of 60 per cent) between plans and commitments, with wary partners and a lack of mutual accountability mechanisms. Whereas the designers of a project usually favour lean, virtual and business-like secretariats, convening and coordination – necessary for success – are resource intensive. Alliance studies support Buse's point that saving on coordination is a false economy. Buse therefore concludes that there is a need for more realistic goals and improved business planning.

The sixth challenge is a wasting of scarce resources through failure to use existing country systems. This results in the duplication both of planning, monitoring and financial management and of service delivery. Buse recommends evaluating GHPs on their use of common systems and linking bilateral financing of GHPs to performance on the use of new aid modalities.

As a seventh and final challenge, Buse points to the sensitive issue of fidelity, loyalty and commitment to one's employer or primary organisation, which can conflict with outside loyalties. It therefore seems advisable to develop rules and incentives to facilitate external relationships by defining tasks and roles (expectations) explicitly, thereby consolidating planning, and by acknowledging and addressing dual accountability.

Buse's findings are further supported by a study by Rama Baru and Madhurima Nundy in 2006 (see Chapter 9 in this volume). For a PPP to be successful, they emphasise the importance of monitoring, accountability and transparency. They also put their finger on another crucial aspect of a partnership when pointing to the need for shared values. A partnership is built on the assumption of equality. If, however, values turn out to be different between partnering agencies, ethical dilemmas may evolve that negatively affect the results of the PPP.

In addition, partners are often not held accountable for the quality of services delivered. One reason could be that the Memorandum of Understanding (MOU) does not detail the required parameters; another might be that monitoring is inadequate. Baru and Nundy criticise the fact that, "even when services are not up to the mark, there is a lack of clarity as to how they can be rectified and made accountable". They go along with Nishtar, who notes that "[t]o hold partners accountable for their actions, it is imperative to have clear governance mechanisms and clarify partner's rights and obligations. Clarity in such relationships is needed in order to avoid ambiguities that lead to break up of partnerships."[37]

The Women's Health Initiative (WHI) against the background of such challenges

The debates alluded to above clearly illustrate the interlinkage of issues that need to be systematically integrated in designing a PPP project that aims to contribute to reaching (especially) MDG5 by the target date of 2015.

It is a major challenge to find convincing ways to respond to women's maternal and reproductive health needs while also incorporating human rights demands into everyday business and ensuring compliance and accountability. Public private partnerships, especially those concerned with public goods, will need to be viewed in light of their effectiveness and potential to be up-scaled in order to contribute credibly to MDG efforts.

The UN Global Compact, with all its strengths and weaknesses, provides a reference framework for the corporate, as well as the governmental and non-governmental, actors who engage in such international efforts and cooperation. There is a need to involve small and medium-sized enterprises more strongly in such efforts in order to be successful in the long run (see Chapters 5 and 6).

A final but equally important question, however, is how UN GC PPP approaches can be assessed with due (but also fair) consideration of the increasingly complex requirements of our globalising world?

"The Women's Health Initiative for Improving Women's Maternal and Reproductive Health in India: A PPP within the Framework of the UN Global Compact" was designed against this background

Figure 0.2   The WHI at the interface of challenges of global concern

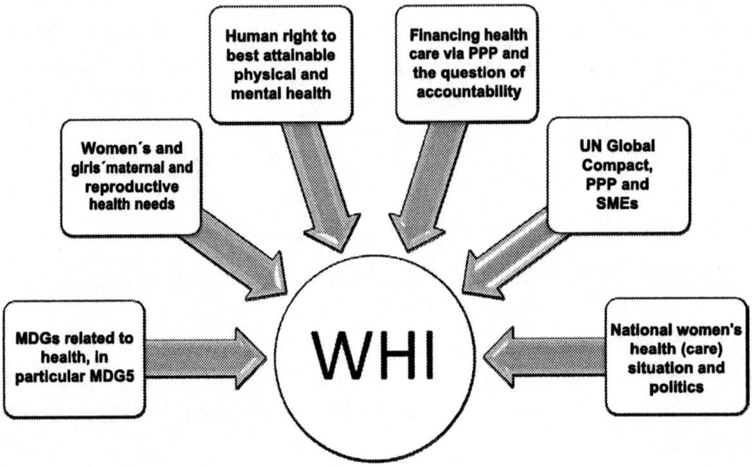

Source: the author.

of challenges and questions (see Figure 0.2). Within the project it was the task of the United Nations University (UNU) to undertake an impartial assessment of the public private partnership at the end of the project. For this reason, UNU developed an assessment model (see Chapter 11 in this volume) that included a self-learning process with two workshops – one learning workshop at the beginning of the project and one stocktaking workshop close to the end of the intervention. Most importantly, however, UNU drew from its very particular structure and mission to serve as a think tank for the exchange of ideas on issues of global concern in organising the final assessment.

Organising a platform for transparency and comprehensive documentation

A comprehensive outcome assessment needs to take into consideration the various national and global challenges outlined above. In addition, it needs to build on outside expert resources. But it is also vital to consult with shareholders in this process.

Inviting the partners to share their perceptions

In order to provide the partners as well as the experts with more scope for their arguments, UNU invited each partner to contribute a chapter in which they could present their particular positions and perceptions from both the management side in Germany and from the implementation side in India.

Inviting the experts to provide in-depth reference chapters

The experts were invited to the workshops and to contribute academic chapters for this book. They thereby had the opportunity to provide information that went beyond their workshop comments, which were additionally collected and summarised by the workshop rapporteur. In their chapters they were asked to tackle the topics of their expertise and thereby support their positions in greater academic depth. At the same time, their contributions were thought to form a useful framework of reference for the other participants and those interested parties who may think of setting up similar projects. Such contributions constitute Part A of this book and also offer the contextual framework for the following case study.

Since from the beginning the project was thought to have the potential for transfer to other countries where maternal mortality is a very serious issue, we invited Moazzam Ali to introduce the situation of maternal and reproductive health in South Asia and Africa (see Chapter 1). The UN Special Rapporteur on the right to the best attainable physical and mental health, Paul Hunt, together with Judith Bueno de Mesquito, was requested to put his finger on the interlinkage of "Poverty, Health and the Human Right to the Highest Attainable Standard of Health" (Chapter 2). A large part of their study concerns Peru, which contributes to widening the scope beyond Asia and Africa (Paul Hunt's 2008 mission report on India can be found in Appendix C). Their chapter is followed by the question of what business can do when partnering in support of the right to health. This topic is discussed by Klaus M. Leisinger, the former UN Secretary-General's Special Adviser on the UN Global Compact and President and CEO of Novartis Foundation (Chapter 3). Adding the perspective of an economist who used to advise the German government on health care issues, Günter Neubauer along with Iris Driessle discuss the financial challenges that make equal access to the best available health care difficult (Chapter 4). They suggest bringing the private sector in via public private partnerships. However, with partnerships increasingly going beyond national borders, international ethical platforms are needed for communication and for creating trust, reliability and accountability (while also lowering risks). Because the UN Global Compact promises to function as such a platform, and because the UN GC shapes this particular partnership project with two partners being UN GC members, Monika Kruesmann discusses the United Nations Global Compact with particular regard to its potential for embracing diversity (Chapter 5). Kruesmann also provides the background for Chapter 6 by Kai Bethke and Manuela Bösendorfer from UNIDO (United Nations Industrial Development Organization) who write on the particular role of small and medium-sized enterprises within the UN GC and their roles in achieving the Millennium Development Goals.

Whereas Section I discusses the overarching themes that frame this UN GC public private partnership, Section II of this volume focuses deliberately on India – the country where this PPP pilot was conducted. Very valuable insights are provided by Suneeta Mittal and Arvind Mathur, who outline "The Health Situation of Women in India: Policies and Programmes" (Chapter 7). Their chapter is followed by a sound overview of "India's Medical System" by Nirmal K. Ganguly and Malabika Roy (Chapter 8). Rama Baru and Madhurima Nundy look at the situation of "Health PPPs in India: Stepping Stones for Improving Women's Health Care?" in Chapter 9. And, finally, Arabinda Ghosh, from the capacity-building department of the government of West Bengal, outlines the features of "Pro-Poor Capacity-Building in India's Women's Health Sector" in Chapter 10.

In Part B we present the case study, and the project participants have the opportunity to put forward their individual perspectives and experiences (see Chapters 12–16: Sybill Storz for KARL STORZ GmbH & Co. KG (KS); Nicolaus von der Goltz for the Federal Ministry of Economic Cooperation and Development – BMZ; Diana Kraft and Jörg Hartmann for GTZ; Peter Laser and Anu Chopra for

KS/GTZ in the field; and Kurian Joseph and Alka Kriplani for private and public medical doctors). Christina Gradl, the first UN GC fellow (funded by KS), was invited to provide an academic discussion of the business model developed by Achim Deja as the "practitioner" for KARL STORZ, with particular regard to its impact on the poor (see Chapter 17). In Chapter 18, Timmermann and Kruesmann discuss the outcome of the PPP intervention from the perspective of 2008, based on data from the GTZ final report (2008), a UNU mission report (2007) and two UNU workshop reports (2005 and 2006).[38]

In Part C, this complex input is tied together and discussed with regard to the impact of the project beyond India – in the spirit of UNU's mission goals – and with policy recommendations for this PPP and others that might take this project as a blueprint for action.

By offering this publication platform to all the stakeholders in this project, UNU aims at creating an additional opportunity for transparency and information sharing as well as constructive further debate on those issues that formed the starting point for the project. And finally, through offering insight into the project results, impact and lessons learnt, this publication shall serve as a useful reference framework on the needs and measures of PPPs for improving women's health and human rights within the framework of the UN Global Compact beyond India.

Notes

1. For up-to-date information, see <http://www.un.org/millenniumgoals/> (accessed 16 June 2009).
2. United Nations General Assembly, *United Nations Millennium Declaration*, UN Document A/RES/55/2, 18 September 2000, <http://www.un.org/millennium/declaration/ares552e.pdf> (accessed 16 June 2009).
3. For the "Official List of MDGF Indicators", see <http://mdgs.un.org/unsd/mdg/Resources/Attach/Indicators/OfficialList2008.pdf> (accessed 24 June 2009). The MDGs have been undergoing continuous adjustment in response to experiences in the field and the research being done. The current official MDG framework supersedes the previous version, which had been effective since 2003. The original eight goals, targets and indicators developed in 2002 were used from 2003 to 2007. That same year, the MDG monitor-

ing framework was revised to include four new targets agreed by member states at the 2005 World Summit and recommended, in 2006, by the UN Secretary-General in his report on the Work of the Organization. In 2007, the General Assembly took note of the Secretary-General's report in which he presented the new framework as recommended by the Inter-Agency and Expert Group on MDG Indicators (IAEG). See the Millennium Development Goals Reports, <http://www.un.org/millenniumgoals/reports. shtml>; and World Bank, "About the Goals", <http://ddp-ext.worldbank. org/ext/GMIS/gdmis.do?siteId=2&menuId=LNAV01HOME1> (accessed 24 June 2009).

4. World Bank, *Global Monitoring Report 2008*, Washington DC: 2008, <http://web.worldbank.org/WBSITE/EXTERNAL/EXTDEC/EXTGLO BALMONITOR/EXTGLOMONREP2008/0,,menuPK:4738069~page PK:64168427~piPK:64168435~theSitePK:4738057,00.html> (accessed 5 June 2009).

5. *The State of the World's Children 2009: Maternal and Newborn Health*, New York: United Nations Children's Fund (UNICEF), December 2008, <http://www.unicef.org/sowc09/docs/SOWC09-FullReport-EN.pdf> (accessed 23 June 2009).

6. See UNICEF, <http://www.unicef.org/sowc09/> (accessed 23 June 2009).

7. *Maternal Mortality in 2005: Estimates Developed by WHO, UNICEF, UNFPA, and The World Bank*, Geneva: WHO, 2007, <http://www.who.int/whosis/ mme_2005.pdf> (accessed 17 June 2009).

8. See United Nations Population Fund, "Maternal Mortality Figures Show Limited Progress in Making Motherhood Safer", <http://www.unfpa.org/ mothers/statistics.htm> (accessed 16 June 2009).

9. MOHFW, 2003, cited in "Country Fact File on Maternal, Newborn and Child Health Situation in India", Centre for Community Medicine, All India Institute of Medical Sciences, New Delhi, <http://www.searo. who.int/LinkFiles/WHD_05_Fact_File_India_Fact_File_india.pdf> (accessed 16 June 2009).

10. "National Health Policy 2002 (India)", para. 2.2.3, <http://www.prsindia. org/docs/bills/1188536430/bill146_20071113146_national_health_ policy_2002.pdf> (accessed 16 June 2009).

11. Until 2002, public health investments were comparatively low. As a proportion of India's gross domestic product (GDP), expenditure actually declined from 1.3 per cent in 1990 to 0.9 per cent in 1999. In the National Health Policy 2002, it was planned to increase national health sector expenditure to 6 per cent of GDP by the year 2010, with 2 per cent of GDP as public health investment. The most cost-effective methods to reduce the various gaps and imbalances are thought to be the extension of primary health care and the facilitation of a preventive and early stage curative initiative. In recognition of this, the National Health Policy 2002 set out an increased allocation of 55 per cent of total public health investment for the primary health sector, 35 per cent for the secondary sector, and 10 per cent for the tertiary sector ("National Health Policy 2002 (India)").

12. K. Srinath Reddy, "Establishing Schools of Public Health in India", *Global Forum Update on Research for Health*, 2, 2005, pp. 149–153, at p. 149.

13. Office of the United Nations High Commissioner for Human Rights, *Claiming the Millennium Development Goals: A Human Rights Approach*, New York and Geneva: United Nations, 2008, p. viii. See also Mary Robinson, "Keynote Address", OECD-DAC Workshop on Development Effectiveness in Practice: Applying the Paris Declaration to Advancing Gender Equality, Environmental Sustainability and Human Rights, Dublin, Ireland, 26–27 April 2007, <http://www.oecd.org/dataoecd/16/29/38610055.pdf> (accessed 23 June 2009).

14. Paul Hunt, "Neglected Diseases, Social Justice and Human Rights: Some Preliminary Observations", Health and Human Rights Working Paper Series No. 4, 2003, p. 5.

15. Ibid., p. 2.

16. Convention on the Elimination of All Forms of Discrimination against Women, <http://www.un.org/womenwatch/daw/cedaw/text/econvention.htm#article12> (accessed 16 June 2009).

17. "Platform for Action", United Nations Fourth World Conference on Women, Beijing, China, September 1995, para. 90; <http://www.un.org/womenwatch/daw/beijing/platform/health.htm> (accessed 16 June 2009).

18. United Nations Population Fund, *State of World Population 2005: The Promise of Equality: Gender Equity, Reproductive Health and the Millennium Development Goals*, New York: UNFPA, 2005, chapter 4, p. 1.

19. *Guidelines for Monitoring the Availability and Use of Obstetric Services*, 2nd edn, New York: United Nations Children's Fund, 1997; available at <http://www.unfpa.org/mothers/indicators.htm> (accessed 16 June 2009).

20. WHO, *Health and the Millennium Development Goals*, Geneva, 2005, especially chapter 1. See also UN Millennium Project Task Force on Child Health and Maternal Health, *Who's Got the Power? Transforming Health Systems for Women and Children*, London: Earthscan, 2005.

21. United Nations General Assembly, *Road Map towards the Implementation of the United Nations Millennium Declaration. Report of the Secretary-General*, UN Document A/56/326, 6 September 2001, para. 100; <http://www.un.org/documents/ga/docs/56/a56326.pdf>

22. See Hunt, "Neglected Diseases, Social Justice and Human Rights" p. 11. The Universal Declaration of Human Rights recognises that everyone has the right to a standard of living adequate for health and well-being, including medical care. This resolution also emphasises that transnational corporations and other business enterprises shall respect and contribute towards the realisation of this right. The relationship between the right to health and the private sector raises important issues and needs further careful attention.

23. International Labour Office, *Tripartite Declaration of Principles Concerning Multinational Enterprises and Social Policy*, 4th edn, Geneva: ILO, 2006, <http://www.ilo.org/wcmsp5/groups/public/---ed_emp/---emp_ent/documents/publication/wcms_094386.pdf> (accessed 17 June 2009); Organisation for Economic Co-operation and Development, *OECD Guidelines*

for Multinational Enterprises, Paris: OECD Publishing, 2008, <http://www.oecd.org/dataoecd/56/36/1922428.pdf> (accessed 17 June 2009); United Nations Economic and Social Council, "Norms on the Responsibilities of Transnational Corporations and Other Business Enterprises with Regard to Human Rights", UN Document E/CN.4/Sub.2/2003/12/Rev.2, 23 August 2003, <http://www.unhchr.ch/huridocda/huridoca.nsf/(Symbol)/E.CN.4.Sub.2.2003.12.Rev.2.En> (accessed 17 June 2009).

24. *A Guide for Integrating Human Rights into Business Management*, <http://www.ohchr.org/Documents/Publications/GuideHRBusinessen.pdf> (accessed 17 June 2009).

25. The Millennium Project Task Force on Child Health and Maternal Health, *Who's Got the Power?*, sees this question as an important starting point for building an accountability system, said Lynn Freedman, one of the coauthors of the report, during the first UNU workshop in Chennai, 2 October 2005.

26. The Canadian Council for Public-Private Partnerships, "About PPP", <http://www.pppcouncil.ca/aboutPPP_definition.asp> (accessed 17 June 2009).

27. One prominent example is the Global Fund to Fight AIDS, Malaria and Tuberculosis.

28. The Global Compact's Ten Principles cover the areas of human rights, labour, the environment and anti-corruption and are derived from the Universal Declaration of Human Rights, the ILO Declaration on Fundamental Principles and Rights at Work, the Rio Declaration on Environment and Development and the United Nations Convention Against Corruption. "The Ten Principles", <http://www.unglobalcompact.org/AboutTheGC/TheTenPrinciples/index.html> (accessed 17 June 2009).

29. *UN Global Compact Bulletin*, January 2009, <http://www.unglobalcompact.org/NewsAndEvents/UNGC_bulletin/2009_01_1.html> (accessed 17 June 2009).

30. See Goldman Sachs Global Investment Research, "Introducing GC Sustain", June 2007; TIMA GmbH, "Business und Ethik – Endoskopie, Infrastrukturservices im Public Business – Nachhaltiges Geschäftsmodell/Wachstumskonzeption", strategy paper, 5 March 2006.

31. "Implementation of General Assembly Resolution 60/251 of 15 March 2006. Report of the Special Rapporteur on the right of everyone to the enjoyment of the highest attainable standard of physical and mental health, Paul Hunt", UN Document A/HRC/4/28, 17 January 2007, para. 30, p. 10.

32. See *The Millennium Development Goals Report 2008*, New York: United Nations, 2008, <http://www.un.org/millenniumgoals/2008highlevel/pdf/newsroom/mdg%20reports/MDG_Report_2008_ENGLISH.pdf> (accessed 23 June 2009); UNICEF, *The State of the World's Children 2009*; and UNFPA, UNDP and the World Bank, *Maternal Mortality in 2005*.

33. Kent Buse and Andrew Harper, "Global Health: Making Partnerships Work: Seven Recommendations for Building Effective Global Public–

Private Health Partnerships", Overseas Development Institute (ODI), Briefing Paper 15, January 2007.

34. The "Paris Declaration on Aid Effectiveness" was endorsed on 2 March 2005. It is an international agreement to which over 100 ministers, heads of agencies and other senior officials adhered and committed their countries and organisations to continue to increase efforts at harmonisation, alignment and managing aid for results with a set of monitorable actions and indicators as well as results and mutual accountability. This declaration was followed by the Accra Agenda for Action (AAA), endorsed on 4 September 2008, and building on the commitments agreed upon in the Paris Declaration. The full text of the AAA is available at <http://www.oecd.org/dataoecd/58/16/41202012.pdf> (accessed 24 June 2009).

35. For a definition, see "What Is a Medium-Term Expenditure Framework (MTEF)?", VIE/96/028: Public Expenditure Review, Phase II, UNDP, 2000, available at <http://www.wemos.nl/Documents/whatis%20mtef.pdf> (accessed 17 June 2009).

36. "Poverty Reduction Strategy Papers (PRSPs) are prepared by governments in low-income countries through a participatory process involving domestic stakeholders and external development partners, including the IMF and the World Bank. A PRSP describes the macroeconomic, structural and social policies and programs that a country will pursue over several years to promote broad-based growth and reduce poverty, as well as external financing needs and the associated sources of financing." International Monetary Fund, "Poverty Reduction Strategy Papers. A Factsheet", April 2008, <http://www.imf.org/external/np/exr/facts/prsp.htm> (accessed 17 June 2009).

37. S. Nishtar, "Public-Private 'Partnerships' in Health – A Global Call to Action", Health Research Policy and Systems, 2(5), 2004, <http://www.health-policy-systems.com/content/2/1/5> (accessed 17 June 2009).

38. Martina Timmermann, "Findings and Recommendations Resulting from Communications with Project Stakeholders and Outside Observers in Delhi, Chandigarh and Chennai 8–15 and 23 April 2007", UNU Mission Report, 25 April 2007, unpublished internal document; "Reaching beyond Boundaries – Women's Health Initiative: A Public–Private Partnership", GTZ Monitoring Report by Dr Nisha Lal and Dr J. Peter Steinmann, New Delhi, May 2008; Monika Kruesmann, "Report of the Women's Health Initiative Workshop, Bonn, Germany, 3–5 December 2006", unpublished manuscript; "Public Private Partnership for Improving Women's and Girls' Reproductive Health Care in India", Workshop I: Background, Method, Potential, held in Chennai, India, 1–4 October 2005, UNU Initial Report December 2005, unpublished manuscript.

PART A

CONTEXTUAL FRAME OF REFERENCE

Section I

MDGs, human rights, the UN Global Compact and public private partnerships

1

Improving maternal health in Asia and Africa: Challenges and opportunities

Moazzam Ali

Introduction

It is estimated that one woman dies every minute from causes related to pregnancy or childbirth worldwide, and 1,600 young women die every day from pregnancy-related complications.[1] That equates to around 529,000 women a year.[2] In addition, for every woman who dies in childbirth, around 20 more suffer injury, infection or disease – approximately 10 million women each year.

Much remains to be done to ensure that women have safe and healthy pregnancies, particularly in the poorest countries, where increased attention in the last decade to this "neglected tragedy" has not yet resulted in a reduction in maternal mortality. In the developing world, complications during pregnancy continue to be the leading cause of maternal death and disability for women of reproductive age (15–49 years)[3] and, overall, they account for more than one-quarter of deaths among women.[4] About 99 per cent of estimated maternal deaths occur in Asia, Africa and Latin America, with only 6,000 occurring annually in the developed world. The burden of maternal

Partnerships for women's health: Striving for best practice within the UN Global Compact,
Timmermann and Kruesmann (eds),
United Nations University Press, 2009, ISBN 978-92-808-1185-8

mortality and morbidity in Asia and the Near East is amongst the highest in the world.[5] Women in developing countries are 30 times more likely than those in developed countries to die from pregnancy-related causes.[6] The lifetime risk for a woman to die because of pregnancy and childbirth in developing regions as a whole is estimated to be 1 in 61 (1 in less than 10 in several countries). For developed regions, it is 1 in 2,800 (1 in more than 5,000 in several countries).[7] In 2005, maternal deaths were unevenly distributed across the world's regions and were not in proportion to the populations of women of reproductive age in those regions. Nearly half of all maternal deaths (270,000) occurred in sub-Saharan Africa, where only 10 per cent of all women of reproductive age in the world resided. South Asia and sub-Saharan Africa together accounted for 458,000 (86 per cent) of maternal deaths globally, though they accounted for only 22 per cent of all women of reproductive age in 2005.[8]

Following the International Conference on Population and Development in Cairo in 1994 and the United Nations Fourth World Conference on Women in Beijing in 1995, recommendations were made for national governments to develop comprehensive strategies that ensure universal access to high-quality, affordable sexual and reproductive health services, including family planning through primary health care systems. A major focus of these strategies to reduce maternal mortality has been on enabling women to reach a hospital in time to save their lives. It is acknowledged that life-threatening complications in pregnancy are generally not preventable or predictable far in advance, with the exception of those complications related to unsafe induced abortion, and that when nothing is done to avert maternal death, natural mortality is around 1,000 to 1,500 per 100,000 births.[9] Hence, the reduction of maternal mortality through quality service provision is a key human rights issue for women and their children.[10]

The "Safe Motherhood Initiative" launched by the World Health Organization (WHO) in 1987 increased international awareness of the need to provide accessible essential or emergency obstetric care (EmOC) to any woman who might require it.[11] The WHO began work in the mid-1980s delineating the basic requirements for the provision of emergency obstetric functions and first published the *Essential Elements of Obstetric Care at the First Referral Level* in 1991.[12] It was recognised that these requirements, considered to be minimum levels in the provision of care at the district or sub-district hospital or health centre level, were seriously deficient in many countries where these services did not exist, even at the teaching hospital level.[13] The "Safe Motherhood Initiative" has emphasised the importance of access to EmOC to manage the common causes of obstetric death, which are haemorrhage, obstructed labour, complications resulting from unsafe abortion, eclampsia and infection.[14]

Once complications in pregnancy become apparent, the mother's chances of survival, and those of her infant, are determined by whatever barriers prevent her from receiving the care that might save her life. For example, the "three-delay" model explains how risks increase over the course of pregnancy and labour. The first delay occurs in recognising warning signs and in the decision to seek care. A second delay is caused by barriers of distance and transportation, that is, the time needed to arrive at the appropriate facility as a result of distance and the availability of transportation.[15] A third delay may occur in receiving care at the facility. At the hospital level, a whole range of barriers can be identified, from dismissive attitudes of some health care providers to shortages of essential drugs and life-saving equipment, depriving patients of prompt and appropriate emergency care.[16] Many women overcome the obstacles of distance and poor transportation only to die after they arrive at a medical facility. Some die because they are too ill to be helped when they arrive; others die for lack of prompt and appropriate care.

The WHO notes that most of these maternal deaths are preventable, even in limited-resource settings, and that information is needed upon which to base actions to reduce these tragic deaths. It also observes that knowing the overall rate of maternal mortality is not enough; it is necessary to understand the underlying factors that lead to deaths.[17]

This chapter examines a number of these underlying factors, with particular reference to social and cultural issues, in an international comparative context. Studies of maternal health and mortality in Asian and African developing countries indicate important and complex relationships between diverse factors influencing women's health, including religion, gender and cultural norms, information access, political structures, and training and investment in health services. Each of these presents both challenges and opportunities for improving maternal health, as the following discussion shows.

The influence of socio-cultural factors on maternal health

Maternal health is influenced by complex biological, social and cultural factors that are highly interlinked. It is further complicated by differences in the provision, availability and accessibility of health services, and it also involves issues of basic human rights.

These factors affect women's health throughout their lives and have cumulative effects. It is therefore important to consider the entire life cycle when examining the causes and consequences of women's poor health. For example, girls who are fed inadequately during childhood may have stunted growth, which leads to higher risks of complications during and following childbirth. Similarly, sexual abuse during childhood increases the likelihood of mental depression in later years, and repeated reproductive tract infections can cause infertility.

In South Asia, Bangladesh has the highest ratio of preference for sons over daughters,[18] followed by Pakistan and India – where many women also believe that bearing sons bring them prestige in society.[19] A substantial body of evidence also shows that there is discrimination against daughters with regard to food allocation and access to health services and they suffer from high mortality, especially during the first four years of life.[20]

Generally, in industrialised countries, the female foetus has better chances of survival than the male foetus.[21] Yet in some developing nations, such as India, Nepal, Bangladesh and parts of the Middle East, life expectancy for males is significantly higher than for their female counterparts.[22] A high sex ratio indicates premature death of females, the causes of which may include poor female access to health care or social factors resulting in basic neglect.[23]

It is a matter of concern that for most women in sub-Saharan Africa, poor pregnancy outcomes are usually thought of only as a medical event, sidestepping the underlying social, operational or reproductive background factors. Such factors have an influence on pregnancy outcomes and on the subsequent physical and mental health of the women. Further, essential to reducing maternal mortality in developing country settings is the need to address factors that also contribute to unplanned pregnancy.[24]

As stated in one study, Malawi has one of the highest maternal mortality ratios (984 deaths per 100,000 live births) in the world. The risks of pregnancy are indicated by the words used to describe a pregnant woman in the Chichewa language: either *pakati* (between life and death) or *matenda* (sick). In Malawi, behaviour at the village level can contribute to maternal mortality; for example, this is demonstrated in the fact that most deaths of pregnant women, as well as births, occur at home, and some behaviours within the community hinder timely and appropriate care-seeking.[25]

In Mozambique, it is a general expectation that pregnant women, even when they are in labour, should continue working right up until the moment they stop to give birth. In addition, fears of witchcraft and evil spirits are so strong that women conceal their pregnancies and delay going to the maternity clinics as long as possible.[26] In Uganda, pregnancy is considered a test of endurance and maternal death is a sad but normal event.[27] In Sierra Leone, there is immense pressure to bear children throughout the reproductive years.[28] However, in Uganda, Botswana and Benin, the attitudes of women towards institutional and non-institutional deliveries are not only socio-culturally determined but also result from women's perceptions that the quality of services offered is poor.[29]

The WHO estimates that 60 per cent of births in developing countries occur outside a health facility, with 47 per cent assisted only by traditional birth attendants (TBAs) or family members, or without any assistance at all.[30] In many developing countries, local tradition and culture are important determinants of the non-use of hospital facilities and the preference for TBAs at delivery. For example, one study observed that the vast majority of people in rural Bangladesh believe childbirth is an act of God and a "natural event". For this reason, they do not expect delivery complications or problems and therefore rely on TBAs for childbirth.[31] Villagers also select TBAs because of tradition, convenience and the special attention they receive. TBAs are invariably known and trusted members of the community and are also highly accessible and affordable.

Doctors, nurses and staff at hospitals and clinics, unlike TBAs, are most likely to be from outside the locality. Rural women, particularly in Muslim countries such as Bangladesh, do not usually converse with unknown persons, particularly males.[32] This behaviour is particularly pertinent because most deliveries at rural health centres are attended by male physicians. This situation acts as an important social and religious barrier to the use of these centres for delivery purposes.

In rural areas, TBA activities aim to speed up the expulsion of the baby, the removal of the placenta and the arrest of haemorrhage. They include the application of heat to the mother's abdomen, maintaining a certain position, external pressure on the abdomen, internal interference through the birth canal, and packing the birth canal to stop bleeding and ensure contraction to normal size. In the case of obstructed labour, action (referral) is delayed.

Traditional medicines are often used to induce labour, to speed up delivery, to relieve discomfort or as abortifacients. This group of medicines is heterogeneous: some cause very strong uterine responses (including rupture), some a marked atony of the uterus. The medicines may cause liver or renal failure or strong haemorrhage. The frequency of use varies from area to area. For southern Tanzania,[33] it has been estimated that 95 per cent of all women had recourse to herbal medicine but only 2 per cent of all maternal deaths were the result of herbal intoxication, although in 8 per cent this played a role. In

Malawi, 7 per cent of maternal deaths were attributed to accidental poisoning from herbal medicines.[34]

In Zimbabwe, the third stage of labour worried the traditional midwives most. They fear maternal death due to a retained placenta, a complication attributed to the lack of moral and spiritual hygiene. In cases of delayed delivery of the placenta, the midwives massage the uterus, give traditional oxytocics or increase abdominal pressure over the uterus.[35] Many TBAs perform vaginal examinations, sometimes very frequently. Hygienic knowledge and practices are, however, mostly insufficient. Contaminated unsterile herbs, leaves and emollients can be inserted into the vagina.[36]

Thus, a higher risk of maternal death in villages could be associated with harmful practices, such as unhygienic practices, the use of traditional medicines in toxic doses, or a lack of skills and knowledge to deal with complicated deliveries, such as an obstructed labour or retained placenta.

Links between religion and maternal health

Religion, being concerned with affairs that are regarded as extraordinary and as having a unique importance in life, is an intrinsic aspect of the culture of all societies, and religious groups exert an influence on civil authorities on issues of reproduction such as contraception, procreation, abortion and infertility therapy.[37] Therefore, it is important that those who practise reproduction techniques learn about different religious attitudes to reproductive health problems.[38]

Some indication of Jewish attitudes toward infertility can be found in the first command from God to Adam: "Be fruitful and multiply". In Judaism, abortion on demand is forbidden, although it may be performed if the mother's life is in danger.

Islam also places a strong and unequivocal emphasis on high fertility, and Muslim social structures universally support this. According to Islam, the procedures of in vitro fertilisation and embryo transfer are acceptable; however, they can be performed only between husband and wife. Islam allows contraception only in certain circumstances, and only in special cases can abortion be performed.

Within Christianity, attitudes toward reproductive practices differ between the various denominations. For example, Roman Catholic doctrine does not accept the practice of assisted reproduction. In the Roman Catholic Church, the suffering of spouses who cannot have children or who are afraid of bringing a handicapped child into the world is a suffering that everyone must understand and take into consideration. The embryo is seen as a human being from conception and abortion is therefore strictly forbidden. According to the Vatican, the primary purpose of marriage is procreation. The contraceptive act destroys the potential for producing new life through sexual intercourse, violating the purpose of marriage and therefore constituting a sin against nature. On the other hand, contraception and assisted reproduction may be practised by Protestants and Anglicans.

Factors impeding access to, and utilisation of, health services

There are various factors that may impede access to, and utilisation of, health services. In many countries, gender inequalities restrict women's access to health care, because they face social constraints in managing their own health and that of their children. Social factors further affect men and women differently.[39] An interest in women's seclusion and restricted mobility is central to much of the discourse concerning gender and health in South Asia.[40] For example, unrestricted, independent mobility is thought to improve health outcomes indirectly via increased exposure to information, development of interpersonal skills and greater self-confidence. Seclusion is thus viewed as an important barrier to improving women's health.[41]

In the developed world, impeded access to screening leads to certain ethnic groups being at higher risk of cervical cancer.[42] Further, childless women have less access to health care, and their social isolation has been reported, including in developing countries such as India.[43]

In many developing countries, female participation in public life is extremely restricted: many women cannot venture beyond the family compound without a male companion.[44] Many report they are unable to go to a health facility unaccompanied, and family members, especially male, must accompany them to these health facilities.[45] In Pakistan's rural areas, for example, it has been found that over two-thirds of women required permission to visit relatives within the village, and less than one-third could go unescorted to a health centre.[46] In such a conservative society, women understandably prefer to be seen by women doctors for gynaecological and obstetric consultations.[47] Thus, the absence of women doctors makes many otherwise accessible health facilities, even those whose services include EmOC, unacceptable socially, and hence these women are deprived of their human rights to equality of treatment and dignity.

The likelihood of women making use of biomedical maternity care resources is conditioned by numerous factors, including the women's socio-economic characteristics, social barriers, great distances to the nearest health resources, lack of transport, cost, poor quality of care, and perceptions of need.[48] The available evidence shows that a significant number of women have no access to modern health services, particularly during pregnancy and childbirth.[49]

Some studies verify that geographical distance to a health facility is a barrier to uptake of services. In Mozambique, most women consider visiting a clinic as taking half the day.[50] Similarly, a situation analysis of a network of 1,288 Family Welfare Centres in Pakistan found that the majority of "service users" lived nearby and travelled to the centre on foot.[51]

Another important obstacle in seeking and utilising adequate medical care during obstetric emergencies is the lack of information about the existence and location of a referral hospital and about the quality of the services available.[52] This lack of knowledge is significantly higher among poor families. A study of maternal health in the southern highlands of Tanzania found that lack of information and the consequent lack of appropriate action, such as visits to a health facility after detection of a problem, were found to be major factors contributing to maternal deaths.[53]

Furthermore, many rural residents exposed to modern health services have negative perceptions of the quality of the services offered by rural health facilities and medically trained personnel. This negative perception is attributed variously to inattentive or discourteous staff behaviour; the lack of qualified or skilled staff; abuse, neglect and poor treatment in hospitals; poor cooperation and a lack of privacy.[54] Such negative perceptions are widely considered important to explaining the under-utilisation of rural public health facilities in developing countries.

Untapped potential: Community participation

Maternal health in some countries has been a low priority for policy-makers, not only because of poor epidemiological data but also because of poor community involvement in decision-making about health priorities.[55] Community participation has been described as the key success factor in maternal health programmes. A randomised community trial in Nepal, for example, successfully used lay workers and regular meetings of pregnant women in communities to improve knowledge, empowerment and early access to maternity services.[56] This approach appeared to be cost-effective in terms of cost per life-year saved.[57]

The success of community mobilisation interventions to reduce maternal mortality depends on understanding women's perceptions of the health problems affecting them. This information can assist in creating more effective and acceptable interventions. In Africa, a study in Malawi also showed that, by collectively sharing experiences, groups of women can identify most maternal health problems, recognise how important they are and move to address them.[58] Women's support groups represent one possible mechanism for achieving goals of empowerment, increased knowledge and even problem-solving around such issues as transport to care. Their voices need to be heard by decision-makers, and the participation of women in finding solutions to the huge risks of pregnancy is possibly the most important part of the solution.

Human resources and skilled attendants

The importance of human resources is common to most health services. Internationally, the primary intervention recommended for reducing maternal mortality is to increase the number of skilled attendants, normally classified as doctors, nurses and midwives, at birth. This technical intervention has been recommended as the sole process indicator to guide progress towards achievement of the Millennium Development Goal of maternal mortality reduction. In the developing world, the lack of a skilled attendant at birth is strongly correlated with maternal and infant mortality.[59]

It has been estimated that 63 per cent of all births globally are attended by skilled health personnel. The figure is 99 per cent in developed regions, compared with 59 per cent in developing countries. Considerable regional variation has been observed: 47 per cent in Africa, 61 per cent in Asia, 80 per cent in Oceania, 88 per cent in Latin America and the Caribbean, and 99 per cent in Europe and North America. Within each region, moreover, variations were found by sub-region and country. In all the sub-regions of Africa, for example, the percentage of births attended by skilled personnel was lowest in East Africa (34 per cent) and West Africa (40 per cent). In Asia, the percentage was lowest in south-central Asia (44 per cent).[60]

As in many other developing African and Asian countries, in Somalia home births remain a strong preference compared with institutional births, and are often the only option for many women.[61] A large proportion of home deliveries take place without skilled attendants; most women in the developing world depend on traditional birth attendants who, for the most part, have had no formal midwifery training.[62] Problems occur when emergency services are needed and women cannot or do not seek those services or identify warning signs. It is likely that many women who need treatment cannot reach a hospital. It is imperative to train and educate the birth attendants about warning signs of trouble in childbirth, so pregnant women can get timely and appropriate attention.

Although skilled attendants are undoubtedly essential, maternal outcomes from deliveries that do take place with such attendants will still be affected by the systems in which they occur. Graham et al. examined the relationship between maternal mortality and skilled attendants at delivery in a number of countries, and found that it was not a simple linear one.[63] They suggest that a range of factors may influence the considerable divergence from a linear relationship. One such factor was the notion of what constitutes a skilled attendant; doctors and trained midwives are commonly accepted as such, but studies in many countries also include other medical staff such as trained attendants, even if they have had little midwifery training. Furthermore, Maine and others have argued that the accessibility of emergency services – both for those delivering with a skilled attendant and for those who are not – also plays a large role in shaping maternal outcomes aside from the use of skilled attendants.[64] Where skilled attendants are present, they require resources, motivation and systems to actually provide mortality-reducing services.

Thus, from a health systems perspective, there are questions concerning how people access attendants, what happens when a skilled attendant is reached and the quality of the care received. Reducing maternal deaths requires all elements of a health system to function in coordination. For example, there is evidence that maternal mortality in Sri Lanka and Malaysia has significantly decreased, partly through a more extensive use of midwives but also because, in both countries, increases in the number of women attended by skilled personnel took place alongside widespread health and social improvements, including greatly increased female education and improved access for the treatment of complications at rural health facilities.[65]

There remains complexity in the relationship between skilled attendance and maternal mortality. As cited in one study, for instance, although Uganda has over three times the rate of skilled attendance as Bangladesh (39 per cent of births as opposed to only 12.1 per cent), estimates of the maternal mortality ratio (MMR) tend to be higher in Uganda: 505 per 100,000 live births compared with recent estimates of 322 and 440 in Bangladesh. There are several possible explanations for this outcome. Assuming that the clinical needs are similar, it could be that the quality of hospital care is lower in Uganda, so emergencies are not referred quickly or treated effectively. It was noted, for example, that only 57 per cent of Ugandan hospitals were able to administer general anaesthesia. In terms of staff to handle complications, there are also significantly more physicians per capita in Bangladesh, which has 20 physicians per 100,000 population, compared with only 5.3 in Uganda.[66]

In Russia and South Africa, skilled attendance is nearly universal (over 95 per cent and 86 per cent, respectively), but the outcomes are worse than might be expected, with MMRs of 40 per 100,000 live births in Russia and 150 in South Africa. For comparison, the EU average was 5.5 and the Central and Eastern Europe was 14.3 in 2000).[67] This is despite excess staff capacity in Russia, which has more than twice the number of midwives per 100,000 people than in several West and East European countries. A South African case study in particular has illustrated how measuring skilled attendance is only a first step in understanding the determinants of maternal health outcomes.[68] According to that country's confidential inquiry into maternal deaths between 1999 and 2001, problems in the care of women by health care workers occurred in more than half of the maternal deaths, with the problems being worst at the primary health care level. Common problems were poor diagnosis and poor monitoring of patients, as well as failure to follow standard protocols. Other studies have also documented the poor quality of care given to women in labour. The most striking example is work by Jewkes et al. that documented physical and verbal abuse of women in midwife obstetric units in Cape Town.[69] This suggests that the context in which staff work, the quality of human resource management and issues around health care worker motivation are as important as whether staff are present or not.

The comparative analysis shows that the success of even the most commonly recommended intervention to prevent maternal mortality – skilled attendance at delivery – relies heavily on how overall systems function, in particular the availability and quality of staff to handle emergencies and the strategic placement of attendants within referral networks. An improvement in the relationship between the traditional sector, traditional birth attendants and modern health services in many countries, especially developing countries, is urgent. Increased attendance and improvement of antenatal care, identification of high-risk cases, early recognition of complicated deliveries, availability of transport to health facilities and appropriate action in health facilities by health workers are important factors in lowering maternal mortality. As no dramatic increase is to be expected in the coverage rate of births by health facilities, the role of the TBA (or other village-level workers) will be critical.

Concerns about the effect of user fees on maternal health

Since the 1980s, governments in many low- and middle-income countries have launched health sector reforms as a long-term effort to strengthen and improve the efficiency of their health systems and to address problems such as resource shortages and poor health outcomes.[70] Health sector reforms in recent years have included the decentralisation of health administration and funding to lower levels, the integration of previously separate health services, the privatisation of services and financial reforms affecting the collection and payment of health sector funds.[71] Empirical studies have often found that reforms can produce negative impacts on maternal service provision and use because the change process can strain working relationships or overload health workers.[72]

One of the most common health sector "reforms" that has been undertaken is the introduction of user fees for public services. User fees were generally introduced to improve drug supplies and help cope with insufficient funding for the health sector. Despite carefully defined exemptions for children and preventive services, including antenatal care, anecdotal evidence suggests that exemptions for maternity services are rarely implemented. The literature also shows that the introduction of user fees has had a negative impact on utilisation levels, including an increase in the number of babies "born before arrival at facility". In addition, there is evidence that, even when preventive services are exempt from user fees, utilisation still falls because preventive care, including antenatal services, is some-times delivered to patients who come to health facilities for curative care. As demand for curative care has fallen following the introduction of user fees, there has been a knock-on effect on the amount of preventive care supplied.[73]

In Bangladesh, official user fees are not charged for maternal services, but unofficial fees have had negative effects on hospital service utilisation. South Africa also used to have user fees, but maternal and child health fees were removed in 1994. In many developing countries, such as Nigeria, Ghana and Sierra Leone, the introduction of user fees has also led to a decline in the utilisation of maternal health services.[74] In Uganda, user fees were introduced in the early 1990s but abolished in 2001; it was found that the effect of user fees was not only to improve the motivation of health workers but also to decrease service utilisation.[75] It was also observed that utilisation among the poor increased much more rapidly after the abolition of fees than beforehand, especially for maternal health services.[76] Moreover, the overall effect of fees on consumers was detrimental because funds were often not invested in quality improvements. Thus, the marked decreases in utilisation of non-emergency services found at many of the sites studied suggests that the potential effects of user fees should be carefully analysed by programme planners before fees are instituted.

It should be noted, however, that studies carried out by Schneider and Gilson in South Africa suggest there was some initial increase in the utilisation of services after the abolition of user fees but that this increase was not sustained. This may be partly explained by the fact that fee collection before the abolition of fees was on a rather haphazard basis, with widespread exceptions for the poor, and hospitals provided services even if women could not pay the fees. This shows that, although fees generally decrease maternal service use, the abolition of fees will not necessarily improve maternal care utilisation or outcomes. In some cases, informal fees may be significantly higher than any official fees charged in the first place.[77]

In both Uganda and Bangladesh, other common barriers to maternal health access that have been identified include socio-cultural norms to deliver at home or with traditional birth attendants, the perceived low quality of care at facilities, and physical accessibility problems. Access barriers work in dynamic and mutually reinforcing ways, and the costs of services are only one component affecting service use, especially as official fees are often meant to improve the quality of care.[78]

In other countries, reforms based on user fees have produced differing results. Investigations into the specific ways in which reforms change the health system environment illustrates, however, that there is no simple linear correlation between reforms and their impact. Instead, outcomes are shaped by the structure of the system and how the reform is initiated. For instance, although user fee introduction may reduce the use of services, abolition may not increase use owing to a number of possible interlinked access barriers, including informal fees and low perceived quality. The impact of changing the user fee system will depend greatly on the structure of payments and the access barriers existing within the system.

Direct and indirect factors affecting maternal health

Many factors contribute to maternal mortality; although some of these are direct effects, other more indirect influences are also apparent. The principal determinants of maternal mortality identified in the literature point to lack of trained personnel, lack of material or equipment, inappropriate physical structures, inadequate patient management (quality services), poor referral systems, long distances to the hospital and lack of transport.[79] In many resource-poor countries, it remains a formidable challenge to remedy all these deficiencies.

An estimated 450 million adult women in developing countries are stunted as a result of protein-energy malnutrition during childhood, and more than 50 per cent are anaemic.[80] Approximately 250 million women suffer the effects of iodine deficiency and, although the exact numbers are unknown, millions may be blind owing to vitamin A deficiency.[81] The highest levels of malnutrition among women are found in South Asia, where approximately 60 per cent of women suffer from iron deficiency anaemia. This proportion rises to 80 per cent among pregnant women in India.[82]

It is also important to recognise the potential effect on maternal health of contextual factors, including socio-economic context, national policies on the provision and cost of health care and socio-cultural norms and practices. The fact that gross national product per capita and health expenditure are strongly associated with maternal mortality suggests that these factors are potentially significant in maternal health care.[83] Furthermore, higher health expenditures per capita have been associated with the improved performance of national health systems.

In developed countries, most deaths are to the result of other direct causes, mainly complications with anaesthesia and caesarean sections.[84] However, evidence shows that in developing countries almost 80 per cent of maternal deaths are directly due to obstetric causes and result from haemorrhage, infection, eclampsia, obstructed labour and unsafe abortion.[85] Many studies confirm the prominent role of haemorrhage as a cause of maternal death in developing countries. Hypertensive disorders are among the leading causes of death in Latin America and the Caribbean. The contributions of sepsis and human immunodeficiency virus (HIV) in Africa, anaemia in Asia, abortion in Latin America and the Caribbean, and other direct causes (related to caesarean section and anaesthesia) and embolism in developed countries seem to be more region specific.[86]

Ensuring EmOC services is not enough

For the approximately 15 per cent of women who experience complications in pregnancy and delivery and in the post-partum period, emergency obstetric care must be accessible to prevent maternal deaths. Access to free care, free transport to care and access to skilled attendance at delivery have been recognised as key factors for reducing maternal mortality.[87] In a review analysis to demonstrate the extent to which recommended levels of emergency obstetric care were available in 23 developing countries (including Nepal, Sri Lanka, Pakistan, Malawi, Mali, Rwanda, Bhutan, Peru, Bolivia, Chad, Senegal and Bangladesh), Paxton et al. found that, in 16 of the 23 countries, less than 50 per cent of the recommended levels had been achieved.[88]

In South Africa, 84.4 per cent of women have a skilled attendant at the time of delivery, which is higher than the rates in Asia (61.5 per cent), elsewhere in Africa (46.7 per cent) and in the Caribbean and Latin America (83.2 per cent).[89] South Africa is above internationally recommended rates for basic essential obstetric care (BEOC), having a rate of 6 BEOC facilities per 500,000 population, compared with a recommended minimum of 4 BEOC facilities. South Africa is also above the recommended level for comprehensive essential obstetric care (CEOC) at 3.2 CEOC facilities per 500,000 population, compared with the recommended 1 CEOC facility. However, women also report difficulties reaching these services, either because they cannot afford transportation or because it is not available. Therefore, despite a reasonably functioning health care system, maternal mortality remains relatively high for a middle-income country.

The South African example highlights that the availability of BEOC and CEOC is not enough to ensure quality maternity services, especially if those services are not always accessible or suffer from poor quality of care. Throughout Africa and in other developing countries implementing BEOC and CEOC, hospital and clinic protocols for the assessment and treatment of women and infants must be reviewed and evidence-based standards implemented. Facilities must also be adequately supplied with essential medicines and supplies. Sensitivity training for hospital staff working with mothers and infants should be explored, and communication with families needs to be enhanced. The underlying health care system problems that place undue stress on health workers and reduce their capacity to deliver quality care cannot be ignored.

Abortion care services

Of the estimated 210 million pregnancies worldwide, 40 per cent are unplanned and approximately 25 per cent end in abortion.[90] One tragic consequence of the reproductive subordination of women is the dilemma of unsafe abortion. Women put their health, social standing, future fertility and lives at risk to end unwanted pregnancies.[91] Despite improvements in technology and access to services and changes in legislation, millions of unsafe abortions are still carried out each year. Of the half a million maternal deaths per year, approximately 13–20 per cent are caused by unsafe abortions, that is, approximately 80,000 women die each year from abortions or their complications.[92]

As cited in one report, the majority of maternal deaths occur from the third trimester of pregnancy to the first week following delivery or abortion. A report based on Demographic and Health Surveys data shows that only 61 per cent of women who delivered in a health facility in 30 developing countries received post-partum care; where births took place at home, the percentage receiving post-partum care tended to be much lower. For example, only 11 per cent of women received post-partum care in Ethiopia, 27 per cent in Bangladesh and 28 per cent in Nepal. Even among those who did seek a post-partum check-up, most did so three or more days following delivery outside of health facilities. This check-up should be within 24 hours of delivery, and all women should receive it.[93]

According to estimates by the WHO, of the 46 million pregnancies that are terminated each year around the world, approximately 60 per cent are carried out under unsafe conditions. Further, more than 18 million induced abortions each year are performed by people lacking the necessary skills or in an environment lacking the minimum medical standards, or both, and are therefore also unsafe. Almost all take place in the developing world.[94] The risk of dying from an unsafe abortion is around 350 per 100,000, and 68,000 women die in this way each year. The tragedy is that each of these deaths is unnecessary because abortion can be provided safely and easily.

Abortion was legalised in 1971 in India; however, because of inadequate access to official services, illegal abortion is three times more common in cities and five times more common in rural areas than legal abortion.[95] In a study of six states in India, it was also noted that the average charges for induced abortion were equivalent to, or more than, three weeks of average per capita income.[96]

Generally, deaths resulting from abortion are high in Latin America and the Caribbean and in some East European countries. The reason for relatively high abortion mortality in Latin America might be that there are fewer deaths from other causes or that it has more restrictive abortion laws than other world regions. Abortion death figures are likely to be biased downwards by under-reporting and misclassification (as haemorrhage or sepsis). It is probably safe to assume that abortion deaths are almost always the result of unsafe abortion methods.[97]

Special attention needs to be paid to the consequences of induced abortion, as many studies indicate that it has become the leading cause of maternal death. More and improved sex education in schools, in conjunction with the increased availability and use of modern contraceptives and the legalisation of induced abortion, is the most important means of reducing abortion-related mortality to almost zero.

A matter of concern: Female infanticide and FGM

The difficulty of changing harmful cultural and traditional practices is also notable in female infanticide. Some countries, such as India, have implemented laws making prenatal diagnosis of foetal sex by ultrasound illegal, with strict licensing of ultrasound equipment.[98] This was intended to address gender-based female foeticide based on prenatal sex determination by ultrasound. However, deep cultural beliefs discriminating against women from before they are born that are not easily changed by the introduction of legislation protecting sexual and reproductive rights still remain.[99]

Female genital mutilation or cutting (FGM/C) has been recognised as both a health and a human rights issue. There are laws prohibiting FGM/C in at least 13 African countries as well as in several developed countries. It is estimated that over 132 million women and girls have experienced female genital mutilation, and that some 2 million girls are at risk of undergoing some form of the procedure every year.[100] The WHO has recognised that genital mutilation has serious and sometimes fatal physical consequences as well as psychological effects, yet more than 90 per cent of women in Djibouti, Egypt, Eritrea, Guinea, Mali, Sierra Leone and Somalia have undergone FGM.[101] Governments and non-governmental organisations, including professional organisations and women's groups, should receive encouragement and material support to work for the elimination of genital mutilation. Laws and clear policy declarations prohibiting the practice may help.

Conclusions

Of all the human development indicators, the maternal mortality ratio shows the greatest discrepancy between developed and developing countries. Poor maternal health, nutrition and quality of obstetric care not only take their toll on women, but are also responsible for 20 per cent of the burden of disease among children less than 5 years old.[102] Most of this loss and suffering is preventable, and therefore provides an opportunity for improving maternal health. Investment in pregnancy and safe delivery programmes is a cost-effective way to meet the basic health needs of women in developing countries. The prevention of unwanted or ill-timed pregnancies is also essential to improving women's health and giving them more control over their lives.

Complications in pregnancy and childbirth are the leading cause of death and disability among women of reproductive age in developing countries. Almost all maternal deaths are potentially avoidable. By now, the leading *medical* causes of maternal deaths – haemorrhage, sepsis, obstructed labour, unsafe abortion and hypertensive diseases of pregnancy – are widely known. It is also widely accepted that the application of existing technology can greatly reduce the number of maternal deaths. EmOC is the most essential service required to control the unnecessary loss of life that takes place from maternal causes. Yet in many places EmOC is unavailable, mainly owing to a deficiency of formally trained obstetricians at the peripheral levels as well as a shortage of anaesthesiologists and inadequate transportation systems for the emergency referral of mothers during labour.

In identifying key factors inhibiting improvements in health outcomes, specific country contexts can further determine many factors influencing maternal health outcomes and service performance. Interventions should thus address not only the medical problems but also the *underlying* causes: the precise mix of social, cultural and political factors that interact in individual countries and communities and result in maternal deaths.

Many of the South Asian and sub-Saharan African countries rank low in terms of gender-related human indices. In countries where women make up half of the population, social and economic burdens will become increasingly onerous in the coming decades if due attention is not paid to capacity-building and to women's health issues. Development remains an incomplete process unless we include both men and women at all levels of social, economic and political functioning. There is a compelling need to change mindsets and to develop a societal vision, one where education for women is seen as a means of social change, where access to health care is not an issue and where women have rights over their own lives and bodies.

The issues of health coverage, costs and quality predominate in developing countries. The ability to ensure the delivery of quality health services remains the health sector's biggest challenge. Reducing maternal mortality requires a diversified and multi-sectoral approach to increasing the availability and accessibility of health care. Services and policies must surmount socio-cultural and economic barriers. Effective services to improve overall maternal health need targeted health and social policies that are informed by reliable and valid epidemiological data. A comprehensive summary of the magnitude and distribution of the causes of maternal deaths is critical to inform reproductive health policies and programmes.

The need for improved maternal health has long been on the international agenda, dating from the launch of the Safe Motherhood Conference in 1987 in Nairobi, which was sponsored by the World Bank, the WHO and the United Nations Population Fund. The United Nations World Summit for Children in 1990 adopted the following as a specific goal: "Access by all pregnant women to prenatal care, trained attendants during childbirth and referral facilities for high-risk pregnancies and obstetric emergencies". Similar aims have been voiced in other major international meetings, including the 1994 International Conference on Population and Development (ICPD), the Fourth World Conference on Women in 1995, their five-year follow-up evaluations of progress and the United Nations General Assembly Special Session on Children in 2002. The core policy framework supporting maternal health is the ICPD Programme of Action (chapter 8), now supplemented by ICPD+5 and the Millennium Development Goals (MDGs). Actions suggested included expanding the provision of maternal and child health services in the context of primary health care. Implementation of the Programme of Action will significantly contribute to attainment of MDG5 (target 6) – improving maternal health and reducing maternal deaths. However, a shortcoming of the international treaty process is the glaring gap between countries' adoption of these global contracts in the international arena and their tardy implementation at the domestic level.[103]

Communities and families appear to be an untapped resource from which both maternal and newborn health could benefit. Support as simple as families telling women to go for care or assisting with resources permitting them to obtain care appears to make a difference. The WHO has described a health promotion approach and a health-promoting settings model that focuses on developing supportive and healthy environments through a holistic and integrated approach to health promotion.[104] This requires full participation and involvement by the relevant communities, families and individuals within these settings in order to realise improvements in health.

Notes

1. United Nations Development Fund for Women (UNIFEM), "A Portal on Women, Peace and Security", <http://www.womenwarpeace.org/issues/reprohealth/reprohealth.htm> (accessed 12 July 2007).
2. J. Desai, "The Cost of Emergency Obstetric Care: Concepts and Issues," *International Journal of Gynecology and Obstetrics*, 81, 2003, pp. 74–82.
3. World Bank, *World Development Report 1993: Investing in Health*, New York: Oxford University Press, 1993.
4. United Nations Population Fund (UNFPA), *Reducing Maternal Deaths: Selecting Priorities, Tracking Progress*, Module 1, Distance Learning System on Population Issues, Pilot Edition, UNFPA, 2001.
5. World Health Organization (WHO), *World Health Day Information Kit: Safe Motherhood*, Geneva: World Health Organization, 1998.
6. UNFPA, *Reproductive Health for Communities in Crisis, UNFPA Emergency Response*, Geneva: UNFPA, 2001.
7. WHO, UNICEF, UNFPA, *Maternal Mortality in 2000: Estimates Developed by WHO, UNICEF, UNFPA*, Geneva: UN Press, 2004.
8. I. Shah and L. Say, "Maternal Mortality and Maternity Care from 1990 to 2005: Uneven but Important Gains", *Reproductive Health Matters*, 15(30), 2007, pp. 17–27.
9. M. F. Fathalla, "Human Rights Aspects of Safe Motherhood", *Best Practice and Research*, 20(3), 2006, pp. 409–419.
10. R. Cook, M. Beatriz and G. Bevilacqua, "Invoking Human Rights to Reduce Maternal Deaths", *Lancet*, 363, 2004, p. 73; S. Thaddeus and D. Maine, "Too Far to Walk: Maternal Mortality in Context," *Social Science and Medicine*, 38(8), 1994, pp. 1091–1110.
11. S. Penny and S. Murray, "Training Initiatives for Essential Obstetric Care in Developing Countries: A State of the Art Review", *Health Policy and Planning*, 15(4), 2000, pp. 386–393.
12. WHO, *Essential Elements of Obstetric Care at the First Referral Level*, Geneva: World Health Organization, 1991.
13. D. Maine, *Safe Motherhood Programs: Options and Issues*, New York: Centre for Population and Family Health, Columbia University, 1993.
14. D. Maine and A. Rosenfield, "The Safe Motherhood Initiative: Why Has It Stalled?", *American Journal of Public Health*, 89, 1999, pp. 480–482; see also Maine, *Safe Motherhood Programs*.
15. Thaddeus and Maine, "Too Far to Walk".
16. The Prevention of Maternal Mortality Network, "Situation Analysis of Emergency Obstetric Care: Examples from Eleven Operations Research Projects in West Africa", *Social Science and Medicine*, 40, 1995, pp. 657–667.
17. WHO. *Beyond the Numbers: Reviewing Maternal Deaths and Complications to Make Pregnancy Safer*, Geneva: World Health Organization, 2004.
18. F. Arnold, *Gender Preference in Children*, Calverton, MD: Macro International Inc., 1997; R. Hussain et al., "The Role of Son Preference in Repro-

ductive Behavior in Pakistan", *Bulletin of the World Health Organization*, 78(3), 2000, pp. 379–388.

19. H. Papanek, *Purdah: Separate Worlds and Symbolic Shelter. Studies of Purdah in South Asia*, Columbia, MO: South Asia Books, 1990.

20. G. Bicego and O. B. Ahmad, *Infant and Child Mortality*, Calverton, MD: Macro International Inc., 1996; see also Arnold, *Gender Preference in Children*.

21. W. Stinson, *Women and Health*, Geneva: World Federation of Public Health, 1986.

22. M. Rutter, "Women's Health in Developing Countries", *Nursing*, 25, 1988, pp. 935–936; see also Stinson, *Women and Health*.

23. Z. A. Sathar, "Child Survival and Changing Fertility Patterns in Pakistan", *Pakistan Development Review*, 31(94), 1992, pp. 699–711.

24. M. Mbizvo, M. Bonduelle, S. Chadzuka et al., "Unplanned Pregnancies in Harare: What Are the Social and Sexual Determinants?", *Social Science and Medicine*, 45(6), 1997, pp. 937–942.

25. M. Rosato, C. Mwansambo, P. Kazembe et al., "Women's Groups' Perceptions of Maternal Health Issues in Rural Malawi", *Lancet*, 368, 2006, pp. 1180–1188.

26. R. R. Chapman, "Endangering Safe Motherhood in Mozambique: Prenatal Care as Pregnancy Risk", *Social Science and Medicine*, 57, 2003, pp. 355–374.

27. G. B. Kyomuhendo, "Low Use of Rural Maternity Services in Uganda: Impact of Women's Status, Traditional Beliefs and Limited Resources", *Reproductive Health Matters*, 11, 2003, pp. 16–26.

28. M. Balley, "Determinants of Fertility in a Rural Society: Some Evidence from Sierra Leone", *Social Science & Medicine*, 28(3), 1989, pp. 285–292.

29. J. Parkhurst, L. Penn-Kekana, D. Blaauw et al., "Health Systems Factors Influencing Maternal Health Services: a Four-Country Comparison", *Health Policy*, 73, 2005, pp. 127–138.

30. WHO, *Coverage of Maternity Care. A Listing of Available Information*, Geneva: World Health Organization, 1996.

31. B. K. Paul, "The Geography of Childbirth in Rural Bangladesh: A Case Study", *The Arab World Geographer*, 3, 2000, pp. 208–220.

32. N. Prendiville, "The Role and Effectiveness of Traditional Birth Attendants in Somalia", *Evaluation and Program Planning*, 21, 1998, pp. 353–361.

33. Ernest Urassa et al., "Operational Factors Affecting Maternal Mortality in Tanzania", *Health Policy and Planning*, 12(1), 1997, pp. 50–57, <http://heapol.oxfordjournals.org/cgi/reprint/12/1/50.pdf> (accessed 26 June 2009).

34. C. H. W. Bullough, "Analysis of Maternal Deaths in the Central Region of Malawi", *East African Medical Journal*, 58, 1981, pp. 25–36.

35. J. Mutambirwa, "Pregnancy, Childbirth, Mother and Child Care among the Indigenous People of Zimbabwe", *International Journal of Gynecology and Obstetrics*, 23, 1985, pp. 275–285.

36. V. A. Bouchier, "Maternity Care in the Sudd, Southern Sudan", *Tropical Doctor*, 14, 1984, pp. 32–33.

37. J. G. Schenker, "Women's Reproductive Health: Monotheistic Religious Perspectives", *International Journal of Gynecology & Obstetrics*, 70(1), 2000, pp. 77–86.

38. M. Ali and H. Ushijima, "Perceptions of Men on Role of Religious Leaders in Reproductive Health Issues in Rural Districts in Pakistan", *Journal of Biosocial Science*, 3(1), 2005, pp. 115–122; see also Schenker, "Women's Reproductive Health".

39. N. D. Ojanuga and C. Gilbert, "Women's Access to Health Care in Developing Countries", *Social Science & Medicine*, 35, 1992, pp. 613–617.

40. S. R. Schuler, S. M. Hashemi and A. P. Riley, "The Influence of Women's Changing Roles and Status in Bangladesh's Fertility Transition: Evidence from a Study of Credit Programs and Contraceptive Use", *World Development* 25(4), 1997, pp. 563–575.

41. J. Cleland, N. Kamal and A. Sloggett, *Links between Fertility Regulation and the Schooling of and Autonomy of Women in Bangladesh*, New Delhi: Sage Publications, 1996.

42. V. M. Taylor et al., "A Randomized Controlled Trial of Interventions to Promote Cervical Cancer Screening among Chinese Women in North America", *Journal of National Cancer Institute*, 94, 2002, pp. 670–677; T. G. Hislop, H. F. Clarke and M. Deschamps, "Cervical Cytology Screening. How Can We Improve Rates among First Nations Women in Urban British Columbia?", *Canadian Family Physician*, 42, 1996, pp. 1701–708.

43. J. C. Bhatia, "Ideal Number and Sex Preference of Children in India", *Journal of Family Welfare*, 24, 1987, pp. 3–16.

44. N. J. Piet-Pelon et al., *Men in Bangladesh, India and Pakistan: Reproductive Health Issues*, Dhaka: Karshaf Publishers, 2000.

45. K. Mumtaz and S. Salway, "I Never Go Anywhere: Extricating the Links between Women's Mobility and Uptake of Reproductive Health Services in Pakistan", *Social Science and Medicine*, 60, 2005, pp. 1751–1765.

46. Z. Sathar and S. Kazi, *Women's Autonomy, Livelihood and Fertility: A Study of Rural Punjab*, Islamabad: PIDE, 1997.

47. A. Green, M. Rana, D. Ross and C. Thunhurst, "Health Planning in Pakistan: A Case Study", *International Journal of Health Planning and Management*, 12, 1997, pp. 187–205.

48. A. Noor, S. Luby and M. H. Rahbar, "Does Use of Government Service Depend on Distance from the Health Facility?", *Health Policy and Planning*, 14, 1999, pp. 191–197.

49. Population Council, *The Gap between Reproductive Intentions and Behavior: A Study of Punjabi Men and Women*, Islamabad: Population Council, 1997.

50. Chapman, "Endangering Safe Motherhood in Mozambique: Prenatal Care as Pregnancy Risk".

51. G. Cernada, A. U. Rob and S. Ameen, "A Situation Analysis of Family Welfare Centres in Pakistan", Operations Research Working Paper No. 4, Ministry of Health, Islamabad, 1993.

52. T. K. Sundari, "The Untold Story: How the Health Care Systems in Developing Countries Contribute to Maternal Mortality", *International Journal of Health Services*, 22, 1992, pp. 513–528.

53. T. G. Price, "A Study of Maternal Health in the Southern Highlands of Tanzania – Preliminary Report on Maternal Deaths in the Southern Highlands of Tanzania in 1983", *Journal of Obstetrics and Gynaecology of Eastern and Central Africa*, 3(3), 1984, pp. 103–110; see also G. Mbaruku, "Reducing Maternal Mortality in Kigoma, Tanzania: INV 58", *Tropical Medicine & International Health*, 12 suppl (1), 2007, p. 19.

54. Chapman, "Endangering Safe Motherhood in Mozambique: Prenatal Care as Pregnancy Risk".

55. Rosato et al., "Women's Groups' Perceptions of Maternal Health Issues in Rural Malawi".

56. D. Manandhar, D. Osrin, B. Shrestha et al., "Effect of a Participatory Intervention with Women's Groups on Birth Outcomes in Nepal: Cluster-Randomized Trial", *Lancet*, 364, 2004, pp. 970–979.

57. J. Borghi, B. Thapa, D. Osrin et al., "Economic Assessment of a Women's Group Intervention to Improve Birth Outcomes in Rural Nepal", *Lancet*, 366, 2005, pp. 1882–1884.

58. C. H. W. Bullough, "Analysis of Maternal Deaths in the Central Region of Malawi", *East African Medical Journal*, 58, 1981, pp. 25–36.

59. N. Chaya and J. Dusenberry, *ICPD at Ten: Where Are We Now? A Report Card on Sexual & Reproductive Health & Rights*, New York: Family Care International, International Planned Parenthood Federation and Population Action International, 2004; <http://www.populationaction.org/cd2015/_pdfs/reportCard/reportCard_final_eng.pdf> (accessed 24 June 2009).

60. Shah and Say, "Maternal Mortality and Maternity Care from 1990 to 2005".

61. Prendiville, "The Role and Effectiveness of Traditional Birth Attendants in Somalia".

62. T. C. Cynthia, "The Effects of Skilled Health Attendants on Reducing Maternal Deaths in Developing Countries: Testing the Medical Model", *Evaluation and Program Planning*, 25, 2002, pp. 107–116.

63. W. J. Graham, J. S. Bell and C. H. W. Bullough, "Can Skilled Attendance at Delivery Reduce Maternal Mortality in Developing Countries?", in V. De Brouwere and W. Van Lerveghe (eds), *Safe Motherhood Strategies: A Review of the Evidence*, Antwerp: ITG Pres.

64. D. Maine, "What's So Special about Maternal Mortality", in M. Berer and T. S. Ravindran (eds), *Safe Motherhood Initiatives: Critical Issues*, Oxford: Blackwell Scientific Publications, 1999.

65. I. Pathmanathan, J. Liljestrand, J. M. Martins et al., *Investing in Maternal Health: Learning from Malaysia and Sri Lanka*, Washington DC: World Bank, Human Development Network, 2003.

66. Parkhurst et al., "Health Systems Factors Influencing Maternal Health Services: A Four-Country Comparison".

67. Ibid.

68. D. McIntyre and B. Klugman, "The Human Face of Decentralization and Integration of Health Services: Experience from South Africa", *Reproductive Health Matters*, 11(21), 2003, pp. 108–119.

69. R. Jewkes, N. Abrahams and Z. Mvo, "Why Do Nurses Abuse Patients? Reflections from South African Obstetric Services", *Social Science and Medicine*, 47(11), 1998, pp. 1781–1795.

70. T. Dmytraczenko, V. Rao and L. Ashford, *Health Sector Reform: How It Affects Reproductive Health*, Washington, DC: Population Reference Bureau PRB MEASURE Communication, 2003.

71. Ibid.

72. McIntyre and Klugman, "The Human Face of Decentralization and Integration of Health Services: Experience from South Africa"; Parkhurst et al., "Health Systems Factors Influencing Maternal Health Services: A Four-Country Comparison"; M. Jowett and T. Ensor, "Investing in Safe Motherhood: Evidence of Cost-Effectiveness in Developing Countries, with Specific Reference to Kenya", paper prepared for DFID-EA, International Programme Centre for Health Economics, University of York, 1999.

73. P. Nanda, "Gender Dimensions of User Fees: Implications for Women's Utilisation of Health Care", *Reproductive Health Matters*, 20(10), 2002, pp. 127–134.

74. The Prevention of Maternal Mortality Network, "Situation Analysis of Emergency Obstetric Care: Examples from Eleven Operations Research Projects in West Africa", *Social Science and Medicine*, 40, 1995, pp. 657–667.

75. Nanda, "Gender Dimensions of User Fees: Implications for Women's Utilisation of Health Care".

76. Ke Xu, B. David, P. K. Evans et al., "Understanding the Impact of Eliminating User Fees: Utilisation and Catastrophic Health Expenditures in Uganda", *Social Science and Medicine*, 62, 2006, pp. 866–876.

77. H. Schneider and L. Gilson, "The Impact of Free Maternal Health Care in South Africa", in M. Berer and T. K. S. Ravindran (eds), *Safe Motherhood Initiatives: Critical Issues*, Oxford: Blackwell Publishers (Reproductive Health Matters), 2001.

78. Parkhurst et al., "Health Systems Factors Influencing Maternal Health Services: A Four-Country Comparison".

79. D. Maine, J. McCarthy and V. M. Ward, *Guideline for Monitoring Progress in the Reduction of Maternal Mortality: A Work in Progress*, Columbia: Columbia Press, 1992.

80. WHO, *Women's Health: Across Age and Frontier*, Geneva: World Health Organization, 1992.

81. J. Leslie, "Women's Nutrition: The Key to Improving Family Health in Developing Countries?", *Health Policy and Planning*, 6, 1991, pp. 1–19.

82. UNICEF, *Malnutrition in South Asia: A Regional Profile*, Katmandu: United Nations Children's Fund, 1997.

83. D. Buor and K. Bream, "An Analysis of the Determinants of Maternal Mortality in Sub-Saharan Africa", *Journal of Women's Health*, 13(8), 2004, pp. 926–938.

84. K. Khan, D. Wojdyla, L. Say et al., "WHO Analysis of Causes of Maternal Death: A Systematic Review", *Lancet*, 367, 2006, pp. 1066–1074.

85. P. Bernstein and A. Rosenfield, "Abortion and Maternal Health", *International Journal of Gynecology and Obstetrics*, 63(1), 1998, pp. 115–122; M. Berer, "Making Abortions Safe: A Matter of Good Public Health Policy and Practice", *Bulletin of the World Health Organization*, 78, 2000, pp. 580–592.

86. Khan et al., "WHO Analysis of Causes of Maternal Death: A Systematic Review".

87. A. Paxton et al., "Global Patterns in Availability of Emergency Obstetric Care", *International Journal of Gynecology and Obstetrics*, 93(3), 2006, pp. 300–307.

88. Ibid.

89. P. Tlebere et al., "Community-Based Situation Analysis of Maternal and Neonatal Care in South Africa to Explore Factors that Impact Utilisation of Maternal Health Services", *Journal of Midwifery & Women's Health*, 52(4), 2007, pp. 342–350.

90. WHO, *The World Health Report 2005. Make Every Mother and Child Count* Geneva: World Health Organization, 2005.

91. Berer, "Making Abortions Safe: A Matter of Good Public Health Policy and Practice", Bernstein and Rosenfield, "Abortion and Maternal Health".

92. R. J. Cook et al., *Reproductive Health and Human Rights – Integrating Medicine, Ethics and Law*, London: Oxford University Press, 2003.

93. Shah and Say, "Maternal Mortality and Maternity Care from 1990 to 2005".

94. Khan et al., "WHO Analysis of Causes of Maternal Death: a Systematic Review".

95. K. Coyaji, "Early Medical Abortion in India: Three Studies and Their Implications for Abortion Services" Journal of the American Medical Women's Association, 55, 2000, pp. 191–194.

96. R. Duggal, "The Political Economy of Abortion in India: Cost and Expenditure Patterns", *Reproductive Health Matters*, 12, 2000, pp. 130–137.

97. Khan et al., "WHO Analysis of Causes of Maternal Death: A Systematic Review".

98. N. Oomman and B. R. Ganatra, "Sex Selection: The Systematic Elimination of Girls", *Reproductive Health Matters*, 10, 2002, pp. 184–188; S. Dorothy, "What Is the Relevance of Women's Sexual and Reproductive Rights to the Practicing Obstetrician/Gynecologist?", *Best Practice & Research Clinical Obstetrics & Gynecology*, 20(3), 2006, pp. 299–309.

99. Dorothy, "What Is the Relevance of Women's Sexual and Reproductive Rights to the Practicing Obstetrician/Gynecologist?".

100. WHO, *Female Genital Mutilation*, Joint statement, WHO/UNICEF/UNFPA, Geneva: World Health Organization, 1997.

101. D. Carr, *Female Genital Cutting: Findings from the Demographic and Health Surveys*, Calverston, MD: Macro International Inc., 1997; A. Tinker, "Women's Health: The Unfinished Agenda", *International Journal of Gynecology & Obstetrics*, 70(1), 2000, pp. 149–158.

102. M. Magadia et al., "A Comparative Analysis of the Use of Maternal Health Services between Teenagers and Older Mothers in Sub-Saharan Africa: Evidence from Demographic and Health Surveys (DHS)", *Social Science & Medicine*, 64, 2007, pp. 1311–1325.
103. Chaya and Dusenberry, *ICPD at Ten: Where Are We Now.*
104. WHO, *Working with Individuals, Families and Communities to Improve Maternal and Newborn Health*, WHO/FCH/RHR/03.11, Geneva: World Health Organization, 2003.

2

Poverty, health and the human right to the highest attainable standard of health

PAUL HUNT AND JUDITH BUENO DE MESQUITA

Introduction

This chapter outlines the contribution of the right to the highest attainable standard of health to the reduction and elimination of poverty. This introduction indicates the importance and scope of the right. We then briefly introduce, in general terms, the key features of a strategy for realising the right to health of those living in poverty.[1] This is followed by a country case study: through the prism of the right to health, it considers ill health, poverty, discrimination and inequality in Peru. The last section adopts a thematic approach: it addresses the contribution of the right to health to the reduction in maternal mortality. As is well known, maternal mortality disproportionately affects those living in poverty.

Thus, the chapter moves from the general to the specific. To grasp the contribution of human rights to poverty reduction and elimination, it is important to move beyond generalities about rights and

Partnerships for women's health: Striving for best practice within the UN Global Compact,
Timmermann and Kruesmann (eds),
United Nations University Press, 2009, ISBN 978-92-808-1185-8

poverty. In our view, the way forward is to examine poverty in relation to *specific* human rights, sectors, countries and themes.[2]

The importance of the right to health

Ill health causes and contributes to poverty by destroying livelihoods, reducing worker productivity, lowering educational achievement and limiting opportunities.[3] Because poverty can lead to diminished access to medical care, increased exposure to environmental risks and malnutrition, ill health is also often a consequence of poverty. Accordingly, ill health is both a cause and a consequence of poverty: sick people are more likely to be impoverished and people living in poverty are more vulnerable to disease and disability.

... Good health is central to creating and sustaining the capabilities that the poor need to escape from poverty. A key asset, good health contributes to their greater economic security. Good health is not just an outcome of development: it is a way of achieving development.

... Ill health is constitutive of poverty if lack of command over economic resources plays a role in its causation.[4] Thus, the right to health has a crucial role to play in relation to poverty reduction. Further, enjoyment of the right to health is instrumental in securing other rights such as education and work.

... Health targets are prominent among the MDGs [Millennium Development Goals] to be achieved worldwide by 2015: among them, the goals of reducing under-five child mortality by two thirds and maternal mortality by three quarters, of halving the proportion of people without sustainable access to safe drinking water and of reversing the spread of HIV/AIDS and the incidence of malaria and other major diseases.[5] The Millennium Declaration also highlights other crucial health issues such as increasing the availability of affordable essential drugs to all who need them in developing countries. The prominence accorded to health targets and issues in the Millennium Declaration underlines the importance of the right to health in relation to poverty reduction.

The scope of the right to health

The right to health is not to be understood as the right to be healthy: the State cannot provide protection against every possible cause of ill health.[6] It is the right to the enjoyment of a variety of facilities, goods, services and conditions necessary for the realization of the highest attainable standard of health. The right includes both health care and the underlying determinants of health, including access to safe drinking water, adequate and safe food, adequate sanitation and housing, healthy occupational and environmental conditions, and access to health-related information and education.

... The right to health includes both freedoms and entitlements. The freedoms include the right to control one's body, including reproductive health, and the right to be free from interference, such as freedom from torture and non-consensual medical treatment.

... The entitlements include a system of health care and protection that is available, accessible, acceptable and good quality. Thus, the right to health implies that functioning public health and health-care facilities, goods and services are *available* in sufficient quantity within a State. It also means that they are *accessible* to everyone without discrimination. Accessibility has a number of dimensions, including physical, information and economic. Thus, "information accessibility" includes the right to seek, receive and impart information concerning health issues, subject to the right to have personal health data treated with confidentiality. "Economic accessibility" means that health facilities, goods and services must be affordable for all.[7] Furthermore, all health facilities, goods and services must be *acceptable*, i.e., respectful of medical ethics and culturally appropriate, and of good *quality*.

... According to international human rights law, the generic right to health encompasses a number of more specific health rights, including the right to maternal, child and reproductive health; the right to healthy natural and workplace environments; the right to the prevention, treatment and control of diseases; and the right to health facilities, goods and services.

Key features of a strategy
for realising the right to health

During his tenure as United Nations (UN) Special Rapporteur on
the right of everyone to the enjoyment of the highest attainable
standard of health Paul Hunt contributed to developing "an analytical framework for 'unpacking' the right to health and making this
fundamental human right easier to grasp".[8] In this section, keeping
this analytical framework in mind, we set out in general terms the
key features of a strategy for realising the right to health of those living in poverty.[9]

First, "States should improve the supply of personal health services
and make them more accessible to the poor" by, for example, targeting delivery to people living in poverty by providing tailor-made
services via outreach clinics for vulnerable groups, "such as women,
the elderly, children, indigenous peoples, minorities, slum-dwellers,
labour migrants and remote rural communities". Second, resource allocation should favour the poorer geographical regions and the lower
levels of service delivery (that is, primary care). Third, priority should
be given to reproductive, maternal (pre-natal as well as post-natal)
and child health care. Fourth, states should identify "diseases and
medical conditions, such as malaria, tuberculosis and HIV/AIDS,
that have a particular impact on the poor and, by way of response,
introduc[e] immunization and other programmes that are specifically designed to have a particular impact upon the poor".[10] Fifth,
they should also ensure "that all services are respectful of the culture
of all individuals, groups, minorities and peoples, and are sensitive
to gender and of good quality". Essential drugs, as defined by the
World Health Organization (WHO) Action Programme on Essential
Drugs, should be provided.

Additionally, "States should improve the supply and effectiveness
of public health interventions to the poor" by "introducing and implementing basic environmental controls, especially regarding waste
disposal", in areas populated by people living in poverty, and by ensuring "the provision of clean, safe and accessible drinking water".
Health service provision should be regulated to promote particular

outcomes, for example, "with a view to eliminating the marketing of unsafe drugs and reducing professional malpractice". States are also responsible for "[p]roviding education and information about the main health problems in local communities, including methods of prevention and control".

Further, states must also reduce the financial burden of health care and health protection on people living in poverty, "for example by reducing and eliminating user fees. This can be done either by moving away from user fees and introducing other pre-payment mechanisms (e.g. national insurance or general taxation) or by keeping user fees and introducing non-discretionary, equitable and non-stigmatizing interventions" for people living in poverty (for example, exemption schemes, direct cash subsidies and vouchers).

Because numerous sectors have an impact on health issues, "States should promote policies in other sectors that bear positively on the underlying determinants of health" and that generate particular benefits for people living in poverty. This could be by, for example, "supporting agricultural policies that have positive health outcomes" for people living in poverty (such as food security); "identifying measures that address the negative impact of agricultural policies" on people living in poverty (such as health and safety risks to agricultural labourers); and "generally promoting income-generating activities" for people living in poverty.

Finally, states must take steps to ensure that all those involved in health care and health protection treat those living in poverty with equality and respect. For example, they should "provide all relevant health staff with anti-discrimination training in relation to disability and health status, including HIV/AIDS".

A graphic example of the highly complex interlinkage of health, poverty, discrimination and inequality faced by a government, and the need for nuanced policy responses, can be seen in one example from Latin America: Peru.

The 2005 report of the Special Rapporteur after his mission to Peru provides a framework of reference for other countries when trying to address, in the context of the right to health, the challenging issues of poverty reduction and elimination, as well as the reproductive and maternal health of women living in poverty. It was this report on Peru that might have influenced the Government of India when inviting the Special Rapporteur for a visit from 22 November to 3 December 2007 to consider MDG5 and maternal mortality in Rajasthan and Maharashtra.[11] In the following section, while focusing on Peru, we suggest that the analysis and recommendations also bear upon poverty reduction and elimination, and the reproductive and maternal health of women living in poverty, in numerous other countries.

The example of Peru: Ill health, poverty, discrimination and inequality

In 2004, the UN Special Rapporteur on the right to the highest attainable standard of health was invited by the Government of Peru to visit the country and report on the right to health. The mission took place in June 2004 and a report was submitted to the United Nations in 2005.[12] The following remarks draw from this report.[13]

The context

The government and people of Peru are confronted with a wide range of grave health problems.

Peru has the highest incidence of pulmonary tuberculosis in Latin America, with 100 cases per 100,000 population, compared with the regional average of 17 cases; and a high incidence of multi-drug-resistant tuberculosis. The incidence of HIV/AIDS in Peru is increasing, and an estimated 72,000 people are currently living with HIV/AIDS. Malaria is widespread, in particular in the jungle (*selva*) region, and Peru's population is vulnerable to other infectious diseases such as leishmaniasis. Thirty percent of the urban population and 60 percent of the rural population still do not have access to safe water or adequate sanitation. Environmental determinants of health, such as unsafe drinking water, inadequate sanitation, as well as air and water pollution, exert a heavy toll on the health of the population. Malnutrition affects the health of up to 25 percent of children under the age of 5, while obesity is also an increasing problem, especially in urban areas. Between 1980 and 2000, internal conflict led to the death or disappearance of an estimated 69,000 people, caused widespread psychosocial health problems, and contributed to a culture of violence that continues to have an impact on health in Peru today.

The impact of poverty and discrimination

Many of the health problems in Peru are inextricably linked to problems of poverty and discrimination, which are among the causes and consequences of ill-health in the country. People living in poverty have poorer access to basic services, such as clean water, sanitation and health care. Ill-health also often impoverishes individuals and families on account of the cost of treatment, or because of its impact on revenue-generating activities. Some diseases, including HIV/AIDS, have given rise to multiple forms of discrimination against those affected, which further impedes the enjoyment of the right to health and other human rights. Poverty and discrimination have perpetuated great disparities in the enjoyment of the right to health between rural and urban areas, between regions and among different population groups.

... While Peru is a middle-income country, and despite its recent robust macroeconomic performance, 49 percent of the population lives in poverty, and 18.1 percent in extreme poverty. Moreover, there are striking inequalities between different regions: in the Andean region (*sierra*), for example, 70 percent live in poverty and 35 percent in extreme poverty. Health disparities between regions are also dramatic. For example, while in metropolitan Lima the infant mortality rate is 17 per 1,000 live births, this figure rises to 71 and 84 in the impoverished rural departments of Huancavelica and Cuzco, respectively. In 2000, the infant mortality rate was 28 per 1,000 live births in urban areas while it was 60 per 1,000 in rural areas. While there has been progress at the national level in reducing maternal mortality, and while chronic malnutrition in children under 5 years of age has been stable in recent years, the national aggregates mask growing inequalities: the situation on both counts has worsened for the poorest quintiles in the country, and chronic malnutrition has reached around 75–80 percent in rural areas. For a middle-income country, this is an astonishing state of affairs.

... Particular population groups are at risk in the context of specific health problems. Women and adolescents are especially vulnerable in the context of sexual and reproductive health. The maternal mortality ratio is reported to be 185 deaths per 100,000 live births in 2000, one of the highest in the Latin American region. The incidence of unsafe abortion and teenage pregnancy are also unacceptably high. Women are also particularly vulnerable to violence: an estimated 41 percent of women have been mistreated or subjected to physical aggression by their husbands or partners. The great majority of people living with HIV/AIDS lack access to antiretroviral drugs. Certain groups of people, including people living with HIV/AIDS and indigenous populations, face various forms of discrimination that are rooted deeply in related stigmatisation and prejudices. Indigenous populations have inferior access to health-care services, including on account of linguistic and cultural barriers.

... A lack of access to health care for poor and marginalised groups has compounded many of these health problems. While the supply of primary care clinics has increased significantly in the past decade, in 2001, 25 percent of Peru's population still lacked access even to primary health-care services. Services for specific health or health-related problems, including psychosocial disabilities and the consequences of violence, are not widely available outside urban centres. Access to information on some health issues and for some population groups, notably information for adolescents on sexual and reproductive health, is also unduly restricted.

... Poverty, discrimination and a lack of adequate targeting of the health needs of particular population groups have all contributed to these health-related vulnerabilities. In these circumstances, the main right to health challenge is to identify policies and implement strategies that (i) are based on equity, equality and non-discrimination; and (ii) improve access to health care, and the underlying determinants of health, of those living in poverty....

... In this context, [it is important to emphasise] that international human rights law proscribes any discrimination in access to health care and the underlying determinants of health, as well as to means and entitlements for their procurement, on grounds including race, sex, disability and health status (including HIV/AIDS), which has the intention or effect of nullifying or impairing the equal enjoyment or exercise of the right to health. Under international human rights law, States also have an obligation to take special measures to remove obstacles to, and promote, the enjoyment of the right to health for vulnerable groups.

A national health policy
to address poverty and discrimination

People living in poverty, and other marginalized groups, face the greatest challenges to the enjoyment of their right to health. A range of [governmental] policies ... aim to address the health problems of the poor and other vulnerable groups. Yet there is currently no comprehensive rights-based pro-poor or equity-based health policy in Peru.

... [t]he Government, in cooperation with all stakeholders, [should] formulate a comprehensive health policy and strategy, underpinned by the right to health, that is specifically designed to address inequity, inequality, discrimination and the situation of those living in poverty (in short, a "pro-poor equity-based health policy"). [This] recommendation anticipates both a health policy and strategy, i.e. not only identification of the goals, but also the measures by which the goals are to be reached. The policy and strategy should be informed by human rights, build upon existing initiatives and attract widespread political support. It is important that the policy has sufficiently broad-based support to survive changes of ministers and Governments. In other words, the goal should be a policy of the State rather than a Government.

... At the time of the mission, Peru's Millennium Development Goals Report was in preparation.... [This Report, which was published in December 2004, provides] much of the context within which the Government should endeavour to formulate its pro-poor equity-based health policy. Other existing policy documents, in particular the Acuerdo Nacional and the Ministry of Health's *Lineamientos de Politicas Sectorial para el Periodo 2002–2012*, will also inform and enrich the process.

... While the pro-poor equity-based health policy should have national scope – clearly establishing a national vision, direction and framework – it must also enable the regions and municipalities to define their own health priorities and approaches within this nationally agreed framework.

... The Government of Peru will have to decide upon the best process by which such a pro-poor equity-based health policy should be prepared. [It is suggested, however, that] the process should be: interdepartmental, but led by the Ministry of Health; national in scope, with substantial input from the regions and municipalities; transparent and participatory (e.g. with substantial input from civil society); provided with adequate financial, research and administrative support; and provided with technical assistance from the key international agencies, in particular PAHO [the Pan American Health Organization]. Whatever process is chosen, it must allow sufficient time for the active and informed participation of all stakeholders – probably between 12–24 months from commencement of the project to finalization of the policy and strategy. Of course, implementation will take much longer.

... Throughout the policy-making process, Peru's development partners must be fully included in the most appropriate manner. This is important for a number of reasons, not least that the partners should be invited to provide substantial funds towards this important policy-making project. If the process is to be participatory, inclusive and well-researched, it will have to be supported by significant resources.... Peru's development partners [should] provide the necessary financial support, enabling the government to both organize a good process and prepare a compelling policy.

... Moreover, at the end of the project, when the pro-poor equity-based health policy and strategy has been devised, the development partners should be invited to contribute substantial resources for its implementation by way of a Common Fund for the health sector. Sectoral Common Funds for the implementation of "country-owned" policies and strategies have been used in other states. They have many advantages for all parties. For example, they provide a common vision and avoid the wasteful administrative costs generated by bilateral funding for multiple individual projects.

... [A] number of the following recommendations address issues that are integral to a pro-poor equity-based health policy. For example, a health policy focused on equity, human rights and poverty reduction will have to encompass ... sexual and reproductive health, and issues of ethnicity and culture. Thus, the pro-poor equity-based health policy can provide cohesion to a wide range of interrelated initiatives.

Sexual and reproductive health

[There are] extremely high rates of maternal mortality, the second main cause of which is unsafe abortion. [It is very important to ensure] access – in particular for poor populations – to a wide range of sexual and reproductive health services, including family planning, pre- and post-natal care, emergency obstetric services and access to information. In particular, women should have access to quality services for the management of complications, whether arising from pregnancy, childbirth or abortion. Punitive legal provisions against women who undergo abortions, as well as against the relevant service providers, should be removed.

... [The government has made a welcome commitment] to taking all appropriate measures to promote sexual and reproductive health. In particular, [it has reaffirmed] its commitment to the Programme of Action of the International Conference on Population and Development. [Also to be welcomed is] the position of the Minister of Health [in 2004] that the government's policies, including those on sexual and reproductive health, should be based on scientific evidence and compliant with legal obligations under the Constitution of Peru, as well as regional and international human rights law.[14]

... [There is], however, [an] urgent need for the development of a comprehensive, intersectoral policy on sexual and reproductive health which focuses on the health needs of women, in particular those that are socially and economically marginalised. In particular, sexual and reproductive health-care laws, policies and programmes should be designed to reach women living in poverty, indigenous peoples and rural populations, with full respect for their human rights. Legislation to promote non-discriminatory access to sexual and reproductive health services should be developed, promoted and implemented. Civil society and women's groups should be involved in the development of policy, legislation, programmes and strategies in relation to sexual and reproductive health.

... Similarly, ... a comprehensive, intersectoral policy on sexual and reproductive health should be developed for – and with the participation of – adolescents. The policy should be grounded in international human rights law and should recognize, in particular, the right of adolescents to access information, education and user-friendly sexual and reproductive health services, including on family planning and contraceptives, risks related to early pregnancy and prevention of sexually transmitted infections such as HIV/AIDS. The right of adolescents to privacy, confidentiality and informed consent should be protected.

... Fulfilling the rights to sexual and reproductive health requires ensuring access to high quality and comprehensive reproductive health information and services, including access to a wide range of safe, effective, affordable and acceptable contraceptive methods. ...

... The rights to sexual and reproductive health include an obligation to ensure access to screening, counselling and treatment for sexually transmitted infections including HIV/AIDS, as well as for breast cancer and cancer of the reproductive system ... [S]trategies for implementing the policy [should] explicitly address gender inequalities, stigma and discrimination; provide comprehensive sexual and reproductive health information, education and services to young people; and ensure access to voluntary testing, counselling and treatment for sexually transmitted infections, including HIV/AIDS.

Finally, the donor community's funding policies for sexual and reproductive health care in Peru (and elsewhere) should stress the need to adopt a rights-based approach to their policies and programmes.

Ethnicity and culture

[D]isparities in access to health services and goods for marginalized groups in Peru, including indigenous peoples and ethnic minorities[, are alarming]. These disparities are rooted in geographic, cultural, economic and linguistic barriers. Indigenous peoples and ethnic minorities are also particularly vulnerable to other particular health problems: in some places, mineral extraction has led to environmental degradation and contamination of their water sources and food supplies; they were disproportionately affected by Peru's internal conflict; and thousands of indigenous women, primarily those living in poverty and in rural areas, are believed to have been sterilized without their consent during the family planning programme carried out during the 1990s. Despite [the gravity of] these ... issues, [they rarely attract the attention they deserve in the Peruvian context].

... Following its consideration of Peru's periodic report in 1999, the Committee on the Elimination of Racial Discrimination (CERD) noted its concerns about the close relationship between socio-economic underdevelopment in Peru and ethnic or racial discrimination against part of the population, mainly indigenous and peasant communities ....[15] ... According to international human rights law, disadvantaged indigenous people have the right to specific measures to improve their access to health services and care, as well as the underlying determinants of health. These services should be culturally appropriate, taking into account traditional preventive care, healing practices and medicines.

... [T]he recommendations of CERD [should be endorsed] and ... the government [encouraged] to implement recommendations bearing on the right to health adopted by the Permanent Forum on Indigenous Issues at its third session ....[16]

Moreover, the government should make every effort to ensure that "[r]esearch is carried out into the economic, cultural, political and linguistic obstacles to the enjoyment of the right to health faced by indigenous peoples and ethnic groups in Peru. This research should involve the active participation of representatives, including women, from Peru's indigenous and ethnic minority communities, and should serve as the basis for developing policies and programmes to address these obstacles."

Whenever possible, all health data should be disaggregated by ethnicity and socio-economic status. Also, all health policies, programmes and projects should "specifically take into account the needs, cultures and traditions of, as well as discrimination affecting, different ethnic groups, and indigenous women". Further, all affected ethnic groups should be able to "participate actively and in an informed manner whenever health policies, programmes and projects are formulated and implemented". Health professionals should be "provided with training to ensure that they are aware of, and sensitive to, issues of ethnicity, culture and gender". "So far as possible, the health facilities, programmes and projects that are in – or serve – a community [should be] available in the mother tongue of most people in that community".

Finally,

[C]entral and regional government, teaching institutions, health professional associations and others [should] actively devise and implement strategies that encourage individuals from all ethnic groups to become health professionals. These strategies should include measures to increase the ethnic diversity of the student body attending existing training programmes. However, in addition, new training courses should be devised for – and by – indigenous and other non-dominant ethnic groups. These courses should include training in the medical traditions and practices of the groups concerned. In this way, these courses will serve several extremely important purposes. Not least, they will help to preserve the invaluable and increasingly threatened traditional knowledge of indigenous peoples.

... The [United Nations] Special Rapporteur on the situation of the human rights and fundamental freedoms of indigenous people and the Special Rapporteur on contemporary forms of racism, racial discrimination, xenophobia and related intolerance should be encouraged to visit Peru.

The contribution of the right to health to the reduction in maternal mortality

Peru is not alone in having a shocking rate of maternal mortality. Adopting a right to health perspective, this section makes some preliminary observations about the catastrophic global scale of maternal mortality.[17]

In 2000, the estimated number of maternal deaths worldwide was 529,000; 95 per cent of these deaths occurred in Africa and Asia. While women in developed countries have only a 1-in-2,800 chance of dying in childbirth – and a 1-in-8,700 chance in some countries – women in Africa have a 1-in-20 chance. In several countries the lifetime risk is greater than 1 in 10. Women living in poverty and in rural areas, and women belonging to ethnic minorities or indigenous populations, are among those particularly at risk. Complications from pregnancy and childbirth are the leading cause of death for women 15–19 years old in developing countries. Globally, around 80 per cent of maternal deaths are due to obstetric complications, mainly haemorrhage, sepsis, unsafe abortion, pre-eclampsia and eclampsia, and prolonged or obstructed labour. Complications of unsafe abortions account for 13 per cent of maternal deaths worldwide, and 19 per cent of maternal deaths in South America. An estimated 74 per cent of maternal deaths could be averted if all women had access to the interventions for addressing pregnancy and birth complications, in particular emergency obstetric care.

... For every woman who dies from obstetric complications, approximately 30 more suffer injuries, infection and disabilities. In 1999, WHO estimated that over 2 million women living in developing countries remain untreated for obstetric fistula, a devastating injury of childbirth.... There is no single cause of death and disability for men between the ages of 15 and 44 that is close to the magnitude of maternal death and disability.

... These deeply shocking statistics and facts reveal chronic and entrenched health inequalities. First, the burden of maternal mortality is borne disproportionately by developing countries. Second, in many countries, marginalized women, such as women living in poverty and ethnic minority or indigenous women, are more vulnerable to maternal mortality. Third, maternal mortality and morbidity rates reveal sharp discrepancies between men and women in their enjoyment of sexual and reproductive health rights.

... An increasing number of countries have made progress in reducing maternal mortality. However, progress has stagnated or been reversed in many of the countries with the highest maternal mortality rates. This is despite longstanding international commitment and initiatives to reducing maternal mortality.

What can the right to health add to policies and programmes to reduce maternal mortality?

Space does not permit an analysis of the right to health norms and obligations that are relevant to maternal mortality. Instead, the following paragraphs signal how the right to health has a constructive contribution to make in the context of maternal health policy-making.[18]

First, "on account of its grounding in law, widespread acceptance by the international community and detailed framework of relevant norms and obligations, the right to health can help legitimise policies and programmes that prevent maternal mortality".[19]

Second, the human rights principles of equality and non-discrimination, which are at the heart of the right to health, "have three important roles to play in policies to reduce maternal mortality.... [T]hey underpin programmes that promote more equitable distribution of health care, including provision in rural or poor areas, or areas with high indigenous or minority populations.... [T]hey underpin prioritization of interventions – such as emergency obstetric care – that can guarantee women's enjoyment of the right to health on the basis of non-discrimination and equality.... [P]olicies which promote non-discrimination and equality – as well as dignity, cultural sensitivity, privacy and confidentiality – in the clinical setting, can improve patient-provider relationships and encourage women to seek health care."

Third, "[t]he right to health includes an entitlement to participate in health policymaking at the local, national and international levels. Participation by relevant stakeholders, including women, will help develop more effective and sustainable programmes, reduce exclusion and enhance accountability".

Fourth, "[m]onitoring and accountability are integral features of the right to health and can help reduce maternal mortality. The right to health demands accountability of various stakeholders, including health-care providers, local health authorities, national governments, international organizations and civil society. Accessible and effective accountability mechanisms – including courts, tribunals, health ombudsmen, impact assessments and policy review processes – can all help enhance access to health care".

Fifth, "[a] right-to-health approach to reducing maternal mortality requires appropriate indicators to monitor progress made, and to highlight where policy adjustments may be needed. The scope of this [chapter] does not permit a detailed analysis of which indicators are needed." However, "a methodology for a rights-based approach to health indicators, including in relation to the reproductive health strategy endorsed by the World Health Assembly in May 2004", is set out in a report to the former UN Commission on Human Rights.[20]

> In short, a policy that is animated by the right to health is likely to be equitable, inclusive, non-discriminatory, participatory and evidence-based. In the context of maternal mortality policies, these features help to empower women and ensure that policies are likely to be sustainable, robust and effective.
>
> ... Interventions to prevent maternal mortality – including family-planning services, skilled attendants at birth and emergency obstetric care, and other sexual and reproductive health services – are also imperative measures to prevent and treat other causes of sexual and

reproductive ill health, including fistula and other causes of maternal morbidity. A right-to-health approach to reducing maternal mortality is therefore also likely to lead to improvements in sexual and reproductive health, including maternal health.

The need for a human rights campaign against maternal mortality

Human rights experts and organisations have to move beyond using only their traditional techniques – such as campaigning, "naming and shaming" and court-based approaches – to engage with health decision-makers to ensure that the right to health informs policies.

Although maternal mortality is one of a small number of right to health issues where human rights experts and health policy-makers have engaged extensively and constructively with each other, and although these efforts deserve applause and further support, there is certainly scope for further interactions at the international, national and local levels.

In the 1990s, for example, violence against women was identified as a violation of human rights, and this helped the global campaign to end violence against women gather momentum. By the same token, the human rights community should be challenged to mount a global human rights campaign against maternal mortality. The human rights community must be urged to remonstrate and demonstrate about maternal mortality just as loudly as it complains about extrajudicial executions, arbitrary detention, unfair trials and prisoners of conscience. Persistently high maternal mortality rates, coupled with the fact that all states are committed to reduce by three-quarters the maternal mortality ratio by 2015, suggest that the time is ripe for such an initiative.

This is not to underestimate the many challenges that would confront such an undertaking. For example, whereas violence against women is always a human rights violation, some unavoidable cases of maternal mortality are not. To take another example, the identity of the human rights violator may not always be clear because responsibility for maternal mortality may be attributable to multiple actors, including family members, health professionals and facilities, the relevant state, and the international community. However, that does not stop many maternal deaths from being a human rights violation – and this violation must be investigated precisely to determine where responsibility lies so as to better ensure accountability, so that the appropriate policy changes are introduced as a matter of urgency.

A human rights campaign against avoidable maternal mortality will inevitably lead to other crucial issues, not least the vital importance of constructing effective health systems that are accessible to all, including girls, women and those living in poverty.

In conclusion, it is encouraging to observe that since the first draft of this paper was written, a human rights campaign on maternal mortality has begun to gain momentum, e.g. the International Initiative on Maternal Mortality and Human Rights (IIMMHR) and also within Amnesty International, with the potential of making a critically important contribution to the right to the highest attainable standard of health for all.

Notes

1. The full formulation of the right to health is "the right of everyone to the enjoyment of the highest attainable standard of physical and mental health". For example, see International Covenant on Economic, Social and Cultural Rights, Article 12. By way of shorthand, we use either "the right to the highest attainable standard of health" or "the right to health".
2. For example, see Office of the United Nations High Commissioner for Human Rights and of the Department of Health Policy, Development and Services, and the Health & Human Rights Team of the Department of Ethics, Equity, Trade & Human Rights, of the World Health Organization, *Human Rights, Health and Poverty Reduction Strategies*, Geneva: OHCHR and WHO, 2008; and L.-H. Piron and T. O'Neill, *Integrating Human Rights into Development: A Synthesis of Donor Approaches and Experiences*, London: Overseas Development Institute, 2005.
3. The remainder of this introduction, as well as the following section, draws extensively from Guideline 8 of the Office of the United Nations High Commissioner for Human Rights (OHCHR), *Principles and Guidelines for a*

Human Rights Approach to Poverty Reduction Strategies, 2006, which is based on the draft by Professors Paul Hunt, Manfred Nowak and Siddiq Osmani; <http://www.unhcr.org/refworld/pdfid/46ceaef92.pdf> (accessed 4 June 2009).

4. See OHCHR, *Human Rights and Poverty Reduction: A Conceptual Framework*, New York & Geneva: United Nations, 2004, p. 8.

5. For a discussion of the health-related MDGs in the context of the right to the highest attainable standard of health, see the Report to the General Assembly of Paul Hunt (Special Rapporteur of the Commission on Human Rights), "The Right of Everyone to the Enjoyment of the Highest Attainable Standard of Physical and Mental Health", UN Document A/59/422, 8 October 2004; available at <http://www2.essex.ac.uk/human_rights_centre/rth/> (accessed 4 June 2009).

6. For an introduction to the right to health, see the Report to the Commission on Human Rights of the Special Rapporteur, Paul Hunt, "The Right of Everyone to the Enjoyment of the Highest Attainable Standard of Physical and Mental Health", UN Document E/CN.4/2003/58, 13 February 2003; available at <http://www2.essex.ac.uk/human_rights_centre/rth/> (accessed 4 June 2009).

7. This is particularly the case for primary health care or health services that are considered part of the core package of services in a given country. The state is not always understood to have an obligation to provide all other health services if this is beyond its resources. This issue has been considered by various national courts, including the South African Constitutional Court in the case of *Soobramoney v Minister of Health* (CCT 32/97), decided on 27 November 1997.

8. See "Report of the Special Rapporteur on the Right of Everyone to the Enjoyment of the Highest Attainable Standard of Physical and Mental Health", UN Document A/63/263, General Assembly, 11 August 2008; available at <http://daccessdds.un.org/doc/UNDOC/GEN/N08/456/47/PDF/N0845647.pdf?OpenElement> (accessed 13 June 2009).

9. The quotations in the following paragraphs come from OHCHR, *Principles and Guidelines for a Human Rights Approach to Poverty Reduction Strategies*, para. 179.

10. For a study on neglected diseases (or "poverty-related" diseases) and the right to the highest attainable standard of health, see "Annex: Report of the Special Rapporteur on the Right of Everyone to the Enjoyment of the Highest Attainable Standard of Physical and Mental Health, Paul Hunt, on His Mission to Uganda (17–25 March 2005)", UN Document E/CN.4/2006/48/Add.2, 19 January 2006; available at <http://www2.essex.ac.uk/human_rights_centre/rth/> (accessed 4 June 2009).

11. "Promotion and Protection of All Human Rights, Civil, Political, Economic, Social and Cultural Rights, Including the Right to Development: Report of the Special Rapporteur on the Right of Everyone to the Enjoyment of the Highest Attainable Standard of Physical and Mental Health. Preliminary Note on the Mission to India, Addendum", UN Document

A/HRC/7/11/Add.4, 29 February 2008; available at <http://ap.ohchr.org/documents/dpage_e.aspx?m=100> (accessed 13 June 2009). Also see Appendix C in this volume.

12. "Report Submitted by the Special Rapporteur on the Right of Everyone to the Highest Attainable Standard of Physical and Mental Health, Paul Hunt: Addendum – Mission to Peru", UN Document E/CN.4/2005/51/Add.3, 4 February 2005; available at <http://www2.essex.ac.uk/human_rights_centre/rth/docs/peru.pdf> (accessed 4 June 2009). Judith Bueno de Mesquita, Lisa Oldring and Paul Hunt prepared the report.

13. However, for brevity, several other important issues in the report cannot be touched upon here, for example the United States–Peru trade agreement, the environment and mental health. In late 2006, the Special Rapporteur revisited Peru and found that the report's basic analysis and recommendations remained valid. The footnotes in the original report have been deleted in the following extracts.

14. At that time, the Minister of Health was Dr Pilar Mazzetti. After the elections of 2006, Dr Mazzetti was replaced as Minister of Health and was appointed Minister of the Interior.

15. "Concluding Observations of the Committee on the Elimination of Racial Discrimination: Peru", CERD/C/304/Add.69, 13 April 1999, para. 12.

16. See Economic and Social Council, "Permanent Forum on Indigenous Issues: Report on the Third Session (10–21 May 2004)", UN Document E/2004/43, E/C.19/2003/23, *Official Records*, 2004, Supplement No. 23; <http://daccessdds.un.org/doc/UNDOC/GEN/N04/384/66/PDF/N0438466.pdf?OpenElement> (accessed 4 June 2009).

17. This section draws from "Report of the Special Rapporteur on the Right of Everyone to the Enjoyment of the Highest Attainable Standard of Physical and Mental Health", UN Document A/61/338, 13 September 2006, available at <http://www2.essex.ac.uk/human_rights_centre/rth/> (accessed 4 June 2009). The footnotes in the original have been deleted in the following extracts.

18. The relationship between human rights and maternal mortality has been explored in several publications, including R. Cook and B. Dickens et al., *Advancing Safe Motherhood through Human Rights*, Geneva: World Health Organization, 2001; L. Freedman et al., *Who's Got the Power? Transforming Health Systems for Women and Children*, UN Millennium Project, Task Force on Child Health and Maternal Health, London: Earthscan, 2005; K. Hawkins et al., *Developing a Human Rights-Based Approach to Addressing Maternal Mortality: Desk Review*, London: UK Department for International Development Health Resource Centre, 2005.

19. UN Document A/61/338, para. 28.

20. "Report of the Special Rapporteur on the Right of Everyone to the Enjoyment of the Highest Attainable Standard of Physical and Mental Health, Paul Hunt", UN Document E/CN.4/2006/48, 3 March 2006, paras 22–61 and Annex, available at <http://www2.essex.ac.uk/human_rights_centre/rth/docs/CHR%202006.pdf> (accessed 4 June 2009).

3

Partnering in support of the right to health: What role for business?

Klaus M. Leisinger

Introduction

To improve the health of underprivileged women and girls in any part of the world is a highly valuable objective. And it is even more valuable if it is done in an exemplary, innovative and cost-effective way that might serve as a "proof of concept" model, to be adapted and applied on a bigger scale elsewhere. Beyond the immediate and local benefits, such programmes also contribute to an increasingly important general endeavour – to respect, protect, fulfil and promote the right to health.

Although it is obvious that states are the most comprehensive duty-bearers in this regard, there is a growing expectation within modern societies that business enterprises will also contribute toward progressively realising the right to health, in a measurable and significant way. This chapter considers this issue and suggests some answers to questions about corporate contributions toward the right to health. It is important to develop a consensus model of what a fair division of responsibility in a global society could be.

Partnerships for women's health: Striving for best practice within the UN Global Compact,
Timmermann and Kruesmann (eds),
United Nations University Press, 2009, ISBN 978-92-808-1185-8

The right to health, being part of the economic, social and cultural human rights catalogue, has gained substantial political importance, as well as theoretical significance, in conjunction with the rising popularity of the "rights-based" rhetoric permeating many political and social movements.[1] Rights-based development policy concepts place the respect, protection and fulfilment of all human rights in the centre of the development debate.[2] With regard to the private sector, rights for which there is a *legal* obligation for a state may constitute a *moral* obligation for a non-state actor. Yet for many business enterprises this remains uncharted territory – dealing with a human rights obligation that includes affirmative steps to respect, protect and fulfil those rights in their sphere of influence.

The "right to health" concept emphasises the link between the health status of a person and issues such as dignity, justice, non-discrimination, gender and participation. Based on the formation of the World Health Organization (WHO) in 1946, the International Covenant on Economic, Social and Cultural Rights in 1966 and other human rights treaties, the "Health for All 2000" objective of the Alma-Ata Conference on Primary Health Care in 1978 and the *United Nations Millennium Declaration* in September 2000, the consensus of international institutional thinking is that every human being is entitled to the highest attainable standard of health conducive to living a life in dignity.[3] This consensus was also the background and justification for establishing the Special Rapporteur of the UN Secretary-General for the Right to Health.[4]

The academic "right to health" debate took off powerfully in 1994 in an article by Jonathan Mann.[5] He discussed the positive and negative impacts of different health policies, programmes and practices on human rights (such as the fact that a state's failure to recognise health problems that unduly affect a marginalised or stigmatised group violates the right to non-discrimination); the health effects of human rights violations (such as torture, imprisonment under inhumane conditions or rape); and the fact that the promotion and protection of health are inextricably linked to the promotion and protection of human rights and dignity (as when dealing with HIV/AIDS).

The interrelatedness and interconnectedness of health and development were prominently acknowledged by the United Nations in the specific and measurable health targets contained in the Millennium Development Goals (MDGs). Although progress can be achieved if political will is mobilised and if best practices are applied, most countries are still far from achieving these goals,[6] particularly the health-related ones on child and maternal mortality and on sanitation.[7]

The poverty context: The state of human development

Despite the fact that the last 50 years have been the most successful ever in the fight against poverty, the state of development in 2006 continued to be characterised by an enormous amount of human misery, demonstrating the staggering challenges ahead:[8]

- 1 billion people are living on less than US$1 a day and 2.5 billion on less than US$2 a day;
- 850 million people – including one in three preschool-aged children – are under-nourished;
- 1.8 billion people do not have access to improved water sources, and 2.9 billion people lack access to adequate sanitation;
- 30,000 children under 5 years of age die every day, mainly from dehydration, under-nourishment and preventable diseases;
- every year more than 500,000 women die in childbirth – one every minute of every day;
- 40 million people are living with HIV/AIDS, 25 million of whom are in sub-Saharan Africa; in 2005, some 3 million people died of AIDS and another 5 million became infected with HIV;
- a regional breakdown shows that sub-Saharan Africa and South Asia remain the regions of the world with the highest levels of absolute poverty.

No other indicators demonstrate the North–South gap in the physical quality of life as dramatically as health-related ones. There is a fundamental relationship between health deficits and poverty.[9] Poor people who lack education on health matters and have limited or no access to adequate nutrition, safe water and sanitation also are not likely to have the purchasing power to pay for basic health services. Four broad mechanisms are responsible for and contribute to the perpetuation of health disparities:[10]

- *stratification* – the very fact that people are poor, and are recognised as such in a hierarchical social environment;
- *exposure* – greater exposure to multiple health risks (malnourishment, unsafe water, lack of health knowledge);
- *susceptibility* – greater vulnerability owing to the mutually compounding effects of multiple health risks; and
- *precariousness* – potentially catastrophic effects of loss of income, land or livestock, school dropouts, or illness-related disadvantages that keep the vicious poverty–illness cycle intact.

The realisation of the *right to health* – however defined – is connected to progress in the realisation of all the civil and political as well as economic, social and cultural human rights contained in the Universal Declaration of Human Rights (UDHR): "the right to food, housing, work, education, human dignity, life, non-discrimination, equality, the prohibition of torture, privacy, access to information, and the freedoms of association, assembly and movement."[11]

Sustainable progress in the status of population health requires more than just appropriate policies and allocations of resources by a ministry of health. It depends on, and is instrumental in, poverty alleviation. Poverty reduction strategies can be successful only if they are backed up by a number of synergistic measures and complementary approaches that respect, protect and fulfil human rights, including but not limited to the right to health. A precondition for this to happen is more "voice" – that is, less discrimination against and more political influence for the poor, as well as more participation in the affairs that affect their daily lives.

Many of the greatest disparities with fatal consequences are the result of discrimination against women and girls.[12] Violations of basic human rights – such as of the "right to say no" to sexual coercion, to unsafe sex and to forced or child marriages; freedom from genital mutilation; and freedom to make and realise reproductive choices, to mention just a few – still result in 500,000 girls and women dying every year (virtually all of them in developing countries) from preventable conditions and injuries related to pregnancy and childbirth. More women than men, and at younger ages, are living with HIV/AIDS – the majority of the people aged 15–24 who are infected with HIV-1 in sub-Saharan Africa are female. Girls and women continue to be discriminated against by a "cultural mindset" (which is sometimes defended by religious fundamentalists on a supposedly religious basis) that results in no or severely impaired access to food, health care, education and employment. A concerted effort to guarantee human rights in a gender-neutral way would not cost a great deal and would save millions of lives.

Contrary to the insinuations contained in widespread criticism about the pharmaceutical industry's patent and price policy, it is rarely the patented high-tech solutions that are needed to combat typical poverty-related diseases. Poverty alleviation in general and especially targeted interventions – better nutrition education for mothers (including on the importance of breastfeeding), mass vaccination campaigns, access to basic antibiotics, bed nets for malaria prevention and condom use programmes to prevent the spread of HIV/AIDS and other sexually transmitted diseases – are highly effective in reducing preventable mortality. The combination of these with well-known and inexpensive basic health interventions would have a dramatic positive impact on the health of the poor.

Bearers of duties

A meaningful discussion of rights must deal with the respective duty-bearers. As with all rights formulated in the UDHR, states are the most comprehensive bearers of duties. In the context of a right to health, however, it is important to mention that, along with environmental, social and economic factors, genetic parameters and the availability of health care, there are also lifestyle issues – and hence the spectrum of different responsibilities spans from the state to the individual.

Individual duties

Although governments should play a stronger role in risk prevention policies, education and social marketing, individuals must accept their share of responsibility for their own health. Individual commitments and corresponding actions cannot be replaced by communities or governments and even less so by the international community. Duties in the context of the right to health begin at home and include healthy nutrition, risk-avoiding lifestyles and refraining from alcohol, nicotine and drug abuse.

Community obligations

Local communities can do much to improve perception and understanding of health risks and to reduce them. Functioning communities regard it as their essential obligation to analyse health-related problems, determine needs, initiate community efforts and mobilise resources that will improve health-related infrastructure (such as supplies of safe water), that will eliminate habitats for vectors that spread diseases, that will provide support and care for the needy and that will train community workers for health, education and other roles. Significant health results can be achieved without many financial resources; even poor communities can achieve a great deal, such as encouraging health-promoting behaviours (breastfeeding, use of mosquito nets, heating of unsafe water) and developing peer pressure against health risks (unsafe sex, excessive alcohol consumption, men's violation of women's reproductive rights).

Nation-state obligations

All human rights are, above all, incumbent on states and their institutions because the human rights regime is based on treaties between states. States thus do have the primary responsibility to respect, protect and fulfil people's right to health. According to the Committee on Economic, Social and Cultural Rights, this means the following:[13]

- Obligations to *respect* include, among other considerations, "refraining from denying or limiting equal access for all persons ... to preventive, curative, and palliative health services" but also refraining from "prohibiting or impeding traditional preventive care, healing practices and medicines" (para. 34).

- Obligations to *protect* include, among other considerations, the duty "to ensure that privatization of the health sector does not constitute a threat to the availability, accessibility, acceptability, and quality of health facilities, goods and services" (para. 35).

- Obligations to *fulfil* require states to, among other things, "adopt a national health policy with a detailed plan for realizing the right to health"; to "ensure provision of health care, including immunization programmes against the major infectious diseases"; "to ensure equal access for all to the underlying determinants of health" (safe food, potable water, basic sanitation, and so on); and to ensure "the provision of a sufficient number of hospitals, clinics and other health-related facilities" as well as a public, private or mixed health insurance system that all can afford (para. 36).

States and their institutions must do away with torture, violence against children and harmful traditional practices that violate human rights and the health of the victims.[14] Once the non-negotiable essentials have been achieved, the continuous battle for the fulfilment of the right to health must be fought on at least three fronts:[15]

- Use non-health interventions to provide health benefits, such as by providing clean water, improving sanitation, offering better primary education and improving governance and basic infrastructure.

- Deliver medical interventions, such as vaccines and drugs, medical examinations, tests and cost-effective treatment – especially to poor people (most benefits from public spending on curative health services go not to the poorest but to the better off).[16]

- Deliver non-medical health interventions, such as training medical personnel, building better health information systems and strengthening systems for procuring and storing information.

Health policy outcomes depend on the efficacy of the public sector and the incentive structures of the given institutional arrangements. Wherever the capacity and efficacy of the public sector are low – and they have been low in many instances – adopting strategies that put a greater workload on public institutions may be the wrong choice.[17] There is mounting evidence that non-governmental organisations (NGOs) and the private sector can in some cases deliver essential and other services to poor people more efficiently than the public sector can.[18]

While poor countries, by definition, do have an overall resource scarcity problem, the *allocation pattern of available resources* remains an ongoing issue. Statistics from the UN Development Programme and the World Bank are readily available to prove that a number of governments in the developing world spend up to five times as much on the military as on health. Violations of the state's obligation to fulfil people's right to health include the failure to adopt or implement a national health policy designed to ensure the right to health for everyone, as well as insufficient expenditure or misallocation of public resources to guarantee minimum levels of primary health care, including essential drugs, which results in non-enjoyment of the right to health by individuals or groups, particularly the vulnerable or marginalised. Although the International Covenant on Economic, Social and Cultural Rights endeavours to guarantee minimum levels of subsistence to people in poor nations,[19] the principle of "free public health care" remains a subject of discussion.

A last important point: the interpretation of economic and social rights cannot be made without regard to the stage of development of a country, its available capabilities and resources, and the competing claims on these resources. Social services in the quantity and quality provided in a mature European nation are and will remain for the foreseeable future well out of reach for any sub-Saharan African or South Asian nation.

Obligations of the international community of states

For the sake of a fair discussion of the right to health in a corporate context, it is important to emphasise that where the duty of the state is neglected – whether because of a lack of resources or because of deficits in governance – first and foremost the international community ought to be called to account. With development assistance in the case of incapability and with a mixture of pressure and incentives in the case of unwillingness, the international community is expected to take joint action to achieve full realisation of the right to health. Richer nations in particular are called on to "facilitate access to essential health facilities, goods and services in other countries, wherever possible and provide the necessary aid when required".[20]

Drawing attention to the legitimate sequence of legal duties for the respect, protection and fulfilment of the right to health is necessary for at least two reasons:

- to avoid pushing the debate to the wrong side, thus absolving primary duty-bearers of their responsibilities, tolerating their non-performance and allowing the blame for mass sickness to be placed on other actors; and
- to avoid the development of unrealistic expectations about sustainable deliverables from the private sector, especially pharmaceutical corporations.

In accordance with Articles 55 and 56 of the UN Charter, international cooperation for the development and realisation of human rights is an obligation of all states. International political consensus sees first and foremost bilateral and multilateral development assistance and specialised UN agencies, in particular WHO, as having a role in realising the right to health at the international, regional and country levels.

A number of binding treaties strive to provide a framework for a new international economic order, based on sovereign equality, interdependence, mutual interest and cooperation among all states. From time to time these have been reinforced, as in the *Millennium Declaration*, when 147 Heads of State and Government recognised "that, in addition to our separate responsibilities to our individual societies, we have a collective responsibility to uphold the principles of human dignity, equality and equity at the global level".[21]

The practical consequences of the commitments made have been less than impressive, however. Although in the past few years official development assistance (ODA) did increase, to 0.33 per cent of gross national income in 2005, it still falls short of the 0.54 per cent that the UN Millennium Project estimates will be necessary to achieve the MDGs. With regard to health issues – which are relevant to three of the eight MDGs – the positive news is that the portion of ODA going to these issues increased considerably, to 15 per cent in 2004.

Compounding the fact that the overall aid level is still too low to meet the basic health needs of poor countries, there are acute problems with achieving reasonable aid effectiveness.[22] We seem to be far removed from averting 8 million deaths annually (which would yield economic benefits in the order of US$360 billion) by properly investing an additional US$31 billion a year in donor assistance for health, as the Commission on Macroeconomics and Health estimated.[23] Newer studies suggest that an even greater effect on the economies of poor countries is possible through improvements in health.[24] A key to this might be the adoption of a rights-based approach by crucial institutions such as the WHO as well as by influential governments such as that of the United States, which continue to resist economic, social and cultural rights, including the human right to the highest attainable standard of health.[25]

Non-state actors' obligations

The discussion about non-state actors is restricted here to the two groups most present in the public debate about health issues: NGOs and the private sector.

Consultations with poor people reveal that they consider governments to be very important but that their actions are rather ineffective and sometimes harmful.[26] Problems of corruption emerge in many cases as a key issue in people's daily struggles – whether it is to get an education for their children, access to justice or police protection, or access to basic health care. In contrast, NGOs – in particular, emergency aid NGOs and religious organisations – rate well in responsiveness and trust. They have a role in facilitating the voices of poor people and they can be helpful in supporting the formulation and implementation of policies that actually benefit the poor. NGOs such as Oxfam were among the first to make human rights an integral dimension of the design, implementation, monitoring and evaluation of health-related programmes. Although NGOs should not be considered the "silver bullet" for solving all grassroots health problems, they are an important link in the chain.

For the private sector, meaningful answers and sustainable corporate commitments require not only differentiating political and civil human rights from economic, social and cultural human rights but also defining the boundaries of corporate obligations in a fair societal distribution of responsibility.[27] Many individuals and major business associations are concerned that, where states are incapable or unwilling to fulfil their duties, their human rights obligations will simply be pushed onto non-state actors, especially multinational business enterprises.

As expressed by the first two principles of the UN Global Compact, the prime responsibility of corporations to respect, protect and contribute toward fulfilment of human rights is in the context of normal business activities, as is the goal of ensuring that the company's activities do not contribute directly or indirectly to the violation of rights, in this case the right to health.[28] Successful pharmaceutical companies can make a particular contribution through the results of their research and development endeavours being used to cure diseases, prevent premature mortality and shorten hospital stays. This is highly relevant in the pharmaceutical industry, and examples here are drawn from this sector.

Sincere corporate commitments in the context of the right to health must be handled carefully in the context of competing dynamics:

- On the one hand, there is a structural tension, as private enterprises – being market oriented and profit driven – run up against limits in cases of market failure; things turn even worse if market failure and state failure come together and create negative synergies for the poor.

- On the other hand, to shrug the "corporate shoulder" and walk away doing nothing in the face of the biggest social problems of humankind is not an acceptable option. The situation presents a challenge and an opportunity for moral leadership and corporate vision to determine how much should be done, in what areas, for whom, in partnership with what stakeholders, over what period of time and so on.

Distinguishing corporate responsibilities

A sustainable corporate responsibility approach will carefully examine and decide on the nature and dimension of corporate obligations. It will also define the boundaries beyond which further corporate contributions are seen as unreasonable by management. As with other corporate social responsibility aspects, corporate obligations to respect, protect and fulfil the right to health encompass responsibilities with differing degrees of obligation. A suitable distinction can be drawn among:[29]

- *essential* responsibilities required of any corporation for the respect of the right to health (the "*must*" dimension);
- additional corporate responsibility standards beyond those usually enshrined in national law, meaning what can reasonably be *expected* by society (the "*ought to*" dimension); and
- special corporate responsibility endeavours such as corporate philanthropy (the "*can*" dimension).

The "must" dimension

With regard to respect for the right to health, as with all other human rights, a company competing with integrity complies in its own sphere of influence with all laws and regulations concerning healthy workplaces, environmental protection and the safety of products and services.

A pharmaceutical corporation is particularly able to make further substantial contributions through cutting-edge research, development and manufacture of high-quality drugs. This helps reduce premature mortality as well as prevent or cure diseases that are susceptible to drug therapy; this in turn improves the quality of life of sick people, avoids costly hospitalisation and allows people to go back to normal working lives instead of being bedridden.

Under constructive political and social conditions ("good governance"), these corporate contributions are of major instrumental value in enabling individuals to lead healthy lives, as well as enabling the state to successfully bear its right-to-health duties. In addition, through the wages paid to staff, employees are empowered to fulfil their economic, social and cultural rights. And through taxes paid, the state is enabled to fulfil its duties.

The "ought" dimension

Responsible companies will deliver more than just the essentials. This is particularly so in countries where legal standards are low or not enforced. Such companies – having appropriate corporate responsibility guidelines in place – will adhere to self-imposed corporate responsibility norms even if local laws and regulations allow lower standards. They will do their best to avoid benefiting from unhealthy working conditions or unsafe workplaces of third parties within their sphere of influence.

For employers in the developing world, it can be regarded as a best practice, particularly for a pharmaceutical company, to establish a comprehensive programme of medical services for their employees that includes free or heavily subsidised facilities for diagnosis, treatment and psychosocial care of workers with HIV/AIDS or other poverty-related diseases such as tuberculosis (TB) or malaria. Other relevant actions may, for instance, include free or heavily subsidised meals, provision of nursery schools for single mothers, free training opportunities using company infrastructure and scholarship programmes for the children of low-income employees.

The best pharmaceutical companies are willing to adapt, on the basis of a proper case-by-case evaluation, the prices of life-saving medicines for patients living in individual or collective poverty (at Novartis, examples of this include cooperation with WHO on malaria, which makes Coartem available at production cost, and the Gleevec patients' assistance programme). And, in an effort to protect participants in clinical trials all over the world, companies are well advised to adhere to the ethical principles of the *Declaration of Helsinki* on clinical trials.[30]

The "can" dimension

Deliverables in the context of the "can" dimension consist of actions that are neither required by law nor well-established industry practice. These can involve corporate philanthropy, including donations of first-class quality medicine.[31] Other examples of engagements in this category are institutions engaging in not-for-profit research on neglected diseases (such as the Novartis Institute for Tropical Diseases, which is focusing on TB and dengue fever). Corporate philanthropy endeavours (expenditures beyond a company's actual business activities without any specific direct corporate advantages and without any financially measurable rewards in return) can have a significant effect on the well-being of poor people – and hence on fulfilment of their right to health.

For many reasons it can make sense to create an independent foundation to take care of challenges on the "can" dimension. At Novartis, the Foundation for Sustainable Development has made significant contributions by investing in projects and programmes of development cooperation and humanitarian assistance and has helped to increase the effectiveness, efficiency and significance of project-related aid. Contributions to the fulfilment of the right to health of people whose purchasing power does not allow them to benefit from health services provided through market mechanisms should help to establish best practices – defined as being innovative, making a positive difference and having a sustainable effect, as well as having the potential to be replicated and to serve as a model for initiatives elsewhere.[32] Last but not least, donations in cases of acute emergencies (such as a tsunami) can play a significant role.

Conclusion: The fulfilment of the right to health as a multi-stakeholder task

Given the extent and complexity of global health problems in the twenty-first century and considering the tragic human misery associated with premature death and preventable diseases, the right-to-health debate is expected to gain in importance. If "medical care" is considered a right, national governments and international institutions are the primary parties with the duty to make all reasonable efforts to respect, protect and fulfil this right. Wherever responsible, *national governments* start to meet this commitment by making informed decisions based on the resources available:

- *Excess mortality and morbidity will be reduced*, for example, by focusing on interventions that can achieve the greatest health gains possible within prevailing resource limits. The vast majority of preventable diseases are the result of a relatively small number of identifiable deficits, and hence a focus on communicable diseases, health awareness programmes, and immunisation programmes can dramatically improve health and reduce premature mortality.

- *Potential threats to health will be countered*, for example, by social marketing, with the goal of changing unhealthy environments and reducing risky behaviour (for example, not only environmental measures against vector-borne diseases such as malaria as well as the promotion of bed nets, the use of condoms and the fight against tobacco addiction but also health education for the prevention of cancer and cardiovascular diseases).

- *More effective health systems will be developed*, for example, by setting priorities according to actual needs and giving incentives to improve health sector performance (given that known and cost-effective interventions against the diseases that cause 50 per cent of preventable deaths among the poor have been given insufficient priority within existing health systems).[33]
- *Expanding the knowledge base will be assured*, simply by investing in this field consistently and coherently.

Second in the line of duty is the *international community*. A reality check shows that many poor countries with high infant and child mortality are not on track with regard to the achievement of the MDGs in general and – even more so – with regard to health. Being already two-thirds of the way through the 1990–2015 time period specified in the MDGs, the general child and maternal mortality goals are projected to remain almost universally unmet, with sub-Saharan Africa lagging behind most significantly.[34] Although part of this can be attributed to lack of good governance, industrial countries have failed to keep the promises they made and are still making. Each dollar going to development assistance still has to fight hard against hundreds of dollars spent for military and protectionist purposes.

And the *private sector*? Is there a right to health that poor people can call on to be sustainably *respected* by companies, particularly pharmaceutical companies? Yes, corporations all over the world and from all sectors have social and ecological legal duties within their normal business activities. Is there a right to health that poor people can call on to be sustainably *protected*? Yes, enlightened corporations strive to make sure that questionable labour standards and environmental practices are avoided in their sphere of influence. Is there a right to health that poor people can call on to be sustainably *fulfilled*? Yes, for those who are employed by the company, through a fair remuneration and by the employers' tax and insurance contributions. But beyond that?

The answer to this key question depends on individual perspectives. There is a widespread moral recognition of deliverables beyond the supply of markets, the respect of law and proper norms, and of the provision of productive employment. Today, many companies, but certainly not a majority of companies, do accept such responsibilities through the "can dimension" of corporate responsibility commitments. On its own, however, this cannot make more than a very limited contribution to overcoming the challenges we all face on a global level.

The huge mortality and morbidity burden can be brought down only with a *concerted strategy* that is supported globally with financial resources and know-how on good practices as well as with national and community efforts to increase the access of the world's poor to essential health services. It is obvious that single actors on their own will face narrow limits with regard to their impact on global development and health problems. Solutions of multifaceted problems of global dimensions must be approached with a multi-stakeholder approach. This is why all actors of society – state and non-state – are called on to contribute to solutions according to their obligations, abilities and enlightened self-interest. The watershed for the credibility of all societal actors will be their willingness to make resources available and to cooperate in a creative way in order to meet all the Millennium Development Goals – and to fulfil the right to health.

Notes

1. Article 1 of the *Declaration on the Right to Development*, adopted by General Assembly Resolution 41/128 of 4 December 1986, reads: "The right to development is an inalienable human right by virtue of which every human person and all peoples are entitled to participate in, contribute to, and enjoy economic, social, cultural and political development, in which all human rights and fundamental freedoms can be fully realized." Respective (vague) duties could be deduced from the wording of Article 3: "States have the primary responsibility for the creation of national and international conditions favourable to the realization of the right to development.... The realization of the right to development requires full respect for the principles of international law concerning friendly relations and co-operation among States in accordance with the Charter of the United Nations." And

"States have the duty to co-operate with each other in ensuring development and eliminating obstacles to development. States should realize their rights and fulfil their duties in such a manner as to promote a new international economic order based on sovereign equality, interdependence, mutual interest and co-operation among all States, as well as to encourage the observance and realization of human rights." See <http://www.unhchr.ch/html/menu3/b/74.htm> (accessed 5 June 2009).

2. For an interesting way to deal with this issue, see UNHCHR, *A Human Rights Approach to Poverty Reduction Strategies*, Office of the High Commissioner for Human Rights, United Nations, 2002, <http://www.unhchr.ch/development/povertyfinal.html> (accessed 5 June 2009); see also OHCHR, *Human Rights and Poverty Reduction. A Conceptual Framework*, New York and Geneva: United Nations, 2004.

3. Article 25.1 of the Universal Declaration of Human Rights (1948) affirms that "everyone has the right to a standard of living adequate for the health of himself and of his family, including food, clothing, housing and medical care and necessary social services". The International Covenant on Economic, Social and Cultural Rights (1966) interprets this in Article 12.1 as "the right of everyone to the enjoyment if the highest attainable standard of physical and mental health". A similar articulation, "the enjoyment of the highest attainable standard of health as a fundamental right of every human being", was enshrined in WHO's constitution over 50 years ago and is part of numerous international treaties and conventions (see WHO, "25 Questions & Answers on Health & Human Rights", Health & Human Rights Publication Series No. 1, Geneva: World Health Organization, July 2002). Last but not least, the Economic and Social Council's General Comment No. 14 on "Substantive Issues Arising in the Implementation of the International Covenant on Economic, Social and Cultural Rights" reaffirms the "right to the highest attainable standard of health" (United Nations Economic and Social Council, UN Document E/C.12/2000/4, 11 August 2000), <http://www.unhchr.ch/tbs/doc.nsf/(Symbol)/40d009901358b0e2c1256915005090be?Opendocument> (accessed 5 June 2009).

4. Professor Paul Hunt served as UN "Special Rapporteur on the right of everyone to the enjoyment of the highest attainable standard of physical and mental health" from 2002 to 2008. He was followed by Mr Anand Grover in June 2008. Paul Hunt's last report was published on 21 March 2008 (A/HRC/7/11), with an annex on his mission to GlaxoSmithKline on 5 May 2009 (A/HRC/11/12/Add.2), available at <http://ap.ohchr.org/documents/dpage_e.aspx?m=100> (accessed 26 June 2009).

5. J. Mann, "Health and Human Rights", *Health and Human Rights: An International Journal*, 1, 1994.

6. United Nations Development Programme, *Human Development Report 2003. Millennium Goals: A Compact Among Nations to End Poverty*, New York: Oxford University Press, 2003; see also *Finance & Development*, 40(4), pp. 12–41.

7. M. Baird and S. Shetty, "Getting There. How to Accelerate Progress Toward the Millennium Development Goals", *Finance & Development*, 40(4), 2003, p. 16.

8. Estimated data, taken from *World Development Indicators 2006*, Washington DC, World Bank Development Data Group, <http://devdata.worldbank.org/wdi2006/contents/index2.htm> (accessed 5 June 2009).

9. K. M. Leisinger, "Health Policy for Least Developed Countries", *Social Strategies*, 16, 1985 (available through the Novartis Foundation for Sustainable Development, Basel).

10. D. Carr, "Improving the Health of the World's Poorest People", *Population Reference Bureau: Health Bulletin*, 1, 2004, p. 14.

11. Economic and Social Council, General Comment No. 14, para. 3. The United Nations Committee on Economic, Social and Cultural Rights is a group of experts nominated by the countries that have ratified the International Covenant on Economic, Social and Cultural Rights.

12. A. Germain, "Reproductive Health and Human Rights", *Lancet*, 3 January 2004,.

13. See Economic and Social Council, General Comment No. 14.

14. WHO, "25 Questions & Answers on Health & Human Rights", p. 10.

15. D. E. Bloom and D. Canning. "A New Health Opportunity", *Development*, 44(1), 2001.

16. For example, see F. Castro-Leal et al., "Public Spending on Health Care in Africa: Do the Poor Benefit?", *Bulletin of the World Health Organization*, 78(1), 2000, p. 70.

17. D. Filmer et al., "Health Policy in Poor Countries: Weak Links in the Chain", World Bank Policy Research Working Paper No. 1874, 1999.

18. R. Hecht et al., "Making Health Care Accountable. Why Performance-based Funding of Health Services in Developing Countries Is Getting More Attention", *Finance & Development*, 41(1), 2004, pp. 16–19. See also World Bank, *World Development Report 2004. Making Services Work for Poor People*, New York: Oxford University Press, 2004.

19. Economic and Social Council, General Comment No. 14, para. 52.

20. Ibid., para. 39.

21. Resolution 55/2 adopted by the General Assembly, *United Nations Millennium Declaration*, UN Document A/RES/55/2, 18 September 2000, <http://www.un.org/millennium/declaration/ares552e.pdf> (accessed 5 June 2009).

22. G. Schieber et al., "Getting Real on Health Financing", *Finance & Development*, 43(4), 2006.

23. WHO, Commission on Macroeconomics and Health, "Foreword", *Macroeconomics and Health: Investing in Health for Economic Development*, Geneva: WHO, 2002.

24. D. E. Bloom et al., "Health, Wealth, and Welfare", *Finance & Development*, 41(1), 2004, pp. 10–15.

25. Human Rights Council, "Implementation of General Assembly Resolution 60/251 of 15 March 2006", paras 49–50.

26. D. Narayan et al., *Voices of the Poor. Can Anyone Hear Us?*, Washington DC: Oxford University Press/World Bank, 2000.

27. K. M. Leisinger, "On Corporate Responsibility for Human Rights", in *Humanism in Business*, Cambridge University Press, 2009, pp. 175–203; see also K. M. Leisinger, "Business and Human Rights", in M. McIntosh et

al. (eds), *Learning to Talk: Corporate Citizenship and the Development of the UN Global Compact*, London: Greenleaf Publications, 2004; K. M. Leisinger, "Corporate Responsibilities for Access to Medicines", *Journal of Business Ethics*, 85, 2009, pp. 3–23. Whereas international human rights law considers it important to address all human rights on an equal footing and holistically, from a corporate point of view the economic, social and cultural rights are considered to be the real challenge and hence a distinction should be made.

28. On 7 April 2008, the Special Representative of the Secretary-General on the issue of human rights and transnational corporations and other business enterprises, John Ruggie, presented his report from his original three-year mandate ("Protect, Respect and Remedy: a Framework for Business and Human Rights", UN Document A/HRC/8/5, 7 April 2008, http:// www.reports-and-materials.org/Ruggie-report-7-Apr-2008.pdf>, accessed 5 June 2009). With regard to the "promotion and protection of all human rights, civil, political, economic, social and cultural rights, including the right to development", the report sets out "a framework for business and human rights" using the key terms "protect, respect and remedy", with "respect" marking the responsibility of corporations to respect human rights, basically in the meaning of "do no harm". The report has been widely acknowledged, but efforts have to continue to define clearly for various sectors which practices express the line between violating and respecting (e.g. the right to health) and which practices would have to be regarded as further support of this right (see the section in the report entitled "The Corporate Responsibility to Respect").

29. This follows Dahrendorf's distinction of norms that – together with expectations and sanctions of others – determine the "homo sociologicus"; see Ralf Dahrendorf, *Homo Sociologicus*, 16th edn, Wiesbaden: VS Verlag, 2006.

30. World Medical Association, *Declaration of Helsinki: Ethical Principles for Medical Research Involving Human Subjects*, adopted by the 18th WMA General Assembly, Helsinki, Finland, June 1964, <http://www.wma.net/e/policy/pdf/17c.pdf> (accessed 5 June 2009).

31. Novartis Foundation for Sustainable Development, <http://www.novartisfoundation.com/pdf/Improving_Access_to_Leprosy_Treatment.pdf> (accessed 5 June 2009).

32. *Interim Report of the Special Rapporteur of the Commission on Human Rights on the Right of Everyone to Enjoy the Highest Attainable Standard of Physical and Mental Health, Mr. Paul Hunt*, UN Document A/58/427, 10 October 2003, p. 13, <http://www.unhchr.ch/Huridocda/Huridoca.nsf/(Symbol)/A.58.427.En?Opendocument> (accessed 5 June 2009).

33. S. Spinaci and D. Heymann, "Communicable Disease and Disability of the Poor" *Development*, 44(1), 2001, pp. 66ff.

34. *The Millennium Development Goals Report*, New York: United Nations, 2005. This has not changed, as the World Bank's *Global Monitoring Report 2009: A Development Emergency* illustrates, available at <http://ddp-ext.worldbank.org/ext/GMIS/home.do?siteId=2> (accessed 26 June 2009).

4

The challenge of equal financial access to the best available health care: Bringing in the private sector

GÜNTER NEUBAUER AND IRIS J. DRIESSLE

Introduction

The challenge of achieving equal financial access to the best available health care can be investigated using a variety of analytical lenses. In this chapter, five such lenses are used, and these shape the structure of the discussion. First, we set the context with reference to economic theory by distinguishing between different types of "goods" and situating "access to health care" as a "good" within that framework. Then we consider the question of what constitutes "best available" health care, including the issue of whether "best available" is to be seen in absolute or relative terms. Leading on from this, we investigate possible ways to equalise access to health care, again within the economic theory framework. There are two main approaches to focus on here: to nationalise the entire health care system, as is the case, for example, in the UK; or to privatise the health care system while still guaranteeing each citizen a minimum of health insurance protection. The following section describes a third possible approach,

Partnerships for women's health: Striving for best practice within the UN Global Compact,
Timmermann and Kruesmann (eds),
United Nations University Press, 2009, ISBN 978-92-808-1185-8

striking a balance between these two extremes: public private partnership (PPP) as a method of equalising access to health care. The final section then provides a viewpoint in which PPP is described as a prospective policy for bankrolling public infrastructure, applicable not only in Europe but also in developing countries such as India.

Equal access to health care as a public good

Economic theory distinguishes between three main types of goods: public goods, merit goods and private goods.[1]

Public goods are characterised as being equally accessible to all citizens, as well as there being no principle of individual exclusion. This means that public goods are allotted to public use because there is no rivalry in consumption and no possibility of excluding consumers. Some typical examples of public goods are the external and internal security of a country, the courts, clean air and clean water.

Merit goods are goods that could be passed into private hands, but for various reasons a decision is made that they ought not to be privatised. Governments typically make such decisions, judging that merit goods can or should be treated like public goods. As a consequence, there is also equal access for all citizens to merit goods, which are offered free of economic barriers and therefore without price. Merit goods are intended to provide the population with the opportunity to obtain and sustain a higher level of welfare. Some typical examples of merit goods are most health care services, such as hospitals or physician care, retirement arrangements and access to school education.

In contrast to these two, private goods are typically produced and distributed by markets. In markets, the existence of prices can exclude some consumers from obtaining private goods. Access to private goods is available only to those consumers who have sufficient purchasing power. At this point the genesis of purchasing power is not determined. Typical examples of private goods are all sorts of products that are purchased at individual expense on the markets, for example, luxury goods, clothes and chocolates, to name just a few.[2]

Health care is typically defined as a merit good. It can be distributed either by public organisations or by private companies. If equal access to health care is intended, governments commonly decide to declare health care to be a merit good and open up access to it by abolishing any barriers. Theoretically, there could also be equal access in a privatised environment if the government subsidised all households with sufficient purchasing power, so that each household was enabled to purchase health care services and health care goods as required, independent from its individual household income.[3]

What is "best available" health care?

The term "best available health care" can be interpreted in an absolute or a relative manner. Speaking in absolute terms, best available health care means the very best health care, free from any local or economic constraints. Excellent health care would be available everywhere and it would be offered to anyone in need.

It is obvious that this kind of interpretation and practice of "best available health care" is not likely to be achievable in reality, and particularly not in poorer countries such as India. Therefore, the relative definition of the term seems to be more suitable. "Relatively best available health care" implies that the best possible health care has to be understood in relation to the prevailing economic and social circumstances. Taking these factors into consideration makes it quite difficult to establish an operational definition of what constitutes the *relatively* best available health care. In some ways it could be measured by economic indicators such as the average percentage of the gross domestic product (GDP), which is sometimes used for health care studies. It could also be defined via the proportion of the poor population that has access to a minimum set of health care services and health care goods. Here again the problem arises of defining "poor" or "minimum set".[4]

Providing the best (relatively) available health care also means that regional and local access to health care institutions is guaranteed to those sectors of the population most in need. Along with claims to provide the best standards of health care goes, for example, the need for a working public transportation system enabling every citizen to seek medical assistance when required. Large cities and other densely populated areas usually offer better access to health care institutions than more rural areas. Apart from any other reason, this is because of the dynamics of efficiency. For the population in rural areas, this results in lower availability and higher transaction costs in health care institutions, compared with the urban population.

In conclusion, relatively equal access to the best available health care has to take into account not only the economic conditions in a country but also social and other factors such as the density of the population and the geographical size of the country.

Ways to equalise health care access

Equal access to health care is a human right postulated internationally and also fixed in the UN Charter.[5] This section will compare three different approaches to this matter and discuss the disadvantages and benefits of each.

A first approach: Nationalised health care systems

In many countries, a national health care system is considered the appropriate way to equalise access to health care for all citizens. Most of these nationalised health care systems are financed out of taxes. Normally, the providers of health care are semi-nationalised; this means that larger institutions like hospitals are owned and run by community authorities. In contrast, physicians, mainly general practitioners, work independently but are strictly regulated through reinvestments and are given standards on how to treat patients. Nationalised health care systems are intended to guarantee equal health care access to the entire population of a country. The rationale is that state-financed health care institutions are obliged to accept every citizen as a patient, whereas foreigners are usually subject to special rules concerning access to health care.

One of the problems of nationalised health care systems is financing. Because the system is financed through taxes, the health care budget is subject to parliamentary debate, and is just one of many budgets that compete for resources within the national finances.

On the one hand, political imperatives determine the size of a country's health care budget, meaning the budget may not in practice match requirements. On the other hand, the size of the budget is also influenced by scarcity of means. The corollary is that nationalised health care systems spend less on health care than more individualised health care systems do.[6]

Where a system is financed out of taxes, the government is obliged to control the spending of that budget. One consequence is the growth of bureaucracy to conduct reviews and ensure expenditure is in accordance with predetermined budget parameters. During the year, fixed budgets imply that any change has to go through parliamentary debates, reducing the elasticity of spending as well as the adaptability of the budget to changing health requirements throughout the plan period.

Another disadvantage of a state health care system is low incentives for the providers of health care to give treatment efficiently. Budgets that are determined at the beginning of the year and that are then fixed throughout the whole planning period do not generate efficiency incentives. Health care providers are instead encouraged to limit their efforts to the size of the fixed budget, and are not able to increase their volume of treatment by reinvestment through more or better work.

Of course, there are various ways to bring more dynamism into fixed budgets. Funding systems as they are established in, for example, the UK provide general practitioners with a clearly defined fund for each citizen who enrols on that practitioner's list. The general practitioner is then free to manage the treatment of the patient within the fund. Referred patients will also be paid for out of the fund. In this way, incentives are created for general practitioners to reduce the number of referrals to other providers in order not to decrease their own surplus and in effect their own income. These experiences in the

UK show, however, that single general practitioners cannot manage the entire procedure all on their own. Management expertise and capacity are required in order to organise the fund-financed approach if there is to be a balanced system of give-and-take. Moreover, there is a clear incentive to general practitioners to under-serve their patients, as this would save costs and increase the general practitioner's own income. Such tensions lead to criticism of this model.

Nationalised health care systems suffer from typical issues of state behaviour within a parliamentary government. Budgets are mainly determined by political debates rather than being based on the actual needs of the population. Bureaucracy hinders communication between the giving and the receiving institutions, provides low or incorrect incentives for the providers of health care and contributes to keeping the efficiency and effectiveness of treatment down. Inside the nationalised system, access to health care is formally equalised, but some people are more equal than others; they know the right people and places and get to see the doctor faster. Outside the system, the market rules and privatised health institutions treat patients upon private payment.

A second approach: Privatised health care systems

An alternative way to equalise health care access is to privatise the health care system while subsidising the consumer. Privatisation of the health care system brings the advantage of higher incentives and is therefore expected to be more efficient and effective than a nationalised health care system. A privatised arrangement provides the actors in the health care market with the possibility of generating a higher income and maximising their individual benefit. To accept this impure motive in health care, fair competition has to be granted. However, there is scepticism about whether or not fair competition can work in this sensitive sector as it can in normal markets. Among the many market defects prevailing in the health care system, one of the most important is the low transparency of services. Further, consumers of health care have a very low price elasticity of demand; people in crucial situations are not free to compare the prices and quality of different providers when they are in need of immediate help.[7]

Another flaw of competitive markets in the health care sector is the principle of excludability in prices. Patients in need, but without the required purchasing power, have only limited access to health care, for example through charity institutions. To rectify this disadvantage, the government has to subsidise citizens with low incomes to ensure they have adequate insurance protection. If the subsidy is directly transferred to the indigent households, it is not possible to ensure the allowance is used in line with the intended purpose. For this reason, the government grant is more often transferred to insurers, or a specific-purpose financing fund has to be established by the state. The latter arrangement is practised in the United States, where the federal government finances a health fund, purchasing the required health services and goods for eligible households.

The constraints on a privatised health care system are set by the scarcity of means. The government and parliamentary committees have to decide the extent of protection to be available and the amount and type of transfers given to households. Scarcity in public budgets is also an important argument, and can be a dominating factor in the volume of benefits dispensed. This is a problem common to both nationalised and privatised health care systems.

Only very few countries try to establish market-driven health care systems. In Europe, as in developing countries, solely market-determined health systems are not accepted. The main hurdle to approval lies in the lack of a guarantee of equal access to health care providers.

In conclusion, the privatisation of health care systems seems not to be a suitable approach for achieving equal health care access for all citizens.

A third approach: Equal access health care through public private partnership

Public private partnership (PPP) is a commonly discussed way to accomplish public tasks by bringing in private enterprises. This assumes that the public institution can delegate certain or all issues to one or several private companies. It is the objective of PPP to combine public responsibility with private efficiency. Public demand is in part or wholly met by private providers. The compensation of these services is regulated by contracts between the public and the private parties.[8]

What is public private partnership in health care?

In this context, health care is subject to public responsibility. The supply of the necessary health care infrastructure, as well as the guarantee of equal access to health care providers, is incumbent on public institutions. Public institutions can ask private companies for assistance to fulfil their duties and responsibilities. Very often, public authorities alone are not capable of establishing the health care facilities needed to service an entire population. In this situation, private entrepreneurship can assist public authorities in meeting demand in a shorter time and/or at a higher level by making investments and/ or taking over certain tasks. Within PPP programmes the respective strengths of public and private partners are combined; the PPP projects are customarily planned, financed and implemented jointly for the profit of the private companies as well as to the benefit of the public. The private partners can establish or expand their business, and the public agencies can accelerate the implementation of demanding projects. Furthermore, bringing the private sector in can provide specialised management capacities, new technologies and expertise in how to access private sector financial resources and, last but not least, it may allow the public agency to streamline its overall involvement (see Figure 4.1).

Normally, PPP is focused on the supply side. Private companies value PPP as a kind of risk-sharing method when entering a new market with the support of public authorities. PPP can also be focused on the financing side and may include models of private–public health care insurance.[9]

Figure 4.1 Public private partnership

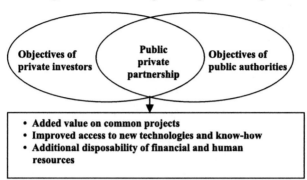

Source: the authors.

Typology of public private partnerships

There are various kinds of PPP. Two common criteria for distinguishing between types are capital investment and management by public and private providers. Different combinations of these can form different types of partnerships.

In the most common type of PPP, both private capital and private management are brought together in order to fulfil a public assignment that is delegated by the public authority to the private company. In this case, the public authority oversees whether or not the private partners fulfil their obligations. Because of a persistent deficit of investment in health care infrastructure and a lack of management know-how, this type of PPP tends to be preferred in newly industrialising countries such as India. In these countries, a growing economy provides good prospects for private companies to pay back credits or to obtain profitable returns on investment. In this way, the accessibility of the health care system even for poor people can be guaranteed by the government.

In another type of PPP, capital investment and management can be arranged differently, with public capital being managed privately. By privatising the management, but not the ownership, of a project and capital, public authorities can seek to encourage increasing entrepreneurial responsibility among public managers, who work together with the private consultants to ensure a mutually successful outcome.

Additional advantages of public private partnerships

There are both benefits and disadvantages to PPPs, and both risks and opportunities exist for the public and the private partners. The risks of PPP for the public partner are the for-profit orientation and imperative of the private partner to generate a positive return on its capital investment. However, public authorities may also have the incentive to calculate a return on investment, which then results in the squandering and misallocation of scarce resources, a fact that has often been neglected in analysis.

Table 4.1 gives an overview of the advantages and disadvantages of PPP. It shows that one important benefit resulting from PPP is the significantly higher efficiency of private investment and private management. Because of the higher efficiency, more people can obtain access to health care. Further, private capital brings in new and better technology and also helps it be used efficiently. Access for all benefi-

Table 4.1   Advantages and disadvantages of public private
               partnerships

Advantages	Disadvantages
Access for all beneficiaries	Profit orientation may affect service
High efficiency	priority
Private capital investment	Investment returns may dominate
Competition orientation	Equality of access may still have to
Sophisticated technology	be publicly guaranteed
Efficient financial investment	
Ethical norms are controlled by public authorities and private competitors	

Source: the authors.

ciaries can be guaranteed only as long as public authorities supervise the PPP or – even better – as long as they are a predominant part of it. Otherwise, there will always be an incentive within the PPP to seek more profitable avenues for investment, entailing a preference for better-paying patients over patients without sufficient purchasing power. The public partner must stipulate equality of access from the very beginning of the partnership.

Public private partnerships in the German hospital care system: A model?

In Germany, hospital services are provided by private for-profit hospitals, private not-for-profit hospitals and public hospitals. All three types of hospital are obliged to accept any patient in need of hospitalisation. Under this framework, private for-profit hospitals cannot refuse admission to any patient and, at the same time, all patients have the right – upon referral – to go to any hospital. This means that, although there are different types of hospital, there is no possibility of price discrimination. All hospitals have to offer equal treatment at equal prices.

A development that can now be observed in the German hospital market is the increasing extent to which public hospitals are being sold to private investors. Private investors commit themselves to maintain health care services at the same standard as the previous public owner offered. Therefore, the private owner is not free to eliminate services or to refuse admission to any patient referred. In the event of the bankruptcy of a private owner, the hospital will be passed back to the former public owner, usually the local community. In this way, private hospitals are a kind of PPP because they fulfil a public task while being financed by private investment and run by private management.[10]

An essential precondition for equal access to hospital services is mandatory health insurance for all citizens, so that no hospital has to bear the financial risk resulting from non-payment. Accordingly, one indispensable requirement for equal access to health care services is an adequate insurance scheme for the entire population. This assertion also applies to developing countries and emerging nations such as India. If it is not possible to implement a mandatory insurance scheme for all citizens, all hospitals can be obliged to accept a predefined ratio of poor patients. This model is, for example, followed in the United States. The fulfilment of the quota of poor patients treated by each hospital again has to be supervised by a public authority.

In less developed countries, such as India, the main aim of PPP is to bring some additional private investment into the general public system. In this case, private investment can top up or complete public investments that are not sufficient owing to resource scarcity. Further, private investors will introduce new technologies into a system. Modern technologies enhance a hospital's attractiveness to wealthier patients but also offer better treatment to poorer patients when access to private hospitals is restricted. The collaboration between KARL STORZ GmBH, the Deutsche Gesellschaft für Technische Zusammenarbeit (GTZ) and the United Nations University (UNU) on a project for improving girls' and women's health (the Women's Health Initiative – WHI) is an excellent example of such cooperation, supporting public authorities while enhancing public access to health care.

PPP does involve the risk that a private partner will withdraw from the financial and/or management engagement if the return on its investment is not satisfactory. The public authority therefore has to give the private investor a fair opportunity to obtain a designated profit and/or has to support the private partner as the preferred partner in up coming projects. At the same time, however, profit must never be achieved through the exclusion of poor patients from health care services, as discussed above.

In Germany, no discrimination against poorer patients, and only limited favouring of privately insured patients, can be observed so far. Privately insured patients help to compensate the hospitals for treating poorer patients via an internal process of redistribution between the different groups of patients. This form of financial reallocation can also contribute to easing the public need to organise redistribution, a means that is also suitable for developing and newly industrialising countries such as India.

Outlook: Public private partnership as a facilitator in financing the best available health care

In Europe and in the United States, public authorities are increasingly calling on private investors to take over formerly public responsibilities and to meet these in a more efficient manner than the public institutions can. Mainly in the United Kingdom but also in Germany, a wide range of public goods are produced by private companies. The supply of goods through private providers is even more common when it comes to the field of so-called merit goods, as described above. The health care sector in particular involves a very broad and also very important field of merit goods. Here PPP can contribute to improving the level of care offered while at the same time limiting the risk of discrimination against poor people.

The main unacknowledged question on private involvement in PPP is empirical. There is a persistent lack of evidence-based data concerning the relative performance of the public and private sectors. Most key criteria such as efficiency, equity, quality of care, transparency or accountability are not available. At least in theory, private engagement promises superior results; but studies are needed to prove this.

As far as the expansion of private finance is concerned, Propper and Green reviewed the consequences of the increasing involvement of the private sector in financing health care in a range of OECD countries. The main conclusions are, first, that an increasing role for the private sector tends to lead to an increase in total health care expenditure; and, second, that health care systems that rely on private financing are less equitable in the sense that contributions are less progressive.[11]

A stable political situation is another important precondition for the creation of PPPs. The less stable the political situation of a country, the less likely it is that private investors will be willing to take the risk of becoming involved in PPP. For less developed countries, in which the political situation is very often not as stable as it is in Europe or North America, the political obstacles to attracting private investors to take over public tasks are greater. In such countries, private companies tend to prefer forms of private investment that offer higher and quicker returns on investment. To encourage private investors to engage in PPP, these countries need to try to stabilise their political situations and frameworks.

The health care sector offers many opportunities for successful PPP. Producers of health care equipment are keenly interested in demonstrating that their products will help developing countries to attain a modernised level of health care. The health care industry has demonstrated its willingness to help other countries to achieve fairer conditions for equal access to health care. Of course, public authorities have to recognise their responsibility to enhance development but, to do this, they can engage in true partnerships with suitable private companies.

Notes

1. N. G. Mankiw, *Makroökonomik*, 4th edn, Stuttgart: Schäffer-Poeschel, 2000.
2. Richard Abel Musgrave, "Multiple Theory of Budget Determination", *FinanzArchiv*, New Series 25(1), 1957, pp. 33–43; and R. A. Musgrave, *Public Finance in a Democratic Society. Vol. 1: Social Goods, Taxation and Fiscal Policy*, New York: New York University Press, 1986.
3. S. G. Karsten, "Health Care: Private Good vs. Public Good", *American Journal of Economics and Sociology*, 54(2), 1995, pp. 129–144.
4. Michael de Looper and Gaetan Lafortune, "Measuring Disparities in Health Status and in Access and Use of Health Care in OECD Countries", OECD Health Working Papers No. 43, DELSA/HEA/WD/HWP(2009)2, Organisation for Economic Co-operation and Development, Directorate for Employment, Labour and Social Affairs, Paris, 9 March 2009; available at <http://www.olis.oecd.org/olis/2009doc.nsf/linkto/DELSA-HEA-WD-HWP(2009)2> (accessed 12 June 2009).
5. United Nations, "The Universal Declaration of Human Rights", 1948, <http://un.org/Overview/rights.html> (accessed 5 June 2009); "United Nations Charter", <http://www.un.org/en/documents/charter/index.shtml> (accessed 5 June 2009).

6. See World Health Organization, "Health Systems Financing", <http://www.who.int/healthsystems/topics/financing/en/> (accessed 12 June 2009); Unto Häkkinen and Isabelle Joumard, "Cross-Country Analysis of Efficiency in OECD Health Care Sectors: Options for Research", Economics Department Working Papers No. 554, ECO/WKP(2007)14, Organisation for Economic Co-operation and Development, Economics Department, Paris, 28 May 2007; available at <http://www.olis.oecd.org/olis/2007doc.nsf/linkto/eco-wkp(2007)14> (accessed 12 June 2009).

7. K. E. Case and R. C. Fair, *Principles of Economics*, 5th edn, Englewood Cliffs, NJ: Prentice Hall, 1999.

8. P. Ullmann et al., "Public Private Partnership (PPP)", Veröffentlichung des Bundesministeriums für wirtschaftliche Zusammenarbeit und Entwicklung (BMZ), Bonn, 2005.

9. D. Budäus, *Kooperationsformen zwischen Staat und Markt –Theoretische Grundlagen und praktische Ausprägungen von Public Private Partnership*, 1st edn, Baden-Baden: Nomos, 2006; and M. Weber and H. W. Alfen, *Public Private Partnership*, Munich: Beck, 2006.

10. G. Neubauer, "Hospital Care System in Germany", *Die BKK* 91(8), 2003, pp. 394–399.

11. C. Propper and K. Green, "A Larger Role for the Private Sector in Health Care? A Review of the Arguments", Working Paper 99/009, Centre for Market and Public Organisation, University of Bristol, 1999. For further information, see Institute for Public Policy Research, "Building Better Partnerships: The Final Report of the Commission on Public Private Partnerships", London: IPPR, 2001; R. Robinson, "Checks and Balances: The Changing Face of Competition", *Health Service Journal*, 8 July 1993, pp. 24–25; C. Scott, "Public and Private Roles in Health Care Systems: Experiences from Seven OECD Countries", Buckingham: Open University Press, 2001.

5

The United Nations Global Compact: Seeking to embrace diversity

Monika Kruesmann

Introduction

There is little debate that contemporary globalisation has dramatically increased the number and complexity of transnational interactions. Whether these are for trade, security, social or other purposes, it is clear that such transactions involve more actors, and more types of actors, on the international stage than ever before. This presents a number of challenges, as well as opportunities, for the global community. One of the greatest challenges is, in the absence of a world government, finding ways to manage and coordinate this multitude of actors and actions effectively.

This is the *raison d'être* of global governance policies and institutions. As a self-identified global governance initiative, the United Nations Global Compact is centrally concerned with finding ways to embrace diverse actors and interests within both its own structures and processes and those of projects conducted under its ethical auspices. Actors here include not only businesses of various types, but governments, civil society groups and non-governmental

Partnerships for women's health: Striving for best practice within the UN Global Compact,
Timmermann and Kruesmann (eds),
United Nations University Press, 2009, ISBN 978-92-808-1185-8

organisations, intergovernmental organisations and academia. The methods by which the Global Compact seeks to embrace and utilise this diversity, as well as the extent to which it is successful, are outlined in this chapter. Understanding this issue helps to clarify and contextualise discussion of the Women's Health Initiative, a project involving varied actors within the ethics of the Global Compact.

The United Nations Global Compact

The United Nations Global Compact (hereafter GC or Compact) was introduced to the world on 31 January 1999, when then United Nations Secretary-General Kofi Annan addressed the World Economic Forum in Davos, Switzerland, and proposed a new form of creative partnership between the United Nations and the private sector. The "Global Compact" would provide a human face to the market by establishing a platform of shared principles to underpin economic activity. Its ultimate aim would be to achieve a more stable global market, in which poor people would have equitable opportunities for advancement. Firms were called on to join the Global Compact by adopting and acting on a specific set of core values in the areas of human rights, labour standards and environmental practices.

In arguing the need for the initiative, Annan explained that, whereas national laws and regulations protect such values in the domestic sphere, there is no commensurate assurance beyond state borders.[1] This is problematic because, as transnational contact and interdependence increase with globalisation, a void of governance emerges where, it was claimed, there are "extensive rules for economic priorities such as intellectual property rights but [a lack of] commensurate measures to protect the environment and human rights".[2] This leaves societies in a state of perpetual instability and insecurity, "vulnerable to backlash from all the 'isms' of our post-cold-war world: protectionism; populism; nationalism; ethnic chauvinism; fanaticism; and terrorism".[3] This vulnerability may put global peace and security at risk; and according to the Global Compact, in the absence of formal interstate regulations, the solution is to establish a voluntary, value-based consensus on standards, ethics and behaviours to guide businesses and underpin the new global economy. Such a consensus can fill the governance void.

To this end, the Compact became operational on 26 July 2000, when it was launched at United Nations Headquarters in New York. In the years since then, more than 4,000 members in 116 countries have joined the initiative, making it the largest of its kind in the world.

Seeking to accommodate diversity

Calling itself a *voluntary corporate citizenship*[4] initiative, the GC connects participants on a common communication platform. There is an emphasis on engaging diverse types of actors and on linking members with each other, seeking to ensure that the scope of those whose interests are taken into account in decision-making goes beyond a small group at the apex of a hierarchy. What are the methods by which the GC seeks to engage with diverse actors, and how successful are these methods?

Open membership

A defining feature of the Global Compact is its open membership approach. This means that membership of the Compact is available to corporations, business organisations, civil society, academic institutions, labour organisations and even cities, under the Global Compact Cities Program.[5] Kofi Annan has emphasised the importance of this approach, not only for the Global Compact but for the United Nations in general, explaining that the Organisation must become more engaged not only with governments, but with "all the new actors on the international scene".[6] The result of this is that the Compact becomes, in essence, a mix of public and private authority.

The practical outcome of this approach can be seen in the Global Compact's membership statistics. The 2008 Annual Report shows that the Compact has approximately 6,500 members. Although the majority of these are businesses (approximately 5,000), there is considerable diversity within this category; in particular, there is an almost even split between "large companies" (having more than 250 employees) and "small and medium-sized enterprises" (having fewer than 250 employees). Of the non-business members, there is a mix of non-governmental organisations (37 per cent); business associations (27 per cent); academic institutions (18 per cent); members of the Global Compact Foundation (7 per cent); cities and public sector organizations (5 per cent); labour groups (2 per cent); CSR organisations (2 per cent); and others (1 per cent).[7]

Public sector actors: The United Nations Organisation

Within this open membership structure, the GC gives particular attention to certain public sector actors, and the creation of links between them and other private and non-governmental groups. Specifically, the United Nations itself is a GC actor, and its central place in the Compact involves participation by the GC Office together with six other UN agencies.[8] Explaining the rationale for UN agency participation, statements by Georg Kell, head of the UN Global Compact Office, highlight a link with the Organisation's institutional legitimacy and external relationships, noting that, "[a]t its core, the Compact is simply a strategy to make the UN relevant by leveraging its authority and convening powers in ways that will actually produce the positive social changes it aspires to create".[9] The remarks below explain how this is the case and why it should be thought necessary.

The United Nations is dedicated to achieving international peace.[10] Its guiding mandates include such items as "Maintenance of international peace and security" and "Promotion of sustained growth and sustainable development";[11] and the work of its agencies is devoted to realising these mandates. Its success as an international organisation is linked to achievement of these mandates; so failings here call into question the United Nations' legitimacy and usefulness as an international actor.

This has been a problem during the past decade, because the Organisation's success in realising its agenda has been inconsistent, leading to calls for fundamental reform.[12] The United Nations itself acknowledged these problems in 1997, with the Secretary-General's report *Renewing the United Nations: A Programme for Reform*[13] being presented to the General Assembly with a comprehensive outline of ways in which the United Nations needed to change in order to re-capture a legitimate role in international governance. Subsequently, the United Nations began to seek ways to renew its legitimacy and effectiveness with a number of measures such as those outlined in the Secretary-General's report.[14]

One element of this reform attempt involved renewing relations with the private sector, which, though strong in the early years of the Organisation's existence, became less supportive during the Cold War years, until, "[t]en years ago, the relationship between the Organization and the private sector was burdened with mistrust".[15] A particular problem was that, throughout the 1990s, civil society groups pressing for environmental protection or human rights and labour campaigns bypassed the Organisation and addressed their concerns directly to corporations, further weakening the United Nations' role.[16]

The Global Compact is an attempt to address this problem and to help the United Nations recapture its legitimacy as an international organisation through working with, and becoming relevant to, diverse groups. By placing this objective at its core, collaboration and cooperation between varied members becomes central to the GC's identity and operation.

Business actors: Facilitating open markets and commercial gain

Moving beyond the United Nations itself, the Global Compact is also fundamentally concerned with private sector actors. Kofi Annan noted in launching and promoting the Compact that its ultimate objective is to build a more inclusive global economy, characterised by open markets.[17] In this view, transnational businesses must be able to pursue their commercial imperatives in a supportive global governance environment, rather than being constrained by regulation or having "local or national communities ... turning in on themselves".[18] The role of the Compact is to help provide such an environment, and in doing this it has a central place for business actors.

The emphasis on including business is articulated in the GC's remarks to prospective new commercial members, where the case for participation is explained; the GC claims that businesses will gain global and local opportunities for business collaboration, improved reputation and increasing brand reputation to consumers, and improved employee morale and operational efficiency.[19] In particular, businesses will benefit from the Compact as "a strong driver of value and success, as you [businesses] come across previously unknown opportunities and build trust in new markets".[20] These comments point to the central place for businesses as actors in the GC's structure and operations.

A concern with accommodating business actors is further evident in the Compact's encouragement of "enlightened self-interest", a term that appears frequently in both official documents and academic commentary on the initiative. "Enlightened self-interest" refers to the idea that, by conducting business in line with Ten Principles of the Compact, corporations can achieve not only good profit outcomes and increased market share but also good social and political outcomes in terms of human rights, poverty reduction and development.

The Compact reports numerous examples of "enlightened self-interest". For instance, Sasol, an integrated oil and gas company based in South Africa and a GC member, discovered that the profitability of its commercial operations was at risk from a lack of appropriately skilled labour. Consequently, it entered partnerships with national training authorities, organised labour and academia to establish a skills development project that has so far trained over 800 learners.[21] One result of this was that numerous (mostly young) people were provided with improved educational opportunities; but the primary motivation for the activity was meeting the company's business needs, a need that the Compact was able to accommodate. This provides evidence of the way the Compact dedicates a space for business actors.

The Global Compact local networks

Attention to the United Nations and to business interests is not, however, sufficient to embrace the level of diversity that effective global governance demands. Social and civil actors, as well as businesses and public sector agencies at the local level, must also be included. This is the objective of the Global Compact Local Networks (Local Networks). Emerging in 2003, the Local Networks have the specific aim of deepening engagement with actors at a local level. In 2007 there were 61 established Local Networks, and approximately 25 more being developed. Local Networks have been established in all major geographical areas, with approximately 4,600 business and other participants from over 120 countries.[22]

Local Networks are "clusters of participants who come together to advance the Global Compact and its principles at the local level".[23] They undertake a variety of activities, including outreach and awareness-raising, organising learning and dialogue events, producing learning materials in local languages, mobilising collective action on priority issues, and motivating participating companies to join partnerships supporting the Millennium Development Goals. These activities are developed and implemented with attention to existing local circumstances and needs, which means the Local Networks help actors to maintain individual priorities and pursue individual interests while engaging with the Compact.

The focus on local needs also means Network members are sometimes able to increase informal participation through engaging with actors that are not GC members, but whose involvement enhances the capacity of governance processes to be inclusive and responsive to local circumstances.[24] Further, Local Networks allow microenterprises to become involved in GC activities, even though capacity constraints mean they are not able to be full members.[25]

The Networks are largely community-focused, and place particular emphasis on making the Compact accessible and relevant to small enterprises and local civil society organisations, as well as to local government and community public sector organisations. As such, they provide further evidence of an ability within the Compact to accommodate diversity of interests and actors in governance.

Public private partnerships

Another programme area of the GC that has grown in recent years is the public private partnerships, an example of which is the Women's Health Initiative. These partnerships constitute a key element of the Compact's activities; in the same way that GC members are explicitly asked to embrace the Ten Principles, they are also asked to engage in partnerships, many of which have been established.[26] Like the Local Networks, public private partnership activities help the Global Compact embrace diversity through flexibility to local circumstances.

Public private partnerships allow different actors in different countries, and in different sectors and levels of social life, to institutionalise rule systems for interaction where diverse interests are not only represented but equal in power relative to each other. Individual PPPs have different internal processes and work programmes according to local conditions, but most are functionally similar in that they achieve goals by pooling resources, skills and expertise, as well as often sharing responsibility for project outcomes. Through these practices, partners have a more collaborative and equal investment in governance and a more equal stake in decision-making than if they were, for example, simply recipients of funding and subject to the conditions of those distributing resources.

To confirm the suggestion that PPPs help the Compact accommodate diversity of interests, formal statements about the importance of partnerships must also be realised in action. There is evidence that statements are translating into practice; the first Annual Review of the Global Compact shows that approximately 75 per cent of members say they engage in partnerships, and provides examples of collaborative work undertaken.[27]

Success in accommodating diversity?

These comments suggest that the Global Compact has had considerable and measurable success in embracing a diversity of actors and interests in its structures and projects. However, there are also criticisms that its success in this regard is incomplete.

For example, the Compact is successful in accommodating diverse types of actors in so far as its open membership approach welcomes members from both the public and private sectors as well as from civil society; and these members are drawn from a wide geographical area. However, its membership remains heavily dominated by business actors. A large majority of members are from business and, of the remainder, almost 60 per cent are either local non-governmental organisations or local business associations. It is therefore doubtful how much significance can be attributed to the muted involvement of, for example, academic institutions or indeed public sector actors apart from the UN Organisation.

In this regard, there is particular doubt about the Global Compact's ability to accommodate public sector actors in the form of states. Possibly the strongest argument that can be made for the accommodation of states is that the Global Compact does not challenge their dominant role in the international system. It accepts state members; it does not seek to challenge the laws of states in relation to business regulations or any other regulation; and it does not try to ignore sovereign borders, attempting rather to better manage interactions across those borders. Further, by maintaining its emphasis on voluntary membership and lack of enforcement mechanisms, the Global Compact does not attempt to alter the anarchic condition of the international system or to impose a higher authority beyond states. These points are significant, but nevertheless show that the accommodation of state actors within the Global Compact is limited.

It is also worthwhile noting that it is not clear that, in terms of inclusive membership, the Global Compact does substantially better than other similar corporate citizenship and corporate social responsibility initiatives. For example, the Organisation for Economic Co-operation and Development (OECD) has established a set of *Guidelines for Multinational Enterprises*, endorsed by the governments of 33 adhering countries. The Guidelines are recommendations on responsible business conduct addressed to multinational enterprises, applying to business operations worldwide. They involve both the public and private sectors, and claim to be "the only multilaterally endorsed and comprehensive code that governments are committed to promoting".[28] Similarly, in 2000 the governments of the United States, the United Kingdom, Norway and the Netherlands came together with private sector and non-governmental organisations to establish the "Voluntary Principles on Security and Human Rights", which aim to provide a guide to how human rights can be promoted and protected worldwide and recognise the important role of business and civil society in achieving human rights protection.[29]

The Global Compact does not need to demonstrate that it does a better of job of accommodating diversity relative to these initiatives in order to be judged successful; but these examples show that it would also be unwise to claim too much for the Compact as a unique or particularly innovative initiative in terms of actor diversity in global governance.

Debate also arises in relation to accommodating other actors. It is true that the Local Networks and the public private partnership initiatives have demonstrated effectiveness in responding to local circumstances. However, the Local Networks are not universally available. Although their numbers are steadily growing, there are many countries in which GC members operate, but in which there is no Local Network or one only emerging. The Local Networks Report, for example, points out that the prevalence of Local Networks varies widely across geographical regions, with Europe having approximately twice as many as any other region. Further, many Local Networks are still "emerging".[30]

Conclusions and future options for development

In conclusion, the Global Compact clearly demonstrates a central interest in accommodating diversity in global governance, and it can be considered somewhat, but not conclusively, successful in this regard. It is successful in that its membership structures, initial statements and key policy platforms acknowledge and support formal accommodation of diverse actors, with particular emphasis on the public sector and the business sector. It is also successful in that the major activities and programmes developed over the course of the Compact's existence are flexible enough and sufficiently locally oriented that they do accommodate a diversity of interests, including not only business actors but also public sector organisations, civil society groups and those that are outside the Compact's formal membership structure.

The Compact is not conclusively successful in accommodating diversity, however, for two key reasons that have become apparent in the course of the analysis. First, the initiative's membership profile does remain weighted in favour of business members and neglects others relative to this in practice if not in policy. Second, although key programmes may be successful in accommodating diverse interests where they exist, these programmes are not universally available and they do not all operate to the same standards of effectiveness. This chapter concludes its discussion of the GC by making suggestions on options for the Compact to develop itself in ways that could allow a firmer and more positive embrace of global diversity.

Deepening engagement with civil society

One possibility may be to deepen engagement with civil society. In particular, the Compact could build on the many synergies between the objectives and activities of civil society advocacy groups and the awareness-raising activities of the Local Networks. Many pressure groups have well-developed communication strategies, which could be leveraged by the Networks to reach wider audiences. Similarly, the Compact could engage more closely with civil society groups by encouraging and helping them to engage in public private partnership projects. In these cases, too, the existing communication networks of the groups could be useful in gathering information with which to develop projects and for reaching out to other private and public sector groups that may be unaware of the networking opportunities provided by Compact membership. In this way, the GC could enhance its reach and the scope of participation and deepen further its ability to accommodate the interests of diverse actors.

Building stronger links with states

As well as building stronger links with civil society, a comprehensively accommodating Compact could give increased attention to state actors, whose pivotal position in the international system is not challenged but is also not fully leveraged. For example, although states provide an important source of funding for the GC through the Global Compact Office, they have little direct input into the development of programmes of activities carried out under the GC's auspices. These are more commonly initiated and delivered by Local Networks or GC members. By engaging state actors, it might be possible not only to attract additional financial support for GC activities but also to give GC actions increased popular legitimacy and prominence and to bring them more closely into line with existing government human rights and business ethics initiatives. This does also involve a risk of decreased GC independence and of difficulties reconciling the Compact's international principles with partisan and local political imperatives; such issues would have to be carefully managed.

Further, one of the strongest criticisms of the GC relates to its lack of enforcement capacity, and the fact that it does not engage with legal regulation; this remains the prerogative of state governments and judicial authorities. One way to counter this criticism could be to strengthen links between the Compact and state actors and to work collaboratively to develop legally binding compliance mechanisms for the Compact's principles. These could be adopted into national law in the same way that other items of international law are adopted, and thereby cement a stronger and more direct relationship between the Global Compact and state actors. This would involve a sharp deviation from a number of the Compact's current pillars, such as its emphasis on voluntarism. However, this does not discount the possibility of change and, as the principle of voluntarism is already undergoing some reform through an increasing emphasis on reporting and accountability, it seems reasonable to suggest that such a development may be possible.

The purpose of outlining these possible future developments is not to advocate one or the other. It is to use the conclusions of the preceding comments to identify areas in which change is possible for the Global Compact and to suggest ways in which this might occur. The Compact's own emphasis on development and evolution means it is reasonable to make such suggestions and useful to be aware of the alterations that could be wrought by changing the Compact's fundamental structures and processes that affect accommodation of diversity.

Notes

1. K. Annan (1999) "Secretary-General Proposes Global Compact on Human Rights, Labour, Environment, in Address to World Economic Forum in Davos", Press Release SG/SM/6881, 1 February 1999, available at <http://www.un.org/News/Press/docs/1999/19990201.sgsm6881.html> (accessed 8 June 2009).
2. G. Kell and D. Levin, "The Global Compact: An Historic Experiment", *United Nations Chronicle*, 40(1), 2003, Academic Research Library, p. 64. In light of the multitude of regulations and standards for human rights and environmental protection, comments on this claim are clearly valid, though it is beyond the scope of this chapter to embark on such a discussion.
3. Annan, "Secretary-General Proposes Global Compact".
4. See the United Nations Global Compact website, <http://www.unglobal compact.org/AboutTheGC/> (accessed 8 June 2009).
5. See the United Nations Global Compact website, <http://www.unglobal compact.org/HowToParticipate/> (accessed 8 June 2009).
6. K. Annan, "A New Mindset for the United Nations", *United Nations Chronicle*, 42(4), 2005, Academic Research Library, p. 5.

7. United Nations, *United Nations Global Compact Annual Review: 2008*, New York: United Nations Global Compact Office, 2008, <http://www.unglobalcompact.org/docs/news_events/9.1_news_archives/2009_04_08/GC_2008AR_FINAL.pdf> (accessed 15 September 2009).

8. United National Global Compact website, "Participants and Stakeholders", <http://www.unglobalcompact.org/participantsandstakeholders/un_agencies/index.html> (accessed 8 June 2009). Other UN agencies are also encouraged to participate.

9. G. Kell and D. Levin, "The Global Network: An Historic Experiment in Learning and Action", *Business and Society Review*, 108(2), 2003, p. 64.

10. This is evident in the Preamble to the Charter of the United Nations (1945), which begins: "We the peoples of the United Nations determined to save succeeding generations from the scourge of war ... [and] promote social progress and better standards of life in larger freedom" (see <http://www.un.org/en/documents/charter/preamble.shtml>, accessed 8 June 2009).

11. United Nations, *Mandating and Delivering: Analysis and Recommendations to Facilitate the Review of Mandates. Report of the Secretary-General*, 2006, available at <http://www.un.org/mandatereview/> (accessed 8 June 2009).

12. See, for example, J. Hainsfurther, "The UN at 63: Is It Still Relevant?", opinion piece published on the website of the International Relations and Security Network, ISN, ETH Zurich, 2 October 2008, <http://www.isn.ethz.ch/isn/Current-Affairs/Security-Watch/> (accessed 20 October 2008).

13. United Nations, *Renewing the United Nations: A Programme for Reform. Report of the Secretary-General*, General Assembly 51st Session, Agenda Item 168, presented 14 July 1997, UN Document A/51/950, available at <http://www.un.org/reform/highlights.shtml> (accessed 8 June 2009).

14. Ibid., pp. 6–8.

15. G. Kell, A.-M. Slaughter and T. Hale, "Silent Reform through the Global Compact", *United Nations Chronicle*, 44(1), 2007, Academic Research Library, p. 27.

16. Ibid.

17. K. Annan, "Open Markets, Open Values", *United Nations Chronicle*, 37(2), 2000, Academic Research Library, p. 46.

18. Ibid.

19. United Nations Global Compact, "How to Participate: Business Participation", <http://www.unglobalcompact.org/HowToParticipate/>, 2008 (accessed 8 June 2009).

20. United Nations, *After the Signature: A Guide to Engagement in the United Nations Global Compact*, 2006, <http://www.unglobalcompact.org/docs/news_events/8.1/after_the_signature.pdf> (accessed 8 June 2009), p. 4. Similar comments were made by Mary Robinson, former UN High Commissioner for Human Rights, in relation to the Global Compact; see M. Robinson, "Internalizing Human Rights in Corporate Business Practices", *United Nations Chronicle*, 37(2), 2000, Academic Research Library, p. 38.

21. *Sasol Sustainable Development Report 2006*, <http://www.sasol.com/sasol_internet/downloads/sasol_SD_rep_06_1165499470408.pdf> (accessed 8 June 2009), p. 30.

22. United Nations, "Local Network Report", New York: United Nations Global Compact Office, 2007, available at <http://www.unglobalcompact.org/docs/news_events/8.1/LNReport_FINAL.pdf> (accessed 10 September 2008), pp. 15–19.

23. Ibid., p. 8.

24. Ibid., p. 29.

25. Ibid., p. 16. The Report notes that the ability of Local Networks to engage microenterprises means some Networks have been able to register more participants than are included on the Global Compact database, although it is also noted that inconsistencies in data collection may affect the accuracy of some statistics.

26. UN Global Compact website, "Partnerships for Development", <http://www.unglobalcompact.org/Issues/partnerships/index.html> (accessed 8 June 2009).

27. United Nations, *UN Global Compact Annual Review: 2007 Leaders Summit*, p. 41.

28. Organisation for Economic Co-operation and Development, *The OECD Guidelines for Multinational Enterprises*, Paris: OECD Publications, 2000, p. 5.

29. International Business Leaders Forum and Business for Social Responsibility, "Voluntary Principles on Security and Human Rights" website, 2008, <http://www.voluntaryprinciples.org/participants/index.php>

30. United Nations, "Local Network Report", pp. 15–17.

6

Small and medium-sized enterprises: Their role in achieving the Millennium Development Goals

KAI BETHKE AND MANUELA BÖSENDORFER

Introduction

The private sector is the main driving force of economic development all over the world and shapes the globalisation process through changing patterns of production, investment and trade. A vibrant private sector flourishing through the combined strengths and linkages between large, medium and small enterprises is an essential prerequisite for fostering dynamic economic development, increasing productivity, maintaining competitiveness, transferring and spreading innovative technologies, and contributing to entrepreneurship development and, consequently, poverty alleviation.

In particular, small and medium-sized enterprises (SMEs) play a crucial role in this process because they foster economic cohesion by linking up with larger enterprises (often in the context of partnerships for development), by serving niche markets and by contributing to the development of productive capacities. Furthermore, these businesses contribute to social cohesion by reducing development

Partnerships for women's health: Striving for best practice within the UN Global Compact,
Timmermann and Kruesmann (eds),
United Nations University Press, 2009, ISBN 978-92-808-1185-8

gaps and disparities, thus spreading the benefits of economic growth to disadvantaged population groups, including women – as specifically provided for in Millennium Development Goal (MDG) 3 – and underdeveloped regions.[1]

Taking into account the facts that SMEs not only make up a predominant share of the private sector but also have very specific characteristics and potentials that distinguish them from larger companies, special attention needs to be given to their role in the development process. The overall incentives for the private sector to become involved in the achievement of the MDGs include:[2]

- Advocacy – firms can serve in a leadership position to change government policies;
- Expansion – companies can provide affordable products and services while expanding into new markets;
- Image – consumers increasingly want to buy from businesses that care about development issues;
- Lobby – firms engaged in corporate social responsibility often take the lead in regulatory and financial reform;
- Lower costs – lower production and transportation costs can be achieved by producing in-market.

There is an opportunity for each and every private sector entity to engage with the international community in supporting the United Nations MDGs. To achieve this, it is necessary to go beyond the scope of individual actors and to push forward forms of cooperation between the public and private sectors and civil society, and thereby complement each other's development resources and competences. In this sense, public private and other multi-stakeholder partnerships have a long tradition in the UN system because they can be an elemental force in strengthening societies throughout the world.

One of the most important prerequisites for making such partnerships with the private sector sustainable and for endowing them with credibility is the concept of corporate social responsibility (CSR), which can be best understood in terms of the changing relationship between business and society. It covers companies' obligations to be sensitive to the needs of their stakeholders – referring to all those who are influenced by business decisions and actions – in their operations and to make a positive contribution to their local communities. Today's keen interest in the role businesses have to play in society has been shaped by a constantly increasing sensitivity to environmental and ethical issues, such as pollution and other forms of environmental degradation, improper treatment of employees, and faulty production and the resulting dangers for consumers.

The past decade has seen a radical change in the private sector's relationship with both the state and civil society. Far-reaching changes in the macroeconomic environment such as globalisation, deregulation, privatisation and a redrawing of the lines between the state and the market have changed the basis on which business is expected to contribute to the public good. Meanwhile, the relationship between companies and the general public has moved on from paternalistic philanthropy to a re-examination of the roles, rights and responsibilities of business in a society.

The United Nations Global Compact (GC) brings companies together with UN agencies, civil society, governments and other partners with the aim of advancing universal environmental and social principles in order to foster sustainable development. Not only does it offer a framework for discussion on possible ways to mitigate the negative repercussions of globalisation on societies and the environment, but it also enhances the CSR compliance of companies by binding them to a system of "voluntary self-obligations" through a set of universal values and standards. The GC initiative represents the endeavour to bring the concept of CSR into line with the dynamics of the discussions around global economic developments.

Every business entity – from a small textile firm to a complex multinational enterprise – has stakeholders and affects society in positive and negative ways. The concept of CSR should therefore be equally valid for large and small companies. Yet, when CSR is discussed in policy circles, academia, the media and a wider civil society, the focus tends to be on the larger companies, and SMEs are often neglected. As a result, the CSR tools, frameworks and justifications for responsible business operations tend to appeal to this larger companies, particularly those that see a benefit deriving from investments in "reputation improvement measures". SMEs are usually affected in a reactive or indirect sense, either as suppliers to larger firms or as the beneficiaries of their philanthropic engagement. As a consequence, many small businesses, in particular those situated in developing countries, are still untouched by and unaware of the entire CSR movement. The bulk of SMEs that have come into contact with CSR issues can usually be found on the receiving end of top-down supply chain standards imposed by larger business partners, with limited or no support to comply with those principles.[3]

The recent emergence of the "business linkages" theme within the CSR context shows that large companies operating in developing countries are increasingly expected to expand their sourcing from SMEs as part of what is expected from a responsible business unit. However, there is a need to regard SMEs as CSR actors themselves in order to make real progress towards sustainable development. In many sectors, their cumulative social and environmental impacts are greater than those of large enterprises. It is therefore essential that SMEs are provided with the capacities to go beyond reactive compliance-based CSR approaches and to engage in the ongoing development of proactive, effective and sustainable CSR modes at all levels.

The concept of CSR frequently accompanies other development interventions and is seen as a way for donor countries to support the development process. However, the aim of having CSR make an essential contribution to the achievement of global development goals will not be reached if SMEs are not incorporated successfully into the global "social" value chain.

The crucial role of SMEs in the achievement of international development targets

Out of 75 million companies across the world, around 90 per cent are SMEs.[4] They are critical to long-term economic stability and the development of a functioning market economy. They are increasingly responsible for the creation of the majority of jobs because they account for 50–60 per cent of employment at the national level, and contribute to the development of a favourable environment for innovation.[5]

In addition, smaller business units improve the overall efficiency of domestic markets because, owing to their very specific characteristics and the resulting constraints these enterprises face, they are forced to make productive use of scarce resources such as capital, and thereby contribute to a large extent to long-term economic welfare. In many cases SMEs are considered to be even more productive than large companies, but they are often impeded in their development prospects by failures of market systems, the poor quality of (state-owned or controlled) infrastructure services, blocked access to distribution channels, weak mechanisms for resolving commercial disputes and the absence of rule-based procedures for (and the complexity of) business licensing, registration and inspections. Furthermore, limited access to credit facilities, the high costs of complying with all kinds of regulations, a limited capacity to market and sell products in foreign markets, restricted access to policy-makers and a variety of other institutional and managerial constraints weigh more heavily against SMEs than large corporations.

Major contributions of SMEs to development targets

- SMEs (partly because of the industrial sub-sectors and product groups covered by them) tend to employ more labour-intensive production processes than large enterprises. Accordingly, they contribute significantly to the provision of productive employment opportunities, the generation of income and, ultimately, the reduction of poverty. It is essentially through the promotion of SMEs that individual countries and the international community at large can make progress towards reaching the Millennium Development Goal of halving poverty levels by the year 2015.

- There is ample empirical evidence that countries with a high share of small industrial enterprises have succeeded in making income distribution (both regionally and functionally) more equitable. This in turn is a key contribution to ensuring long-term social stability by alleviating ex-post redistributional pressure and by reducing economic disparities between urban and rural areas.

- SMEs are key to the transition from agriculture-led to industrial economies as they provide simple opportunities for value-adding processing activities, which can generate sustainable livelihoods. In this context, the predominant role of women is of particular importance.

- SMEs are a seedbed for entrepreneurship development, innovation and risk-taking behaviour and provide the foundation for long-term growth dynamics and the transition towards larger enterprises.

- SMEs support the building up of systemic productive capacities. They help to absorb productive resources at all levels of the economy and contribute to the creation of resilient economic systems in which small and large firms are interlinked.

- Such linkages are of increasing importance also for the attraction of foreign investment. Investing transnational corporations seek reliable domestic suppliers for their supply chains. There is thus a premium on the existence of domestic supporting industries in the competition for foreign investors.

- SMEs, as amply demonstrated in information and communication technologies, are a significant source of innovation, often producing goods in niche markets in a highly flexible and customized manner.[6]

Especially with regard to women's empowerment and the implementation of MDG3 (to promote gender equality and fight discrimination), the contribution of the female workforce and their importance for SME development has to be outlined. Women comprise between a quarter and a third of SME operators across the world.[7] However, their productivity is often hampered by legislative, regulatory and administrative barriers, and in particular market distortions relating to the participation of men and women in private sector development. As a consequence, women are more likely to be involved in the informal sector of the economy.

As CSR also deals with those issues, the proper implementation of this concept in small businesses has the potential to make a valuable contribution to gender equality and fighting discrimination against women in the workplace. Nowadays there is a general consensus that CSR will remain an important force with a high potential to have a positive impact on the development agenda only if SMEs can be effectively engaged in this movement.

The concept of corporate social responsibility: Realisation and practical implications in the SME sector

Although there is no universally agreed definition of the CSR concept, many see it as the private sector's way of integrating the economic, social and environmental imperatives of their activities (the "Triple Bottom Line", or TBL). As such, CSR stands for the business quest for sustainable development.

In this sense it is important to draw a distinction between CSR and charitable donations or philanthropy. Even though the latter will directly enhance the reputation of a company and strengthen its brand, the concept of CSR goes beyond charity and requires that responsible businesses take into full account their impact on all stakeholders when making decisions, requiring them to operate in an economically, socially and environmentally sustainable way.

This involves internal factors such as the quality of management, in terms of people and processes, and the nature and extent of a company's impact on society at the various levels. Apart from integration into corporate structures and processes, CSR also involves the

**Figure 6.1   Mapping corporate social responsibility:
Issues and stakeholders**

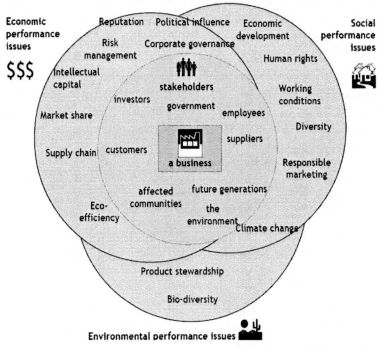

Source: P. Raynard and M. Forstater et al., *Corporate Social Responsibility – Implications for Small and Medium Enterprises in Developing Countries*, Vienna: UNIDO, 2002, Figure 2, p. 6.

development of innovative and proactive solutions to societal and environmental challenges, as well as collaboration with both internal and external stakeholders to improve a company's performance in that respect.

Even though the individual impacts of SMEs are small, the cumulative social and environmental impacts of such a large body of economic actors are enormous. This is not always a consequence of the fact that they simply constitute a large number of enterprises and of their overall economic significance. It is often the case that SMEs are overrepresented in industrial sectors with high environmental impacts,[8] and that those businesses are not subject to the same regulatory requirements and enforcement processes that aim at mitigating the negative impacts of large enterprises. Therefore, the need for monitoring the social and environmental performance of SMEs and ensuring their compliance is crucial to the objective of achieving significant progress towards sustainable development.

In general, SMEs have a greater understanding of local social, cultural and political contexts, have more linkages with local civil society and show an enhanced commitment to operate in a specific area. Family-owned businesses in particular often exhibit strong ethical and philanthropic approaches and thus already practise some kind of "silent social responsibility".

However, enormous difficulties appear when smaller businesses are asked to apply highly sophisticated CSR concepts. The general lessons and approaches of CSR cannot be simply transferred to (imposed on) smaller business units. Taking into consideration that SMEs do not share many of the concerns underlying calls for enhanced ethical business standards and the considerable resource constraints they face, approaches have to be modified in a way that fits their particular needs and capacities and does not adversely affect the economic viability of those firms.

In seeking to resolve this problem and find a way to assist SMEs in meeting social and environmental standards without losing their competitiveness, the TBL approach is finding increasing and widespread international acceptance within the corporate world. The TBL approach encompasses an expanded spectrum of values and criteria for measuring organisational and societal success, meaning that the traditional reporting framework of a company is widened to take into account its environmental and social performance in addition to its financial performance. The concept of reporting against the three components or "bottom lines" of economic, environmental and social performance is directly tied to the goals of sustainable development and corporate social responsibility. It should be seen as an attempt to align private enterprises with the objective of sustainable global development by providing them with a more comprehensive set of working objectives than just the profit focus as a stand-alone vision. TBL reporting, if properly implemented, will provide companies with information that will enable them and their stakeholders to assess how sustainable their operations are. The general view is that, for an enterprise to be sustainable, it must be financially secure, it has to minimise its negative environmental impacts to the greatest extent possible and it needs to act in accordance with societal expectations.

The importance of enrolling SMEs in the Global Compact

Out of the almost 2,900 businesses enrolled in the Global Compact, only about 45 per cent are SMEs. Bearing in mind the large number of this type of company worldwide, there is a need to be more proactive in reaching out to SMEs. In addition, there is a general consensus that SMEs need more assistance in getting incorporated in the Global Compact framework. Therefore, efforts need to be undertaken to encourage those businesses to join the initiative, while at the same time developing more tools and resources to facilitate the implementation of the targeted core principles.

In this respect the United Nations Industrial Development Organization (UNIDO) is currently engaged in a project to elaborate a UN Global Compact Operational Guide for SMEs, for which UNIDO will serve as a project coordinator. Recognising the importance of small businesses in the GC in order to yield a significant impact, especially at the country and regional levels, this project aims to adapt current CSR provisions to the needs and requirements of SMEs in order to increase the level of participation of those companies in the network. The main target areas in this respect will encompass the business case for SMEs (for those connected to international markets via supply chains as well as for strictly local firms); new outreach mechanisms in order to increase the spread at country and local levels; more efficient training and learning modalities; and an adaptation of the integrity measures to the nature and capacities of SMEs (referring to the scope and methodology of reporting).

During the projects on the TBL concept and its applicability in small businesses, UNIDO also began to develop a tool that assists SMEs to better evaluate their performance and identify areas of weakness, to monitor and track their progress in the TBL and to report on their efforts and successes to business partners and other interested stakeholders. With these objectives in mind, UNIDO developed the Responsible Entrepreneurs Achievement Programme (REAP), a software tool that enables companies, in particular SMEs, to implement CSR practices in a cost-effective manner through benchmarking, analysing and improving company performance in the financial, environmental and social areas. It can be seen as an operative guide for businesses for both the analysis of the baseline situation and the documentation of the changes and improvements achieved. The programme is based on the Ten Principles of the UN Global Compact and is designed to prepare reports that enterprises can use to demonstrate to clients, business partners and other stakeholders the efforts undertaken to improve CSR concepts. REAP creates a stable and solid ground for broad implementation of responsible business practices, responsible supply chain management and a national and local business-related policy framework geared towards sustainable industrial development.

REAP is equally useful for multinational enterprises that plan to implement a responsible supply chain management system for their global suppliers and partners. In this respect, UNIDO is currently undertaking comprehensive training efforts – also with a view of increasing the GC membership by targeting companies and business networks in underrepresented sectors and regions in the network, in particular small and medium-sized enterprises.

Successfully integrating SMEs into the CSR movement involves the requirement to identify synergies between social and environmental improvements, on the one hand, and productivity gains, technology upgrading, innovation and market access, on the other. SMEs, in particular those operating in developing countries, need to be provided with adequate tools to monitor and report on their particular CSR performance and to strive for continuous improvement. Only if SMEs are able to link economic benefits to enhanced CSR performance can a critical mass of SMEs be incorporated and the CSR movement itself become more sustainable.

The importance of integrating SMEs into multi-stakeholder partnerships and other forms of cooperation involving the business community

Umbrella organisations, as well as large corporations, have the potential to play a pivotal role in advocating CSR standards and the GC concept to SMEs, underlining the importance of all kinds of partnerships in that respect. In order to confront the challenges arising from future developments in that sphere, it is equally important to get other relevant actors engaged in partnership activities such as SMEs, local community organisations or non-governmental organisations (NGOs).

The gradual convergence of public and private sector interests explains why, for instance, public private partnerships (PPPs) are increasingly regarded as a vehicle for effectively promoting economic and social development around the world. The surge in global interest in PPPs goes hand in hand with the increasing importance of global value chains and a general recognition that governments often lack the financial resources, administrative capacity and technological know-how to ensure the effective implementation of policies.

Nowadays, involving the private sector and linking up with its huge resource base has become a strategic necessity for the UN system. However, the driving rationales of such partnerships clearly extend beyond the mere objective of attracting additional funding to the United Nations, indicating the importance of leveraging UN development programmes by improving market access, developing new technologies and providing specialised expertise and know-how.

In this context, the question of the sustainability of such partnerships arises, as the objectives of development cooperation meet market-oriented philosophies and acting. This emphasises the ever-growing necessity on the part of the businesses engaged in such partnerships (either as the recipient or the provider of development assistance) to respond to societal demands for greater accountability to its stakeholders in terms of environmental sustainability and social responsibility. Forming a partnership between business and those groups that are affected by its operations constitutes an integral part of this new concept of corporate strategy orientation, the TBL approach.

Particular reference must be made to the significance of business linkages between SMEs and large companies and the role of global value chains, which assume great importance with regard to the diffusion of CSR practices. In this context, the United Nations has an important function in terms of facilitating the building of business relations between SMEs and large companies (or multinationals) that promote economic prosperity while at the same time improving social and environmental performance. Through multi-stakeholder partnerships encouraged and supported by framework initiatives such as the GC, as well as by individual agencies such as UNIDO, the United Nations system is well placed to facilitate the implementation of socially responsible business practices in SMEs operating in developing countries and countries in transition. Within the framework of UNIDO, the relationship with the private sector, which was initially focused on the mere procurement of know-how and technology for individual development projects, has reached a point where projects are designed and implemented jointly.

The establishment of multi-sector partnerships is also the central focus of the UNIDO Business Partnership Programme, which involves large corporations as well as business representative organisations, research institutions and NGOs, and aims at supporting SMEs situated in developing countries to meet the steadily increasing pressures and expectations in terms of aligning quality, productivity and social responsibility. UNIDO found that pooling different types of expertise and know-how, if properly coordinated, allows a wider perspective on development issues. At the same time, the business case for CSR is of enormous importance for SMEs. There is a need to demonstrate clearly that business benefits derive from such partnership approaches in order to make SMEs responsive to a broader CSR agenda, because such companies can be won over to far-reaching ethical business concepts only if they expect significant advantages from positioning themselves as socially responsible enterprises and from joining the UN Global Compact.

Project approach in the context of global development targets and the potential for replicability

The project approach chosen for the "Women's Health Initiative (WHI) for Improving Women's and Girls' Reproductive and Maternal Health in India" demonstrates that pooling the resources of different partners can make a viable contribution to the achievement of international development targets. The initiative provides a good example of effective cooperation between private, public and international stakeholders within the framework of one of the eight Millennium Development Goals.

In order to make progress towards the goal of reducing by 50 per cent the number of people living in extreme poverty by 2015, it will be necessary to stimulate the growth of the private sector in developing countries, including the SME sector. There is a high potential for replication of that concept, having the public sector providing resources and improving framework conditions, the private sector contributing with know-how and technologies, and international organisations shaping the global context and spreading knowledge and experience. The role of different partners may vary depending on the nature and context of the initiative. In some cases, partnership can be valuable in helping to facilitate relationships and ensuring the successful delivery of technical skills and know-how from larger companies to SMEs. Multinationals, for instance, can have substantial impact by engaging with and supporting SMEs in developing countries, particularly in states where they have operations or in regions that constitute important supply or distribution markets. In addition, they can cooperate with UN agencies and other development organisations at the policy level by providing important inputs that enable governments to create a regulatory framework conducive to private sector development and growth.

In order to safeguard the credibility as well as the sustainability of partnerships with private sector players, it is important to select the partners carefully and to ensure that they comply with a certain set of ethical standards in their business operations. By engaging in initiatives such as the UN Global Compact, which require companies to report their performance in terms of CSR to the general public, the level of trust towards those companies and consequently confidence in the emerging partnerships increase.

Because CSR encompasses many issues that constitute a primary focus of the MDGs, such as promoting gender equality, ensuring environmental sustainability and developing partnerships for development, this concept needs to be incorporated into the activities of actors engaged in development cooperation, particularly the private sector, in order to contribute to the global quest for sustainable development.

Notes

1. See United Nations Industrial Development Organization (UNIDO), "Service Module 4: Private Sector Development – Overview", <http://www.unido. org/index.php?id=5558> (accessed 17 June 2009). For a more recent and detailed documentation of UNIDO's approach in India, see *Country Programme of Technical Cooperation in India 2008-2012. Towards Inclusive Growth: Strengthening the Competitiveness and Productivity of Industrial Enterprises*, United Nations Industrial Development Organization, May 2008; available at <http:// www.unido.org/fileadmin/user_media/Publications/Pub_free/country_ programme_of_cooperation_between_India_and_UNIDO_2008-2012. pdf> (accessed 17 June 2009). The programme aims "at raising the competitiveness of industrial enterprises through industrial policy advice, investment and technology promotion; through technology-oriented initiatives to increase productivity, quality, energy efficiency, occupational health and safety; and the environmental sustainability of industrial production".
2. World Bank, "Business Action for the MDGs: Private Sector Involvement as a Vital Factor in Achieving the Millennium Development Goals", 2005, pp. 4–5; available at <http://www-wds.worldbank.org/servlet/main?menuPK=

64187510&pagePK=64193027&piPK=64187937&theSitePK=523679&e ntityID=000160016_20060615171816> (accessed 17 June 2009).

3. International Institute for Environment and Development (IIED), "Small and Medium-Sized Enterprises (SMEs) and Corporate Social Responsibility: A Discussion Paper", 2005, <http://www.iied.org/pubs/pdfs/G00193.pdf> (accessed 17 June 2009).

4. The Global Development Research Centre (GDRC) offers valuable materials related to SMEs under "Resources for Small and Medium Enterprises", <http://www.gdrc.org/sustbiz/for-sme.html> (accessed 17 June 2009).

5. W. Luetkenhorst, "Corporate Social Responsibility and the Development Agenda: Should SMEs Care?", SME Technical Working Paper No. 13, UNIDO, 2004, <http://www.unido.org/fileadmin/user_media/Publications/ Pub_free/Corporate_social_responsibility_and_development_agenda.pdf> (accessed 17 June 2009).

6. P. Raynard and M. Forstater et al., *Corporate Social Responsibility – Implications for Small and Medium Enterprises in Developing Countries*, Vienna: UNIDO, 2002, pp. 2–3; available at <http://www.unido.org/fileadmin/ import/userfiles/puffk/corporatesocialresponsibility.pdf> (accessed 17 June 2009). See also Luetkenhorst, "Corporate Social Responsibility and the Development Agenda"; Jane Nelson, *Building Linkages for Competitive and Responsible Entrepreneurship – Innovative Partnerships to Foster Small Enterprise, Promote Economic Growth and Reduce Poverty in Developing Countries*, Corporate Social Responsibility Initiative Report No 8, UNIDO and John F. Kennedy School of Government, Harvard University, 2007; available at <http://www. unido.org/fileadmin/import/68647_CSRI_ReportNo.08_Linkages.pdf> (accessed 17 June 2009).

7. International Finance Corporation, *Women in Enterprise Development*, Regional Forum on Engendering SMEs, 2–3 October 2005, Dhaka, Bangladesh.

8. IIED, "Small and Medium-Sized Enterprises (SMEs) and Corporate Social Responsibility: A Discussion Paper".

Section II

Women's health needs and
health care in India

7

The health situation of women in India: Policies and programmes

Suneeta Mittal and Arvind Mathur

Introduction

Women's health status is intrinsically linked with their status in society. The goal of improving women's health remains a major development task in India. The consequences of biological and social factors affecting women's health are pervasive and cumulative. For instance, inadequate nutrition for a young girl can result in stunted growth, increasing the risk that as a woman she will experience delivery-related complications and have low-birth-weight babies. Early and high levels of fertility exacerbate many of the health problems of Indian women. Complications during pregnancy and delivery are a major cause of death and disability among women of reproductive age. Quality reproductive health services, particularly maternal health and family planning, can save and improve lives while addressing women's needs. Highly cost-effective interventions are available, substantially reducing the risks of ill health and death associated with women's low socio-economic status and reproductive roles. Multi-pronged approaches are urgently needed that reduce gender inequities, strengthen social programmes, ensure the availability of

Partnerships for women's health: Striving for best practice within the UN Global Compact,
Timmermann and Kruesmann (eds),
United Nations University Press, 2009, ISBN 978-92-808-1185-8

good-quality maternal health services and expand partnerships for health services.

The status of girls' and women's health in India

The health of female children

Indian society has strong patriarchal practices with a high degree of "son preference" and persistent gender discrimination. Women in India start life on an unequal playing field, as is illustrated by the masculine sex ratio at birth. Over the past century, India has seen a steady decline in the sex ratio from 972 women per 1,000 men in 1901 to 933 women per 1,000 men in 2001. State-level data indicate widespread regional variations, with a sex ratio of 861 in Haryana but 1,058 in Kerala.

Abortion was legalised in 1971 with the Medical Termination of Pregnancy Act.[1] The Act (revised in 2002) allows induced abortions for any of the following reasons:

1. the pregnant woman has a serious disease or medical condition that would endanger her life if the pregnancy were to continue;
2. the foetus has a substantial risk of a medical or physical handicap;
3. the pregnancy resulted from rape;
4. the socio-economic conditions of the mother would endanger the health of the newborn child;
5. the pregnancy occurred as a result of contraceptive failure.

As a result of this last point, abortion is in practice available on demand. However, the provision of contraceptive failure does not apply to unmarried women. Studies estimate that between 100,000[2] and 500,000[3] female foetuses may be lost every year owing to sex-selective abortions. It is estimated that 5–6 million abortions occur in India every year, and that twice as many illegal and unsafe abortions take place; some estimates place the number of illegal abortions at 10 times that of legal procedures. Studies show that later-term unsafe abortions include up to 11 per cent sex-selective-related procedures.

The 1970s saw the availability of modern techniques such as amniocentesis, chorionic villi sampling and ultrasonography for determining the sex of the foetus. The increasing availability and aggressive marketing of these tests were linked to their excessive use for sex determination and subsequent sex-selective abortion. Intervention by women's groups and health activists led to the enactment of the Pre-Natal Diagnostic Techniques (Regulation and Prevention of Misuse) Amendment Act in 1994.[4] The legislation calls for compulsory registration of clinics or laboratories that employ prenatal diagnostic procedures that could be used to assess the sex of a foetus; that no prenatal diagnostic procedures are to be used unless there is a likelihood of genetic disease or harmful conditions in the baby; and that the person conducting the test will not communicate the gender of the foetus in any way. However, despite the legislation in place, there are many indications that the law is circumvented and an illegal sex test market thrives in India, particularly in the north Indian states of Punjab and Haryana.[5]

Gender differentials in child mortality are particularly evident. For instance, India's first National Family Health Survey (NFHS-1) reported that female child mortality was 42 per 1,000 in 1992–1993, compared with male child mortality of 29.4 per 1,000.[6] Pervasive discrimination in the care of female children is apparent in the gender differentials in nutritional status; girls are more likely to be malnourished than boys in many parts of the country.[7] Discriminatory breastfeeding practices are also seen, with infant girls being breastfed less frequently, for a shorter duration and over shorter periods than boys.[8] Differences in health-seeking behaviour are evident both for preventive health care (immunisation) and curative health care (treatment of illness), which is related to the increased fragility of the female child in India and its impact across generations.[9]

The health of adolescent girls

"Adolescence" spans the ages between 10 and 19 years, and is characterised by rapid physical and psychological growth and development. The period is critical as it presents the last opportunity to correct the nutritional and health lags of childhood. Adolescents constitute a sizeable 22 per cent of the Indian population and, although adolescent mortality rates are lower than for other age groups, gender discrimination, the lower nutritional status of females, early marriage and early childbearing contribute to a significant difference in mortality rates between adolescent females and males.[10] About 13 per cent of female deaths below the age of 24 years are attributed to pregnancy and childbirth-related causes.[11] Sizeable proportions of late adolescent girls (15–19 years) are acutely malnourished (low mean body mass), have inadequate caloric intake and are stunted, which puts them at risk of complicated childbirth.[12] Deep-rooted gender discrimination is considered to influence the much greater proportion of adolescent girls being under-nourished (45 per cent) than boys (20 per cent).[13] Anaemia among adolescent girls is widespread (55 per cent) and, when exacerbated by pregnancy, it heightens obstetric risks and reproductive failures.

Early childbearing is associated with adverse health consequences such as maternal mortality, pregnancy complications, damage to the reproductive tract, peri-natal and neo-natal mortality, and low birth-weight of the baby.[14] Of adolescent girls aged 15–19 years, 50 per cent are already married and face double the risk of maternal death compared with women older than 20.[15] Susceptibility to medical complications (owing to immature growth), lower utilisation of maternal health services and poor nutrition are linked to higher maternal mortality among adolescents. Studies report a higher rate of peri-natal mortality, spontaneous abortion and stillbirth among adolescent mothers, compared with women aged 20–29 years.[16]

Adolescents who marry between 15 and 19 years of age have high fertility and will bear on average 6–7 children over the course of their lives.[17] A study in rural Maharashtra revealed that married adolescent girls are expected to conceive within the first year of marriage. Health care is sought promptly for illnesses that interfere with domestic chores, whereas menstrual disorders and symptoms of reproductive tract infections (RTI) and sexually transmitted infections (STI) often go untreated under a culture of silence and shame.[18] Sexual victimisation of adolescent girls is also a complex issue with serious health ramifications such as STI/RTI and HIV/AIDS. The available data indicate that a high percentage of rapes occurs in the 10–16 year-old age group.[19] Increasing alcohol abuse, in both domestic and non-domestic settings, has been cited as one of the major contributors to adolescent rape in India.[20] According to a study by the Centre of Concern for Child Labour,[21] girls below 14 years constitute 30 per cent of the nearly 900,000 prostitutes in the country. Cultural myths related to virginity and a lack of negotiation skills increase their risk of pregnancy and of contracting sexually transmitted diseases including HIV and AIDS.

Women's health

Fertility is an important predictor of maternal health, and high fertility levels are associated with high maternal mortality.[22] The total fertility rate (TFR) signifies the total number of children a woman will produce in her lifetime. The 2005–2006 National Family Health Survey (NFHS-3) shows there was a decline in the TFR from 6.4 in the 1950s to 2.7 in 2006.[23] However, India's goal of achieving a TFR of 2.1, which would put the country on the road to population stabilisation, is still distant. Although some states such as Kerala, Tamil Nadu, Himachal Pradesh, Goa, Maharashtra, Andhra Pradesh and Punjab have already achieved a TFR of less than 2.1, it is postulated that states such as Rajasthan, Madhya Pradesh, Bihar, Uttar Pradesh, Chattisgarh and Uttaranchal, which account for more than 40 per cent of the total population, will take 18 to 45 years to achieve similar levels.[24]

Use of family planning methods can significantly improve maternal and child health in India. However, female sterilisation accounts for about 77 per cent of the use of modern contraceptive methods; and male sterilisation in fact fell from 2 per cent to 1 per cent

**Figure 7.1 Distribution of modern contraceptive methods,
2005–2006 (per cent)**

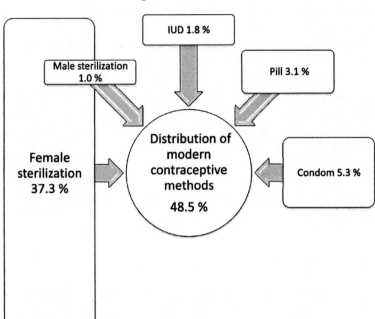

Source: Government of India, National Family Health Survey 3, <http://www.
nfhsindia.org/nfhs3.html> (accessed 16 June 2009).

between NFHS-2[25] and NFHS-3.[26] Condom use, though still very
low, has increased to 5.3 per cent from 3.1 per cent. Use of intra-
uterine devices (IUD) and oral contraceptive pills (OCP) accounts for
2–3 per cent. Data show that sterilisation, which dominates contraceptive practice, is adopted by women who already have very large
families.[27] Considerable demand already exists for temporary methods, both for controlling spacing and for limiting births. In order to
bring about reductions in fertility levels, these methods will have to
become more widely known, available and adopted.

Of the 5–6 million abortions estimated to be performed annually, only 0.6 million are performed in registered facilities; the
rest are often performed by unskilled providers in unauthorised facili-

ties. Approximately 9 per cent of maternal deaths are attributable to abortion.[28] As previously mentioned, abortion is legal under specific conditions in India. However, despite the enactment of liberal policies for abortion, the majority of women are compelled to resort to unsafe abortions owing, in part, to a lack of awareness of suitable providers. An International Centre for Research on Women (ICRW) study in rural Madhya Pradesh revealed that more than 50 per cent of the women surveyed used potentially unsafe procedures such as folk methods, stress on the body, vaginally invasive procedures and ingestion of pills.[29] Further, 35 per cent of women reported severe complications, including haemorrhage and incomplete abortions.

Each year, approximately 30 million women in India experience pregnancy, of which 27 million result in live births.[30] India has the highest burden of maternal mortality in the world. Moreover, for every maternal death in India, 30 more women suffer from pregnancy- and delivery-related injuries, infection or ill health. Based on data available through the Sample Registration System, maternal mortality was estimated to be 301 per 1,000 in 2001–2003. This corresponds to a projected maternal mortality rate (MMR) of approximately 195 in 2012, which indicates that both the national goal of reducing MMR to 100 by 2012 (National Rural Health Mission) and the Millennium Development Goal (MDG) of reducing it to 109 by 2015 are likely to be missed. With two-thirds of maternal deaths occurring in the Empowered Action Group (EAG)[31] states and Assam, the pace of interventions in these states will have to be stepped up in order to reduce maternal mortality.

The most common direct causes of maternal death in India are haemorrhage and sepsis, followed by obstructed labour/malpresentation, pre-eclampsia and unsafe abortion (Figure 7.2).[32] Most of these can be prevented in a hospital or first referral unit (FRU) with emergency obstetric care facilities and skilled medical providers. Anaemia is the biggest indirect cause of maternal mortality, and can be addressed through good-quality antenatal care and improved nutrition.

The links between proper antenatal care and maternal mortality are well recognised. Universal screening of pregnant women can

Figure 7.2   Causes of maternal mortality in India

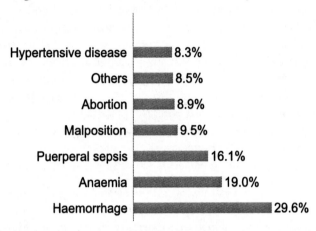

Source: Office of the Registrar General, India, *Sample Registration Bulletin*, 33(1), 1999.

ensure a favourable health outcome for the baby and the mother. However, antenatal coverage remains grossly inadequate, and half of all mothers do not receive the recommended minimum of three antenatal care visits, and nearly four in five pregnant women do not consume the recommended dosage of iron folic acid tablets.[33] A majority of women are anaemic in India (56 per cent), and continue to be so during pregnancy (58 per cent). There are concerns about the significant increase in anaemia levels from 50 per cent to 58 per cent from NFHS-2 to NFHS-3.

One in three women (33 per cent) in India is under-nourished, as measured by having a below-average body mass index.[34] Energy, fatty acids and micronutrient deficiencies before conception or even in early pregnancy have been associated with low infant birth-weight. Additional caloric requirements during pregnancy, along with existing cultural norms of dietary restrictions during pregnancy, further exacerbate the already compromised nutritional status of the average Indian woman. Average weight gain during pregnancy among Indian women is only 7 kilograms, compared with 12 kilograms in developed countries. Women in India are conditioned to tolerate ill

**Figure 7.3 Distribution of births by type of medical
attention at delivery, 2006 (per cent)**

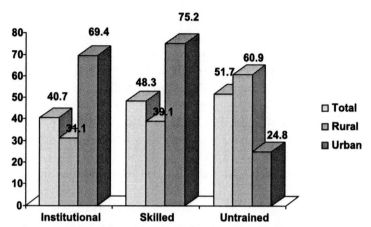

Source: International Institute for Population Sciences, World Health Organization and World Health Organization India – WR Office, *Health System Performance Assessment: World Health Survey 2003 India*, Mumbai: IIPS, 2006.

health and suffering, even when a genuine need is there for health
care, and pregnancy and childbirth are culturally not considered to
be conditions necessitating health care.

By itself, good quality antenatal care, which screens pregnant
women for risk conditions, cannot reduce the major burden of
delivery-related complications. Deliveries assisted by a skilled birth
attendant can reduce these risks substantially; however, more than
half of all births are still assisted by an untrained provider and only
41 per cent of women have institutional deliveries (see Figure 7.3).[35]
The National Population Policy goal of increasing the proportion
of institutional deliveries to 80 per cent by 2010 is unlikely to be
achieved within the next three years.

It is estimated that more than 60 per cent of maternal deaths occur
in the post-partum period; haemorrhage, pregnancy-induced hypertension complications, and obstetric infections are the most common causes of death.[36] Nearly half of post-partum deaths have been
found to occur within one day of delivery, and 80 per cent within

two weeks. Post-partum visits by any health-care provider within two days of birth were reported by only 28 per cent of rural Indian mothers.[37]

There is increasing evidence of the extent and significance of gynaecological morbidity in India, particularly among poor women. A study conducted in rural Maharashtra in the mid-1980s revealed that as many as 92 per cent of the 650 women clinically examined showed the presence of at least one gynaecological disease, with an average of 3.5 conditions per woman.[38] A multi-centre study in four culturally and geographically distinct communities based on self-reported histories and clinical examinations revealed unacceptably high levels of gynaecological morbidity, though they were appreciably lower than in the Maharashtra study.[39] More than two in every three women reported at least one condition across the sites, and between one-quarter and one-third of women showed clinical signs of one or more gynaecological morbidities. Cervicitis, vaginitis and pelvic inflammatory disease – all reproductive tract infections – were among the most frequently occurring morbidities. In Bombay, genital prolapse (18.2 per cent) and cervical erosion (18.5 per cent) were quite prominent.

Another nationwide study found that 24.4 per cent of women reported at least one gynaecological problem but only 14.2 per cent sought care for reported problems.[40] Low levels of care-seeking were attributed more to personal reasons such as a lack of time (48.3 per cent) or an inability to go alone (23.2 per cent) than to inadequate facilities/infrastructure (13.4 per cent) and other extrinsic factors. A study of gynaecological morbidity in a Delhi slum showed a high prevalence of bacterial vaginosis (41 per cent), chlamydia (29 per cent) and candidiasis (19 per cent).[41] A study among 385 women in Karnataka revealed a high burden of reproductive tract infections, the most common being bacterial vaginosis and mucopurulent cervicitis.[42] Approximately one-quarter of the women had clinical evidence of pelvic inflammatory disease, cervical ectopy and fistula. The growing extent of RTI/STI and other gynaecological morbidities and their potentially devastating consequences, such as post-abortion and puerperal sepsis, ectopic pregnancy, fetal and peri-natal death, cervical cancer, infertility and the increased risk of HIV transmission, are now a reality with which Indian health services have to grapple.

There are serious concerns about the upward trend in Caesarean-section rates in India, particularly in private facilities. Although Caesarean-section rates nationally are not high (7 per cent of women who had recently had a baby reported Caesarean deliveries in 1998–1999), an analysis of NFHS-2 data suggests a considerable rural–urban disparity (5 per cent and 15 per cent, respectively). Caesarean-section deliveries are particularly high in states with high literacy rates, such as Goa and Kerala (20 per cent and 29 per cent, respectively). Whereas the World Health Organization (WHO) recommends an optimal Caesarean-section rate of 10–15 per cent, there are recent reports that rates may be as high as 65 per cent in private hospitals in Delhi.[43] The economics of Caesarean sections, along with the time factor associated with normal deliveries, may be linked to these alarming statistics. Childbirth through Caesarean section has a four times higher incidence of maternal death than vaginal deliveries.[44] Even elective Caesarean sections have a 2.84-fold greater chance of maternal death.[45] The immediate risks of Caesarean section include potential anaesthesia-related complications and postoperative complications. A first-birth Caesarean section has a 30 per cent chance of causing placental disruption in a subsequent pregnancy.[46] Other long-term consequences of Caesarean section include reduced fertility and increased risk of ectopic pregnancy.

The AIDS pandemic has added another dimension to the poor health scenario and is affecting women in increasing numbers. Though the "feminisation" of the HIV/AIDS epidemic in India is not as apparent as in sub-Saharan Africa, it is a cause of great concern, particularly in a society where gender imbalances affect consistent condom use and where homosexuality is stigmatised. Female sex workers constitute 0.55 per cent of the adult female population but, as may be expected, have higher prevalence rates of AIDS (8.44 per cent) than the general female population (0.60 per cent). Targeted interventions, which include condom promotion and STI prevention and presumptive treatment, aimed at high-risk groups such as female sex workers have, to a large extent, successfully increased condom usage and limited the spread of infections. Indian women account for around 2 million of the 5.2 million (or 39 per cent) of the people globally estimated to be living with HIV and AIDS.[47] The surveillance data indicate that, in high-prevalence states, the epidemic is moving gradually from urban areas to rural areas and from high-risk groups to the general population. Importantly, a significant proportion of new infections are occurring in women whose husbands or partners have multiple sex partners.

Gender differences in seeking treatment for opportunistic infections and anti-retroviral therapy are significant, revealing the increased vulnerability of infected women.[48] Although awareness about HIV/AIDS increased from 40 per cent in 1998–1999[49] to 57 per cent in 2005–2006,[50] only a fraction (34.7 per cent) are aware that consistent condom use can reduce the chances of getting HIV/AIDS. The biological vulnerability of women (male to female transmission during sex is about twice as high as female to male transmission) is compounded by other socio-cultural and economic factors such as gender inequality in the power to negotiate condom use, a lack of awareness about the means of protecting against infection, poverty, early marriage, trafficking and sex work, and lack of education.

Approximately two-thirds (63 per cent) of married women in India have experienced spousal violence.[51] A multi-centre study of nearly 10,000 households revealed that 40 per cent of the women experienced at least one form of physical abuse and 26 per cent reported severe physical abuse. Of the women who experienced severe physical abuse, 50 per cent reported being beaten three or more times in their lifetime and at least once during pregnancy.[52] These data indicate the pervasiveness of domestic violence in India irrespective of age, educational level, social strata, duration of marriage and family composition.

The policy environment

Past efforts

Women's health has been on the national agenda for several decades but has undergone significant shifts in programme emphasis. India inherited a predominantly urban, hospital-based and curative health care system at the time of independence. Post-independence, efforts began to create a three-tiered primary health care infrastructure for providing basic health care, including maternal health care. Though public health is constitutionally the responsibility of the states, the central government has been financing national disease control, family welfare and reproductive and child health programmes. All the programmes discussed in this chapter are largely funded by the central government. Health polices and programmes are designed at the central level with input from state governments and other stakeholders, including civil society and donor agencies. However, flexibilities exist with regard to the implementation of specific strategies at the local level by state governments.

In 1951, the family planning programme was launched with an emphasis on population control. The demographic orientation of the family planning programme led to the neglect of maternal health services. This was changed in 1977 with the Family Welfare Programme, which integrated maternal and child health interventions, focusing on fertility control. However, family planning and immunisation promotion activities continued to be the mainstay of the Family Welfare Programme in the 1980s and early 1990s, and scant attention was paid on the ground to maternal health.

A global call for a renewed focus on maternal mortality following the International Safe Motherhood Conference in Nairobi in 1987 led to the reorientation of the national programme and the evolution of the World Bank and UNICEF-assisted US$300 million national Child Survival and Safe Mother (CSSM) programme in 1992, with the objective of improving the health status of infants, children and pregnant women. Under the safe motherhood component, focus was placed on the training of trained birth assistants (TBAs), the strengthening of antenatal care and tetanus immunisation for mothers, the provision of aseptic delivery kits and the strengthening of first referral units to deal with high-risk and obstetric emergencies. However, the programme had several limitations. Despite the identification of 1,748 referral units and the provision of equipment kits "E" to "P",[53] not even half of these units were fully operational owing to a lack of skilled workers to use them, particularly anaesthetists and gynaecologists, a lack of adequate infrastructure and a lack of medicines. Training tended to focus on child survival and neglected maternal health, including the importance of emergency obstetric care (EmOC). Identification of mothers at risk of problems and of complications during pregnancy tended to be uneven, and community awareness-building was limited.[54]

In spite of various policy goals aimed at reducing maternal mortality, there was neither encouragement nor any monitoring of deliveries conducted in health facilities or by skilled health staff (doctors and midwives). Maternal deaths remained unregistered, unaudited and unaccounted for, and virtually forgotten. This seems to have given an implicit message to the health system that maternal health was not a priority, even though policy statements and programme objectives included reduction of the MMR. The neglect of maternal care was further compounded by exclusive reliance on interventions such as antenatal care (specifically only on tetanus toxoid vaccination and iron supplementation) to the neglect of intra-natal care and of EmOC training for TBAs. Such activities also gave programme managers a false sense of security that the problem of maternal mortality was being addressed when in fact maternal mortality was still high and not declining.

Following the recommendations of the International Conference on Population and Development in Cairo in 1994, the Reproductive & Child Health Programme (RCHP) was launched in 1997 with much broader objectives.[55] With a budget of about US$250 million, the programme was an attempt to integrate the CSSM interventions with existing reproductive and child health services. In particular, a new component for the management of RTIs and STIs was incorporated in the programme. The RCHP espoused the principles of client satisfaction in delivering comprehensive and integrated high-quality health services. The objective of the RCHP (1997–2004) was to improve reproductive health, including maternal health and child health, focusing its strategies on enhancing maternal and newborn health in four broad areas, namely strengthening facilities and upgrading the skills of a variety of providers, enhancing institutional delivery and mobilising community support, promoting skilled attendance at home and at the sub-centre level, and advocating post-partum and essential newborn care.[56] Several schemes were implemented to improve EmOC: the provision of additional Auxiliary Nurse Midwives (ANMs) to improve coverage in selected districts; the provision of public health or staff nurses in selected disadvantaged districts; the operationalisation of FRUs by engaging the services of laboratory technicians, private anaesthetists and safe motherhood consultants; the provision for referral transport with selected *panchayats*; and additional honorariums to staff for night deliveries at selected primary health centres (PHCs).

The RCHP also sought to strengthen essential and emergency obstetric care facilities at the sub-district and district levels by expanding existing rural health services to include facilities for institutional delivery. In addition, arrangements were made in both rural and urban areas for expanding access, as part of the public health system, to the services of a sizeable private sector (maternity homes, hospitals and physicians) and, in some areas, non-governmental organisations (NGOs). Attention was also paid to ensuring that supplies of medicines are regular and that appropriate equipment is available and functioning. Operationalisation of the RCHP happened as a composite of individual schemes with suboptimal linkages among them. For example, some PHCs and community health centres (CHCs) were renovated and others were staffed, and some villages received transport money. Given that the RCHP had many components (family planning, maternal health, child health, adolescent health, RTI/STD, etc.), the focus on EmOC was diluted. For the first time in the national programme, three post-partum visits were recommended; yet, in the absence of any goal for post-partum care, it is not surprising that scant attention was in practice paid to this period by either the health workers or the mothers themselves.

Overall, the impact of these general and specific interventions in reducing MMR has not been encouraging. Access to affordable and efficient maternal health care, particularly in rural areas and urban slums, has remained elusive despite the CSSM programme (1992–1997) and the RCHP (1997–2004). Each programme and policy statement has set ambitious goals in terms of reducing maternal mortality. However, these somewhat unrealistic goals have had to be continuously revised. For example, the CSSM proposed achieving a maternal mortality ratio of 200 per 100,000 live births by the year 2000. This goal was revised by the RCHP, which set itself the equally difficult goals of attaining an MMR below 100 per 100,000 live births by 2010 and of skilled attendance at all births.[57]

In 2000, India established a National Population Policy,[58] which provides a framework for achieving the twin objectives of population stabilisation and promoting reproductive health within the wider context of sustainable development. The National Population Policy advocates a holistic, multi-sectoral approach to population stabilisation, with no targets for specific contraceptive methods except for achieving a national average total fertility rate of 2.1 by the year 2010. This policy resulted in a shift in implementation from centrally fixed targets to target-free dispensation through a decentralised, participatory approach. The target-free approach was recast as a community needs assessment approach.

The Tenth Five Year Plan (2002–2007) outlined efforts in three broad areas: meeting the unmet need for contraception, reducing infant and maternal mortality and enabling families to achieve their reproductive goals.[59] Goals set in the Tenth Plan advocated an ambitious agenda to make pregnancy safe, including the achievement of skilled attendance at 80 per cent of all deliveries by 2007, institutional deliveries for 65 per cent of all births, at least three antenatal check-ups for 90 per cent of pregnant women, and universal achievement of complete immunisation for pregnant women. It aimed to attain a maternal mortality ratio of 200 per 100,000 live births by the year 2007. The Tenth Plan also emphasised the need to enhance the number of functioning first referral units and community health centres by:

(a) posting specialists (obstetricians, gynaecologists and paediatricians) in these facilities;

(b) providing funds for hiring specialists, including anaesthesiologists, on a contract basis;

(c) improving access to blood banks; and

(d) establishing links with private and NGO sector institutions in providing essential and emergency obstetric care.

"Around-the-clock" delivery services were to be available in 50 per cent of all primary health centres in addition to all community health centres, first referral units and district hospitals; and emergency obstetric care was to be available at all first referral units and district hospitals. Finally, the Tenth Plan advocated that at least one trained birth attendant must be available in each village and must receive training in clean delivery practices.[60]

Ongoing and planned initiatives

The second phase of the five-year Reproductive and Child Health Programme (RCH-II)[61] – launched in April 2005 with a US$360 million credit from the World Bank – similarly advocates enhancing provider skills and expanding the pool of physicians. To meet the shortfall of specialists, RCH-II advocates the training of MBBS (Bachelor of Medicine and Bachelor of Surgery) doctors in anaesthesiology and obstetric management skills for EmOC at FRUs and district hospitals. It also proposes the establishment of blood storage units at FRUs and blood banks in district hospitals to address treatment delays for pregnancy-related complications. To encourage institutional deliveries, all CHCs and at least 50 per cent of all PHCs will provide "around-the-clock" delivery services. Apart from improving access to skilled delivery care and EmOC and continued emphasis on the coverage and quality of antenatal care, the programme will aim to increase coverage of post-partum care.

The planning and implementation of the maternal health strategies of RCH-II are guided by the principles of :

• evidence-based interventions;

• continuum of care from community to facility;

• health systems approach; and

- integration of maternal health interventions with neo-natal and child health and family planning interventions.

Probably the most significant point of departure from previous programmes is the strong focus on using evidence for designing RCH-II strategies. Population stabilisation, as a means of improving maternal health, will be achieved through a range of strategies that aim to expand contraceptive choices based on evidence that every additional method can increase the contraceptive prevalence rate by 1.2 per cent. This will include training of medical officers to provide a quality sterilisation service; skill-based clinical training of Lady Health Visitors (LHVs); and ANMs for spacing methods, including IUD insertion and removal, lactational amenorrhea method (LAM), standard days method (SDM) and emergency contraception (EC); the training of district hospital/CHC/PHC staff to offer LAM, SDM, EC and injectables; and engaging the private sector to provide quality family planning services. Efforts will also be made to reverse the skewed acceptance of female sterilisation methods and increase the proportion of no-scalpel and conventional vasectomy.

Earlier programmes that rested on the hypothesis that obstetric complications could be prevented or predicted by good care during pregnancy and delivery focused on antenatal care and TBA training. However, both these approaches were found to have no effect in reducing maternal mortality in the absence of a functioning health care system. The risk-screening approach was based on the understanding that obstetric complications could be predicted and that high-risk women could be monitored and treated. However, studies indicated that maternal mortality could be lowered through this approach only in a setting with already low levels of MMR. Based on evidence contradicting these two approaches, the centre of attention in RCH-II has shifted from unfocused antenatal care, TBA training and risk assessment to improving access to high-quality delivery care through skilled attendance at birth and access to EmOC.

The programme recognises that TBAs, even after training, do not fulfil the criteria for a skilled attendant, and that scarce resources should be spent not on training TBAs but rather on making skilled birth attendants available, with the back-up of a functioning health system and facilities for EmOC. It is proposed that a cadre of community skilled birth attendants in the private sector be trained in midwifery by the government. Although the core task of providing skilled birth attendance in public facilities and in the community will continue to be with the government, options will be explored for engaging the private sector in the provisioning of EmOC, particularly for families living below the poverty line. The role of ANMs will also be extended after systematic training to administer life-saving drugs for managing basic obstetric emergencies when doctors are not available.[62] Apart from monitoring maternal health outcomes, such as ANC coverage, anaemia levels, skilled birth attendance and institutional deliveries, for the first time the proportion of mothers who receive post-partum care from a health care provider within two days of delivery will be monitored. This is expected to generate much-needed attention to the critical post-partum period.

Management of unwanted pregnancy through early and safe abortion services as envisaged under the Medical Termination of Pregnancy (MTP) Act is an important component of RCH-II. The Act allows for decentralisation of approval of MTP facilities at district level, and punitive measures and actions against MTPs performed by unqualified persons or in unregistered facilities. The Act also validates the use of Mifepristone (RU486) followed by Misoprostol as an established and safe method for terminating early pregnancy. This is recommended for use up to the first 7 weeks of gestation (49 days of amenorrhea) in a facility with provision for safe abortion services and blood transfusions.[63] The use of manual vacuum aspiration techniques is also being piloted in two districts of eight states as a safe and simple technique for the termination of early pregnancy in settings such as the PHCs.

In 2003, the Janani Suraksha Yojana (JSY) was launched with the amalgamation of previous maternity protection schemes such as the National Maternity Benefit Scheme.[64] The objectives of JSY are to reduce maternal and infant mortality through the promotion of institutional deliveries and to protect the female foetus and child. Pregnant women living below the poverty line are eligible for assistance, which includes financial assistance for institutional delivery (Rs 1,000 for a girl and Rs 500 for a boy) and Caesarean-section deliveries, transport assistance for travel to health centres for delivery, and compensation to TBAs facilitating an institutional delivery. The compensation has been revised upwards recently.

Another scheme for safe motherhood and family planning services operational since 2004 is the Vande Mataram health scheme, which envisages increased involvement of the private sector in achieving national maternal health goals. Each enrolled gynaecologist and obstetrician voluntarily provides free antenatal and family planning services to pregnant women on a fixed day each month.

The National Rural Health Mission (2005–2012) (the Mission) is the overarching programme of the Government of India,[65] and seeks to provide effective health care to rural populations, particularly the poor, women and children, through a synergistic approach to complement RCH-II, taking account of the various factors that affect health, such as nutrition, sanitation, hygiene and safe drinking water. The Mission spans the duration of the Eleventh Plan and is expected to address gaps in the provision of effective health care to rural populations, with a special focus on 18 states with weak public health indicators and/or poor health infrastructure. Improving women's health through access to quality public health services, population stabilization and gender balance is one of the key goals of the programme. The Mission is an articulation of the government's commitment to increase public health spending from 0.9 per cent of India's gross domestic product (GDP) to 2–3 per cent of GDP. Under the Mission, quality will be assured through minimum norms set for infrastructure, personnel, equipment, drugs and management at sub-centre, PHC, CHC and district hospital levels. Among other strategies, the Mission proposes improved capacity and numbers of skilled health care workers, including the identification and training of a village-level accredited social health activist to act as an interface between the community and the health system as well as a strengthened public health care infrastructure. The Mission aims to achieve an MMR of 100 per 100,000 and a TFR of 2.1 by 2012.

The passing of the Domestic Violence Act (DVA) 2005 is an important milestone in the history of the women's movement in India. The DVA provides scope for protective injunctions against violence, dispossession from the matrimonial home and an alternative residence as well as scope for claiming financial protection, including maintenance. For the first time, the broad definition of domestic violence – physical, mental, economical and sexual – brings under its purview the invisible violence suffered by a large section of women and entitles them to claim protection from the courts.

Health expenditure

According to the *National Health Accounts*, in 2001–2002 total health expenditure in India was 4.6 per cent of GDP. Of that expenditure, 20.5 per cent was public expenditure, 77.2 per cent was private expenditure and the remaining 2.3 per cent consisted of external support.[66] Overall, per capita health expenditure for the year was Rs 1,021. Table 7.1 provides the details of expenditure on overall health care in India. Households are the main source of health expenditure as they account for 72 per cent of the total. The central government contributes 6 per cent, and states give a larger share of 13 per cent. Donor assistance accounts for less than 2 per cent of total health finances in the sector.

The National Health Accounts also provide a ratio of private to public sector expenditure on health, and in most of the states across India private sector expenditure outweighs public sector expenditure on health (see Figure 7.4). This is critically important because health-related expenditure is considered to be the second largest cause of indebtedness. In addition, this affects women's abilities to access health care services. Most often the decision lies with the husband because women do not have economic independence and decision-making freedom. This also indicates the rampant growth of the private sector in India and its potential role, or further role, in improving access to health care services.

Table 7.1   The financing of health care in India: Health expenditure by financing source

Source	Expenditure (Rs '000)	% distribution
Public		
Central government	67,198,262	6.3
State government	132,709,065	12.5
Urban local bodies and *Panchayat Raj*	18,042,955	1.7
Total	217,950,282	20.5
Private		
Households	764,840,500	71.9
Firms[a]	55,460,000	5.2
NGOs and Indian funding agencies	NA	
Total	820,300,500	77.2
External support		
Aid to central government (MOHFW budget)	16,483,158	1.6
Material aid to central government (MOH)	825,937	0.1
Aid to state government (state budgets)	2,389,522	0.2
To NGOs	5,161,353	0.5
Total	24,860,003	2.3
Total	1,063,110,785	100.0

Source: Ministry of Health and Family Welfare, *National Health Accounts, India – 2001–02*, New Delhi: MOHFW, 2005.
Notes: NA = not available.
[a] From National Commission on Macroeconomics and Health, *Financing and Delivery of Health Care Services in India*, New Delhi: Ministry of Health and Family Welfare, Government of India, 2005.

The way forward

Improving women's health requires a robust and sustained commitment by the government. As a signatory to the *Millennium Declaration*,[67] India is committed to working towards maternal health goals as well as gender equality and empowerment. The recent paradigm shift in the national health programme from demographic-oriented vertical approaches to an integrated life-cycle approach is a step in that direction.

Figure 7.4   Ratio of public to private expenditure on health in major states

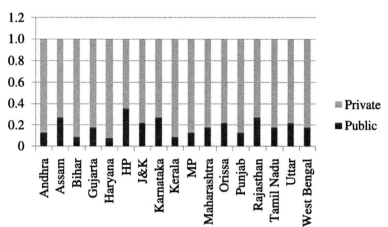

Source: MOHFW, *National Health Accounts, India – 2001–02*, New Delhi, 2005.

Increase public health spending on primary health care. In 2001–2002, total expenditure on health was 4.6 per cent of the gross domestic product (GDP). Public health spending was only 20.5 per cent of total expenditure, whereas 77.2 per cent was private expenditure and the remaining 2.3 per cent external support.[68] The bulk of health expenditure (72.0 per cent) is borne by households through out-of-pocket expenses. There are concerns that only 20 per cent of total expenditure is on primary health care. Reproductive and child health spending accounted for only 11.3 per cent of total health spending, whereas curative care services accounted for a mammoth 74.0 per cent of the national health expenditure. Public spending on primary health care has been spread too thinly for these services to be effective. National consensus on mechanisms for predictable, sustained and increased funding will need to be strengthened. Budgetary allocations for primary health care, particularly for operationalising FRUs for institutional deliveries and EmOC, will need to be prioritised to have an impact on maternal health.

Focus on poorly performing states. There is evidence that the bulk of the maternal morbidity and mortality burden lies in certain states, which are slowing down national progress. These states need to be systematically mentored to deliver positive maternal health outcomes. At the same time, clear objectives and expected outcomes will need to be monitored at the state and district level.

Building human resources for health. India's vision of achieving maternal health goals and MDGs will be severely diminished unless there is an equitable presence of skilled health care workers in the required numbers. Apart from restructuring recruitment and transfer policies, providing incentives and career development opportunities, and reducing inter-state differences in health workforce availability, there is an urgent need to improve the skills of the current workforce and increase the number of trained and motivated public health workers available to the public sector.

Research for evidence-based planning. In India, public health research output is inordinately low and not commensurate with the magnitude and distribution of the disease burden. Unless dynamic, relevant and good-quality research in various aspects of maternal health is available, public health policies will not be guided by local evidence.

Expanding partnerships. Although the primary onus for providing basic health care remains with the government, the pro-rich public health system does not ensure equitable availability of services. Partnerships with civil society and the private sector can improve accessibility to services, ensure quality of service delivery, help establish accountability mechanisms and maintain political momentum for maternal health care.

Health technology. Low-cost interventions that are effective in low-resource settings are available for substantially reducing the risk of maternal ill health and death. However, with increasing evidence of gynaecological morbidity in India, there is a demand for making available new techniques to bring about improvements in women's health. Minimally invasive technologies, such as endoscopes, with wide application in obstetrics and gynaecology could be introduced for early diagnosis of gynaecological pathologies and for reducing the risks associated with invasive surgeries.

Acknowledgement

We gratefully acknowledge the huge contribution of Ms Anju Dadhwal, National Consultant, WHO-India, in bringing the chapter to its final shape.

Notes

1. Medical Termination of Pregnancy Act, available at <http://mohfw.nic.in/MTP.htm> (accessed 9 June 2009).
2. F. Arnold et al., "Sex-Selective Abortions In India", *Population and Development Review*, 28, 2002, pp. 759–785.
3. P. Jha et al., "Low Male-to-Female Sex Ratio of Children Born in India: National Survey of 1.1 Million Households", *Lancet*, 367, 2006, pp. 211–218.
4. The Pre-Natal Diagnostic Techniques (Regulation and Prevention of Misuse) Amendment Act, 2002, available at <http://mohfw.nic.in/PNDT%20-%20%20(act%202002).htm> (accessed 9 June 2009).
5. R. Patel, "The Practice of Sex Selective Abortion in India: May You Be the Mother of a Thousand Sons", Department of Maternal and Child Health, University of North Carolina, 1996, <http://cgi.unc.edu/research/pdf/abortion.pdf> (accessed 9 June 2009).
6. International Institute for Population Sciences (IIPS), *National Family Health Survey (MCH and Family Planning), India, 1992–93*, Mumbai: IIPS, 1995; see <http://www.nfhsindia.org/nfhs1.html> (accessed 17 June 2009). The first National Family Health Survey was launched by the Ministry of Health and Family Welfare (MOHFW), Government of India, in 1991. The main objective of the survey was to collect reliable and up-to-date information on fertility, family planning, mortality, and maternal and child health. Data collection was carried out in three phases from April 1992 to September 1993. NFHS-1 was a major landmark in the development of a demographic database for India.
7. F. Arnold, M. K. Choe and T. K. Roy, "Son Preference, the Family-Building Process and Child Mortality in India", *Population Studies*, 52(3), 1998, pp. 301–315; A. Sen and S. Sengupta, "Malnutrition of Rural Children and the Sex Bias", *Economic and Political Weekly*, 18(19–21), 1983, pp. 855–864; A. Pebley and S. Amin, "The Impact of a Public-Health Intervention on Sex Differentials in Childhood Mortality in Rural Punjab, India", *Health Transition Review*, No. 1, 1991, pp. 143–169; S. S. Wadley, "Family Composition Strategies in Rural North India", *Social Science and Medicine*, No. 37, 1993, pp. 1367–1376; A. Asfaw, S. Klasen and F. Lamanna, "Intra-Household Gender Disparities in Children's Medical Care before Death in India", Institute for the Study of Labor (IZA) Discussion Paper No. 2586, January 2007, available at <http://ssrn.com/abstract=964967> (accessed 16 June 2009).

8. J. B. Wyon and J. E. Gordon, *The Khanna Study*, Cambridge, MA: Harvard University Press, 1971; A. A. Kielmann, C. De Sweemer, R. L. Parker and C. E. Taylor (eds), *Child and Maternal Health Services in Rural India: The Narangwal Experiment*, vol. I, Baltimore, MD: Johns Hopkins University Press, 1983; M. Das Gupta, "Selective Discrimination against Female Children in Rural Punjab, India", *Population and Development Review*, 13(1), 1987, pp. 77–100, <http://gbytes.gsood.com/files/dasgupta-punjab.pdf> (accessed 15 June 2009).

9. See P. Arokiasamy and J. Pradhan, "Gender Bias against Female Children in India: Regional Differences and Their Implications for MDGs", *IIPS Newsletter*, Mumbai: IIPS, 2005.

10. Central Statistical Organization, *Women and Men in India 1998*, Delhi: Government of India, 1999, p. 10.

11. S. Bezbaruah and M. K. Janeja, *Adolescents in India: A Profile*, New Delhi: UNFPA, 2000, available at <http://www.un.org.in/adolescentsfinalbook-800kb.pdf> (accessed 9 June 2009).

12. United Nations Population Fund (UNFPA) Country Support Team for Central and South Asia, *The South Asia Conference on Adolescents, New Delhi, India, 21–23 July 1998*, Kathmandu, Nepal: UNFPA CST for CASA, 1999, <http://www.unfpa.org.np/pub/adol.pdf> (accessed 9 June 2009).

13. Department of Women and Child Development, *India Country Paper*, Delhi: Government of India, 1999.

14. S. Kulkarni, "The Reproductive Health Status of Married Adolescents as Assessed by IIPS, ORC MACRO, India", in S. Bott et al. (eds), *Towards Adulthood: Exploring the Sexual and Reproductive Health of Adolescents of South Asia*, Geneva: WHO, 2003, pp. 55–58.

15. S. Mehta, "Responsible Sexual and Reproductive Health Behaviour Among Adolescents", Theme Paper prepared for UNFPA-sponsored South Asia Conference on Adolescents, 21–23 July 1998, New Delhi.

16. D. W. Khandait et al., "Maternal Age a Risk Factor for Still Birth", *Indian Journal of Public Health*, 44, 2000, pp. 28–30.

17. B. D. Bhatia and R. Chandra, "Adolescent Mother – An Unprepared Child", *Indian Journal of Maternal and Child Health*, 4(3), 1993, pp. 67–70.

18. A. Barua and K. Kurz, "Reproductive Health-Seeking by Married Adolescent Girls in Maharashtra, India", *Reproductive Health Matters*, 9(17), 2001, pp. 53–62.

19. K. Kabir, "Exploitation of and Violence Against Adolescents", Theme paper for the UNFPA-sponsored South Asia Conference on Adolescents, 21–23 July 1998, New Delhi, India.

20. UNFPA, *The South Asia Conference on Adolescents*.

21. Centre of Concern for Child Labour, "Child Prostitution in India", New Delhi, 1998, cited in *The Times of India*, 10 November 1998, <http://www.preda.org/archives/research/cpr/ecpat990501.html> (accessed 15 June 2009).

22. C. Shen and J. B. Williamson, "Maternal Mortality, Women's Status, and Economic Dependency in Less Developed Countries: A Cross National Analysis", *Social Science & Medicine*, 49, 1999, pp. 197–214.

23. The 2005–2006 "National Family Health Survey, India" (NFHS-3) is the third in the NFHS series of surveys. It provides information on population, health and nutrition in India and each of its 29 states. NFHS-3 provides trend data on key indicators and includes information on several new topics. For the first time, NFHS-3 also provides information on men and unmarried women. The NFHS-3 fieldwork was conducted by 18 research organisations between December 2005 and August 2006. For further reference, see <http://www.nfhsindia.org/nfhs3.html> (accessed 15 June 2009).

24. See National Population Stabilisation Fund website at <http://www.jsk. gov.in/indias_population.asp> (accessed 9 June 2009).

25. International Institute for Population Sciences (IIPS) and ORC Macro, *National Family Health Survey (NFHS-2), 1998–99, India*, Mumbai: IIPS, 2000. NFHS-2 is considered an important step to strengthen the database for implementation of the Reproductive and Child Health approach adopted by India after the International Conference on Population and Development (ICPD) in Cairo. The principal objective of NFHS-2 was to provide state and national estimates of fertility, the practice of family planning, infant and child mortality, maternal and child health, and the utilisation of health services provided to mothers and children. In addition, the survey included information on the quality of health and family welfare services and provided indicators of the status of women, women's reproductive health and domestic violence. Another feature of NFHS-2 is measurement of the nutritional status of women. See <http://www. nfhsindia.org/nfhs2.html> (accessed 15 June 2009).

26. India's Family Welfare Programme (starting in 1966/67) placed heavy emphasis on sterilisation as the major method of family planning. This "time-bound", "target-oriented" and "incentive-based" approach contributed to the predominant focus on female sterilisation by providers. With an expanded basket of contraceptive choices being promoted by the government as well as the popularisation of a two-child norm, there is increased acceptance of reversible contraceptive methods.

27. K. B. Pathak et al., "Accelerating India's Fertility Decline: The Role of Temporary Contraceptive Methods", *NFHS Bulletin*, Mumbai: IIPS, February 1998, p. 9.

28. SRS-based abridged life tables, 1992–1996 and 1993–1997, published by the Office of the Registrar General, India, New Delhi, 2000 (*SRS Analytical Studies Report*, No. 1, 2000)]. See also SRS-based abridged life tables, 2000–2004, published by the Office of the Registrar General, India, New Delhi, 2007 (*SRS Analytical Studies Report*, No. 1, 2007); SRS-based abridged life tables, 2001–2005, published by the Office of the Registrar General, India, New Delhi, 2007 (*SRS Analytical Studies Report*, No. 3, 2007).

29. International Centre for Research on Women, "The Impact of Unmet Family Planning Needs on Women's Health", *Information Bulletin*, December 2004.

30. *Maternal Mortality in India, 1997–2003: Trends, Causes, and Risk Factors*, Office of the Registrar General India, in collaboration with Centre for Global Health Research, University of Toronto, 2006.

31. EAG states: Bihar, Jharkhand, Orissa, Madhya Pradesh, Chattisgarh, Rajasthan, Uttar Pradesh and Uttaranchal.

32. Registrar General of India, *Sample Registration Bulletin*, 33(1), 1999, New Delhi: Office of the Registrar General.

33. International Institute for Population Sciences (IIPS), World Health Organization (WHO), and World Health Organization India – WR Office, *Health System Performance Assessment: World Health Survey 2003 India*, Mumbai: IIPS, 2006.

34. NFHS-3.

35. IIPS, WHO and WHO India, *Health System Performance Assessment*.

36. X. F. Li et al., "The Postpartum Period: The Key to Maternal Mortality", *International Journal of Gynecology and Obstetrics*, 54(1), 1996, pp. 1–10.

37. NFHS-3.

38. R. A. Bang et al., "High Prevalence of Gynaecological Disease in Rural Indian Women", *Lancet*, 1, 1989, pp. 85–87.

39. K. Latha et al., "Prevalence of Clinically Detectable Gynaecological Morbidity in India: Results of Four Community Based Studies", *Journal of Family Welfare*, 43(4), 1997, pp. 8–16, available at <http://www.gendwaar.gen.in/Other/Oct15.htm> (accessed 9 June 2009).

40. I. P. Kambo et al., "Self-Reported Gynaecological Problems from Twenty Three Districts of India: An ICMR Task Force Study", *Indian Journal of Community Medicine*, 28(2), 2003.

41. S. Garg et al., "Reproductive Morbidity in an India Slum: Need for Health Action", *Sexually Transmitted Infections*, 78(1), 2002, pp. 68–69, available at <http://www.sti.bmj.com/content/vol78/issue1/> (accessed 9 June 2009).

42. J. C. Bhatia et al., "Levels and Determinants of Gynaecological Morbidity in a District of South India", *Studies in Family Planning*, 28(2), 1997, pp. 95–103.

43. A. Ghosh, "City's Private Hospitals Love the Knife", *The Times of India* (New Delhi), 5 April 2007.

44. M. A. Harper et al., "Pregnancy Related Death and Health Care Services", *American Journal of Obstetrics and Gynecology*, 102, 2003, pp. 273–278.

45. S. N. Mukherjee, "Rising Cesarean Section Rate", *Journal of Obstetrics and Gynecology India*, 56(4), 2006, pp. 298–300.

46. M. Lyndon-Rochelle et al., "First-Birth Cesarean and Placental Abruption or Previa at Second Birth", *Journal of Obstetrics and Gynecology*, 97, 2001, pp. 765–769.

47. "2007 estimates suggest national adult HIV prevalence of approximately 0.34 percent, amounting to 1.8 to 2.9 million people living with HIV in India. One third of the AIDS cases are among the youth in the age group of 15–29 years, who are the future of the country. Women and youth are disproportionately affected, with women accounting for about 39% of all infections despite the fact that more than 90% of them are in monogamous relationships." See National Aids Control Organisation, *Mainstreaming HIV and AIDS for Women's Empowerment*, Government of India, 2008, avail-

able at <http://www.nacoonline.org/upload/Publication/IEC%20&%20 Mainstreaming/mainstreaming%20hiv%20and%20aids%20for%20 women.pdf> (accessed 16 June 2009).

48. P. Basanta and S. Ramamani, "Gender Impact of HIV and AIDS in India", NACO, NCAER and UNDP, 2006.

49. NFHS-2.

50. NFHS-3.

51. Ibid.

52. L. Visaria, "Violence against Women in India: Evidence from Rural Gujarat", in *Domestic Violence in India 1: A Summary Report of Three Studies*, Washington, DC: International Center for Research on Women and The Centre for Development and Population Activities, 1999.

53. Laparotomy set, minilaparomoty set, IUD insertion set, vasectomy set, normal delivery set, vacuum extraction set, uterine evacuation set, anaesthesia equipment, reagents and equipment for blood tests, neo-natal resuscitation set, donor blood transfusion set.

54. D. V. Mavalankar, "Promoting Safe Motherhood: Issues and Challenges", in S. Pachauri (ed.) *Implementing a Reproductive Health Agenda in India: The Beginning*, New Delhi: Population Council, 1999, pp. 519–538.

55. Reproductive & Child Health Programme, Department of Family Welfare, Government of India, <http://mohfw.nic.in/dofw%20website/aided%20 projects/rchp%20frame.htm> (accessed 9 June 2009).

56. Ministry of Health and Family Welfare (MOHFW), "RCH II and Family Planning Programme Implementation Plan (PIP)", Draft, Department of Family Welfare, MOHFW, Government of India, New Delhi, 2003.

57. MOHFW, *India Country Report: Fifth Asian and Pacific Population Conference on "Population and Poverty in Asia and Pacific" Bangkok*, New Delhi: Ministry of Health and Family Welfare, Government of India, 2002.

58. See "National Health Policy – 2002", para. 2.28, available at <http://www. mohfw.nic.in/np2002.htm> (accessed 9 June 2009).

59. *Tenth Five Year Plan 2002–2007*, available at <http://www.planning commission.nic.in/plans/planrel/fiveyr/10th/default.htm> (accessed 9 June 2009).

60. MOHFW, *India Country Report*.

61. Reproductive and Child Health Phase II Programme (RCH-II), National Rural Health Mission, Government of India, available at <http://www. mohfw.nic.in/NRHM/RCH/Index.htm> (accessed 9 June 2009).

62. RCH-II, Document 2, *The Principles and Evidence Base for State RCH II Programme Implementation Plans (PIPs)*, available at <http://www.whoindia.org/ LinkFiles/Child_Health_in_India_PIP_Doc_Chapter01.pdf> (accessed 9 June 2009).

63. "Maternal Health Programme", <http://mohfw.nic.in/dofw%20website/ MATERNAL%20HEALTH%20%20PROGRAMME%20%20.htm> (accessed 9 June 2009).

64. See MOHFW, "Janani Suraksha Yojana: Guidelines for Implementation", <http://www.mohfw.nic.in/layout_09-06.pdf> (accessed 9 June 2009).

65. "National Rural Health Mission (2005-2012): Mission Document", <http://www.mohfw.nic.in/NRHM%20Mission%20Document.pdf> (accessed 9 June 2009).
66. MOHFW, *National Health Accounts, India – 2001–02*, New Delhi, 2005, available at <http://www.mohfw.nic.in/NHA%202001-02.pdf> (accessed 9 June 2009). 67. United Nations General Assembly, *United Nations Millennium Declaration*, A/RES/55/2, 18 September 2000, <http://www.un.org/millennium/declaration/ares552e.pdf> (accessed 16 June 2009).
68. MOHFW, *National Health Accounts, India – 2001–02*.

8

India's medical system

NIRMAL KUMAR GANGULY AND MALABIKA ROY

Introduction

Good population health is an important contributor to economic growth and productivity. According to the World Health Report (WHR) 2000,[1] health systems consist of all the people and actions whose primary purpose is to improve health. The health status of a population is thus determined by the health system's performance. The WHR 2000 identified three fundamental objectives of a health system: improving the health of the population, responding to people's expectations, and providing financial protection against the costs of ill health. India, with a population of over 1.1 billion, is the world's largest democracy. It has 29 states and six Union Territories; 70 per cent of its population resides in rural areas, although in recent decades migration to larger cities has led to an exponential increase in the urban population. The national sex ratio is 944 females to 1,000 males. India's median age is 24.66 years and the population growth rate is 1.38 per cent per annum, with 24.1 births per 1,000 population.[2] Provision of first-rate health care accessible to all is thus a formidable task. This chapter considers the current status of the health system in India, discusses its limitations and details some of the measures taken at the national level to address these issues.

Partnerships for women's health: Striving for best practice within the UN Global Compact,
Timmermann and Kruesmann (eds),
United Nations University Press, 2009, ISBN 978-92-808-1185-8

The health system in India

The provision of public health services in India had its foundations in the Bhore Committee Report of 1946,[3] which recommended integration of preventive and curative services at all administrative levels, development of primary health care centres and changes in medical education to include training in preventive and social medicine.

Over the years since independence in 1947, the health system has developed into a three-tier system of primary, secondary and tertiary health care. The primary health care system is part of the rural health care infrastructure; secondary and tertiary health, with some exceptions, are mainly urban oriented. Simultaneously, there has been strong growth in private for-profit health care institutions, non-profit voluntary organisations that provide health care, and an informal private health care provision by unregistered health practitioners.

Public health care

The provision of health care by the public sector is the shared responsibility of the national (Centre), state and local governments. The states are responsible for the delivery of health care and are largely independent in this regard. The Centre's responsibility consists mainly of policy-making, planning, guiding, assisting, evaluating and coordinating the work of the state health ministries. The Centre drives national programmes such as the tuberculosis control programme, leprosy eradication programme, and so on, which are usually administered vertically (that is, directly by the national government without reference to other initiatives). Local governments by and large have no financial authority, except in large cities, although some states are now strengthening local governments by providing financial authority as part of health sector reforms.

The Centre is usually unable to effectively integrate these vertical, centrally sponsored schemes with the provision of general health services. This leads to a decline in health system effectiveness, and over time the Central schemes become disconnected from local health problems and community priorities as well as from structural mismatches owing to lack of coordination between Centre and state-run institutional structures. Other problematic factors are unrealistic and non-evidence-based goal-setting, a lack of strategic planning and inadequate funding. Because of India's vastness and diversity, it will be difficult to combat the rising trend of communicable diseases such as malaria, tuberculosis (TB) and HIV/AIDS without the active participation of communities. However, to make the community responsive, it is important to provide not only functional delegation but also fiscal devolution, including expenditure decision-making with revenue responsibilities.[4]

The organisation of public health care services

At the national level, health care services are the responsibility of the Union Ministry of Health and Family Welfare. The Ministry has two departments – the Department of Health and Family Welfare and the Department of AYUSH (Ayurveda, Yoga and Naturopathy, Unani, Siddha and Homoeopathy). The Directorate General of Health Services (DGHS), acting as a technical advisory wing to the Department of Health, is headed by the Director General. Technical inputs from the Deputy and Assistant Commissioners are provided for implementation of the Family Welfare Programme. The Secretary overseeing both departments heads the executive wing. Both the executive wing and the technical departments under the Union Minister of Health and Family Welfare are supported by a state-level and a deputy-level minister.

At the state level, health care services are the responsibility of the state Department of Health and Family Welfare. Each state department is headed by a Minister with a Secretariat under the charge of a Secretary/Commissioners (Health and Family Welfare). This Secretary invariably belongs to the cadre of the Indian Administrative Service. By and large, the organisational structure adopted by the state follows the pattern of the central government. The State Directorate of Health Services, as the technical wing, is an affiliated office of the State Department of Health and Family Welfare and is headed by a Director of Health Services. However, the organisational structure of the State Directorate of Health Services is not uniform throughout the country. Each programme officer (with responsibility, for example, for family welfare, malaria, tuberculosis, leprosy, blindness or mental health) below the Director of Health Services deals with one or more subject(s). Every State Directorate has supporting areas comprising both technical and administrative staff. The area of medical education, which was integrated with the Directorate of Health Services at the state level, has a separate identity as a Directorate of Medical Education and Research. This Directorate is under the charge of the Director of Medical Education, who is answerable directly to the Health Secretary/Commissioner of the state.

These organisational structures at the state and national level implement the delivery of primary, secondary and tertiary health care services in the public sector's rural health care infrastructure. The government has built up a large three-tiered system of rural health care infrastructure for delivery of primary health care nation-wide, which consists of sub-centres, primary health centres and community health centres designated as "first referral units" (FRUs). These are established on the basis of population norms as shown in Table 8.1.

Sub-centres

The sub-centre is the first contact point between the primary health care system and the community. It is manned by one female Auxiliary Nurse Midwife (ANM)/Multipurpose Health Worker and one male Multipurpose Health Worker. Sub-centres are responsible for maternal and child health, family welfare, nutrition, immunisation, control of diarrhoea and acute respiratory infections, and control of communicable disease programmes. Basic drugs are available for treating minor ailments and for taking care of the essential health needs of women and children.

Primary health centre (PHC)

The PHC is the first contact point between the village community and the Medical Officer. It is manned by a Medical Officer and 14

Table 8.1   Population norms for rural health centres

	Population norms	
Centre	Plain area	Hilly/tribal area
Sub-centre	5,000	3,000
Primary health centre (PHC)	30,000	20,000
Community health centre (CHC)	120,000	80,000

Source: Ministry of Health and Family Welfare, Annual Report 2005–06, Delhi: Government of India, 2006.
Note: The most peripheral unit of the health system in the public sector is the sub-centre, which covers a population of 5,000 (3,000 in hilly and tribal areas). The next in the hierarchy is the PHC and then the CHC. The CHC acts as the first referral unit for the PHC and the sub-centre.

other staff, including paramedic and supporting staff. It has 4–6 beds and acts as a referral unit for 6 sub-centres. It provides curative, preventive, promotive and family welfare services. The male Health Supervisor and one Lady Health Visitor (LHV)/Female Health Supervisor in each PHC are responsible for supervision of the male Multipurpose Worker and ANM, respectively. The overall supervisor of the sub-centre and the PHC is the Medical Officer.

Community health centre (CHC)

The CHC is manned by four medical specialists, that is, a surgeon, a physician, a gynaecologist and a paediatrician, supported by 21 paramedic and other staff. It has 30 indoor beds with one operating theatre, X-ray and labour room, and laboratory facilities, and serves as a referral centre for four PHCs. It provides facilities for emergency obstetric care and specialist consultations. The CHCs act as a first referral unit for primary health care.

The primary health care institutions also form the delivery point for the provision of services in rural areas under the centrally sponsored disease control programmes, which currently include the National Vector Borne Disease Control Programme, the National

Tuberculosis Control Programme, the National Leprosy Eradication Programme, the National AIDS Control Programme, the National Programme for Control of Blindness and the Reproductive and Child Health Programme.

Secondary health care

Secondary care is provided by district hospitals. Each hospital caters for a population of approximately 500,000, and is expected to provide specialist care addressing those diseases/conditions needing a wider range of technology and expertise. This is a middle-level hospital, and serves as a link between the state on one side and the primary-level structures of the CHC, PHC and sub-centre on the other. It receives information from the state level and transmits this to the periphery with suitable modifications to meet local needs. In doing so, the district hospital adopts the functions of a manager and manages general, organisational and administrative issues in relation to health service provision.

The district officer with overall control of both health and family welfare programmes is designated as the Chief Medical and Health Officer (CM and HO) or as the District Medical and Health Officer (DM and HO).

The major functions of district health administrations are to undertake preventive and promotive health activities in an integrated manner. Hospitals must provide access to medical care and family welfare services as well as to statutory health requirements such as medico-legal work, post-mortems, medical examinations, certificates and supervision of jail hospitals and so on. The district health administration is also responsible for organising pre-service entry training for para-professionals and paramedics as well as in-service training for health personnel working at the PHCs and sub-centres in the district.

Health administrators at district hospitals are also responsible for implementing programmes according to policies laid down and finalised at state and national levels The number of officers involved here, their specialisation and their status in the cadre of State Civil Medical Services differs from state to state. Consequently, the control and hierarchy of reporting of these programme officers also varies.

Tertiary health care

Tertiary health care centres are medical college hospitals and other specialty hospitals with facilities for various medical specialisations. They do not include teaching hospitals or super-specialty hospitals (teaching hospitals with higher medical and surgical specialisations such as endocrinology, gastroenterology, cardiology, oncology, neonatology and cardio-thoracic surgery), and they are mainly situated in urban areas. Although these hospitals are expected to be referral hospitals from secondary health care institutions, they usually run independently and no functioning referral system exists.

In addition to the above, there are urban family health posts and urban health and family welfare centres. The current status of the public health care infrastructure is indicated in Table 8.2.

Table 8.2   Public sector health care infrastructure

1. Sub-centres	142,655
2. Primary health centres	23,109
3. Community health centres	3,222
4. Dispensaries (Indian system of medicine)	22,442
5. Urban family welfare centres	1,083
6. Urban health posts	871
7. Number of hospitals: Rural	2,450
Urban	10,284

Sources: Ministry of Health and Family Welfare, *Annual Report 2005–06*, Delhi: Government of India, 2006; Ministry of Health and Family Welfare, *Health Information of India*, Central Bureau of Health Intelligence, Directorate General of Health Services, Delhi: Government of India, 2002.

Health-related activities of other government departments

In addition to health services delivered by the Ministry of Health and Family Welfare, several other government ministries and departments also provide health and support services.

The Ministry of Women and Child Development operates the Integrated Child Development Services (ICDS) scheme, which was launched in 1975 especially for child welfare in pursuance of the National Policy for Children. The ICDS provides an integrated package of early childhood services, including supplementary nutrition, growth monitoring, education for families to adopt better feeding practices and better nutrition during pregnancy, breastfeeding, weaning foods and balanced nutrition. The ICDS also assist ANMs in administering Vitamin A and iron supplementation in the early years of development (up to 6 years) and promoting holistic child development through pre-school education. A scheme for adolescent girls has been approved in some blocks as a special intervention for girls aged 11–18 years.

Health service delivery is primarily through a local village-level worker known as an Anganwadi Worker (AWW), and Anganwadi Centres are located in the villages. One AWW per 1,000 residents in non-tribal areas and one per 700 people in tribal areas is the accepted norm. The programme covers 5,652 designated areas, with 0.7 million Anganwadi Centres reaching 49.9 million beneficiaries.[5] Evaluations carried out by various agencies indicate that the effectiveness of the programme for reducing malnutrition is poor, presumably because the most vulnerable children (aged less than 2 years) are excluded from the programme. However, the AWW, who is usually a resident of the village, liaises with the ANM for immunisation and antenatal services and thus forms a useful link between the community and the formal health system.

The Ministry of Defence and Ministry of Railways have an independent health system to cater for their staff. In addition, several public sector undertakings have their own health services for their staff.

The functioning of public health institutions

Despite the existence of a huge infrastructure, primary health care institutions are underutilised; but there is overcrowding at the secondary and tertiary health care levels.[6] The functional problems of public health systems include:

1. Coverage: The average number of villages, as well as the population covered by the primary health care institutions, is in practice greater than the mandated ratio set by official norms. Furthermore, urban areas lack an organised primary health care structure as exists in rural areas.

2. Manpower:
   a. There is a shortage of critical staff in sub-centres, especially of male health workers. The shortage of medical officers in PHCs and of specialists (especially anaesthetists) in CHCs is pronounced in the under-served rural, hilly and tribal areas. Also, resident women doctors are not available in most of the PHCs.
   b. There is a problem with lack of productivity and accountability of the supervisory cadre of male and female health assistants, who provide a link between the doctor and the ANM. There is also a problem of staff absenteeism.
   c. These problems may be related to poor motivation of staff, owing to a lack of clear career progression opportunities and an inadequate reward system.

3. Shortages of equipment and medicine.

4. Mismatches between services and available human resources.

5. Irregular payments of salary to staff in peripheral health institutions, especially in poorly performing states.

6. Poor quality of services.

7. Under-funding of public health institutions.

8. Inadequately defined referral linkages from primary to secondary and higher levels of care for optimal utilisation of resources.

9. Absence of continuing education, in-service training and skill upgradation.

Health sector reforms

In order to improve the functioning of the health system, during the 1990s several states attempted innovations in delivery of health services.[7] States such as Gujarat and Karnataka handed over the management of PHCs to non-governmental organisations (NGOs). Many states are also appointing doctors/specialists on a part-time basis to fill labour force gaps in primary health care institutions. In addition, states contract out services such as maintenance of hospital premises to the private sector. Madhya Pradesh, Rajasthan, Haryana and West Bengal have levied user charges and promoted financial autonomy for health institutions, while Kerala, Madhya Pradesh and Karnataka decentralised health services through budget transfers to local bodies. Finally, health innovations are apparent in the improved availability of drugs through centralised drug procurement schemes.

The impact of these interventions needs to be researched. Attempts to engage the private sector in service provision under the national health programmes, with the primary aim of expanding access, have been far from satisfactory. Where some success has been achieved in the areas of cataract blindness and especially for the care and support of people living with HIV/AIDS, this is more a result of the partnership with the non-profit and NGO sectors. One small study on the impact of levying user charges suggests that the number of poor accessing public facilities actually decreased, particularly for inpatient services.[8]

Private health care

The private sector has been providing a significant proportion of health care since the 1950s. Evidence from studies carried out as early as 1963 indicated that most episodes of illness in rural areas

Figure 8.1   Share of public and private sector delivery

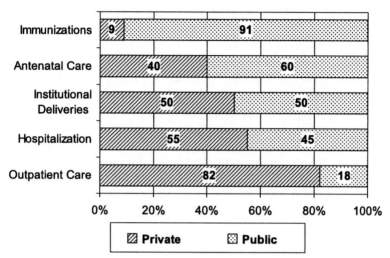

Source: A. Mahal et al., "Who Benefits from Public Health Spending in India", National Council for Applied Economic Research, New Delhi, 2000.

were treated by private providers, and only 10 per cent were treated by public providers.[9] This leads to the poor seeking private health care from unqualified practitioners, which can lead to undesirable outcomes.

To meet the growing demand for hospital care, the government extended substantial subsidies to the private sector. For example, the government allocated land to the private sector on condition that subsidised care would be provided to the poor, but this scheme failed owing to the lack of a regulatory framework and accreditation.

There are no reliable data on the number of hospitals, beds, clinics/ dispensaries or practitioners in the private sector. One study using various assumptions estimates that 850,000 doctors are working in the private sector. The private sector caters for most (82 per cent) outpatient visits, with no significant variations by income group. The range is 79–85 per cent from poorest to richest quintile, by urban and rural, gender, caste or tribe.[10] The share of public and private sectors in the delivery of health care is given in Figure 8.1.

It has been estimated recently that 93 per cent of hospitals and 64 per cent of beds in India are in the private sector; 80 per cent of the private sector belongs to the sole proprietorship category. Specialty and super-specialty care constitutes only 1–2 per cent and corporate hospitals constitute less than 1 per cent. These are mainly run by trusts or by private or public limited companies. Most of the investment in these large hospitals is in high technology, which is viewed as a competitive strategy. Unexpectedly, private hospitals are less frequently located in urban centres than are public hospitals: about 31 per cent of private sector hospitals and 29 per cent of private beds are in rural areas, whereas 25 per cent of public sector hospitals and 10 per cent of public beds are in rural areas.[11]

Voluntary health agencies

Until the mid-1960s voluntary effort in health care was confined to hospital-based care. The National Health Policy of 1983 called for service coverage to be expanded through the voluntary sector to improve public access, as indicated in Table 8.3.

Voluntary health agencies are involved in the provision of services such as family planning, reproductive and child health, AIDS control,

Table 8.3   Growth of voluntary hospitals and beds

	1983				1987			
Ownership	No. of hospitals	%	No. of beds	%	No. of hospitals	%	No. of beds	%
Voluntary	569	8	53,513	11	935	10	74,498	13
Total	7,398	100	512,474	100	9,603	100	573,578	100

Source: GOI, Central Bureau of Health Intelligence, Directorate General of Health Services, Ministry of Health and Family Welfare, "Directory of Hospitals in India", 1985 and 1988; <http://www.cbhidghs.nic.in/index2.asp?slid=878&sublinkid=665> (accessed 24 June 2009).

ICDS and so on. These agencies safeguard and supplement government work by providing guidance, criticism and expertise to explore ways and means of doing things differently; supplementing health education; undertaking demonstration projects; and mobilising public opinion for health legislation. There are no reliable data on the number of currently functioning voluntary agencies. According to a rough estimate, more than 7,000 voluntary organisations contribute to basic health care delivery and community development, rehabilitation services for disadvantaged groups such as those with leprosy or other disabilities, blindness control, polio eradication, management of blood banks and support during disasters and epidemics.[12] The voluntary sector has a high presence in the rural areas.

Unqualified rural medical practitioners

The urban concentration of qualified practitioners and facilities and the limited spread of voluntary sectors has given rise to a number of rural medical practitioners in rural areas. An estimated 1 million unqualified practitioners manage about 50–70 per cent of primary consultations here, mostly for minor ailments.[13]

The National Rural Health Mission

In order to improve access and quality of care in rural areas, the Government of India has launched the National Rural Health Mission (NRHM),[14] with a special focus on 18 selected states with poor demographic and health indicators. The NRHM is intended to run for seven years (2005–2012), and seeks to provide accessible, affordable, accountable, equitable and effective quality health care, especially to the vulnerable rural population. Realising the need for coordination with other departments and agencies that contribute to aggregate population health outcomes, the NRHM provides an overarching umbrella that accommodates existing national government programmes, including those focused on water supply and sanitation.

Figure 8.2   Approaches of the National Rural Health Mission

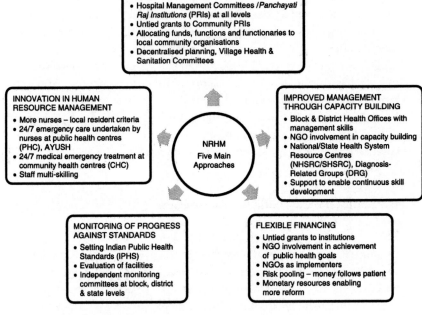

COMMUNITY-LEVEL FOCUS
- Hospital Management Committees /*Panchayati Raj Institutions* (PRIs) at all levels
- Untied grants to Community PRIs
- Allocating funds, functions and functionaries to local community organisations
- Decentralised planning, Village Health & Sanitation Committees

INNOVATION IN HUMAN RESOURCE MANAGEMENT
- More nurses – local resident criteria
- 24/7 emergency care undertaken by nurses at public health centres (PHC), AYUSH
- 24/7 medical emergency treatment at community health centres (CHC)
- Staff multi-skilling

NRHM Five Main Approaches

IMPROVED MANAGEMENT THROUGH CAPACITY BUILDING
- Block & District Health Offices with management skills
- NGO involvement in capacity building
- National/State Health System Resource Centres (NHSRC/SHSRC), Diagnosis-Related Groups (DRG)
- Support to enable continuous skill development

MONITORING OF PROGRESS AGAINST STANDARDS
- Setting Indian Public Health Standards (IPHS)
- Evaluation of facilities
- Independent monitoring committees at block, district & state levels

FLEXIBLE FINANCING
- Untied grants to institutions
- NGO involvement in achievement of public health goals
- NGOs as implementers
- Risk pooling – money follows patient
- Monetary resources enabling more reform

Source: compiled by the authors.

The NRHM aims to achieve the goals and objectives of the National Health Policy 2002, the National Population Policy 2000 and the UN Millennium Development Goals, and to increase public outlays on health from the current 0.9 per cent to 2–3 per cent of gross domestic product (GDP) between 2005 and 2012.[15] The NRHM also plans systemic correction of the health system to ensure increased outlays are utilised effectively for sustainable health outcomes. A schematic representation of the main approaches of the NRHM is given in Figure 8.2.

The NRHM hopes to provide effective health care to rural populations by establishing village-level workers (termed "accredited social health activists", ASHA) – one in each village of 1,000 residents;

constructing village health plans formulated by a local team headed by the Health & Sanitation Committee of each *Panchayat*; and strengthening the CHCs and rural hospitals accredited under the Indian Public Health Standards (IPHS) for curative care. The NRHM will integrate all vertical health and family welfare programmes to optimise utilisation of funds and infrastructure and strengthen the delivery of primary health care. Additional attention will be given to improving access to health care for rural people and marginalised groups, especially poor women and children, revitalising local health traditions and mainstreaming AYUSH into the public health systems. The structure of the NRHM is represented in Figure 8.3.

NRHM implementation since 2004

Strategies adopted by the NRHM since its inception include training and enhancing the capacity of local bodies (*Panchayati Raj Institutions*, PRI) to own, control and manage public health services, and promoting access to improved health care at household level through the village-level ASHA. Additional strategies include the promotion of public private partnerships (PPP) for achieving public health goals, as well as pooling effective and viable risks and social health insurance to provide health security to the poor by ensuring accessible, affordable, accountable and good-quality hospital care. The implementation of the Reproductive and Child Health initiatives (RCH-II) and other disease control programmes has also been adopted.

Achievements

The huge infrastructure created since India's independence has resulted in significant improvements in the health status of the population.[16] At the national level, life expectancy went up from 36 years in 1951 to 66 in 2001. The infant mortality rate has been halved from 146 per 1,000 live births to 58 per 1,000 live births in 2004. The crude birth rate (births per 1,000 people per year) has been reduced

Figure 8.3 Structure of the NRHM

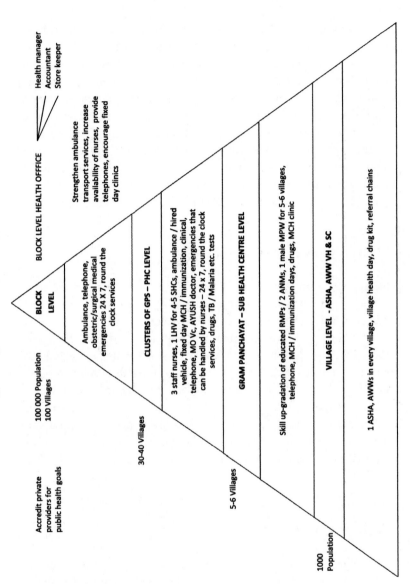

Accredit private
providers for
public health goals

100 000 Population
100 Villages

BLOCK
LEVEL

BLOCK LEVEL HEALTH OFFICE

Health manager
Accountant
Store keeper

Strengthen ambulance
transport services, increase
availability of nurses, provide
telephones, encourage fixed
day clinics

Ambulance, telephone,
obstetric/surgical medical
emergencies 24 X 7, round the
clock services

30-40 Villages

CLUSTERS OF GPS – PHC LEVEL

3 staff nurses, 1 LHV for 4-5 SHCs, ambulance / hired
vehicle, fixed day MCH / immunization, clinical,
telephone, MO Vc, AYUSH doctor, emergencies that
can be handled by nurses – 24 x 7, round the clock
services, drugs, TB / Malaria etc. tests

GRAM PANCHAYAT – SUB HEALTH CENTRE LEVEL

5-6 Villages

Skill up-gradation of educated RMPs / 2 ANMs, 1 male MPW for 5-6 villages,
telephone, MCH / immunization days, drugs, MCH clinic

VILLAGE LEVEL - ASHA, AWW VH & SC

1000
Population

1 ASHA, AWWs in every village, village health day, drug kit, referral chains

Source: the authors.

from 40.8 in 1951 to 24.1 in 2004 and the crude death rate (number of deaths per 1,000 people per year) has dropped from 25.0 in 1951 to 7.5 in 2004. Significant improvement has taken place in the reproductive health of the population. The couple protection rate (the percentage of eligible couples effectively protected from childbirth by one or another contraceptive method) increased from 1.4 per cent in 1970/71 to 56.3 per cent in 2005/06, and the total fertility rate (the average number of children that would be born to a woman over her lifetime) declined from 6.0 to 2.7 in 2005/06.

India's advantage

The bio-pharma sector, comprising mainly vaccines, therapeutic drugs, animal biologicals and diagnostics, recorded growth of 31.88 per cent and grossed more than US$1 billion in 2005/06, and it is the largest contributor to the size of the biotech industry, followed by diagnostics.[17] Local firms, both public and private, are playing a leading role in promoting health biotechnology. There are over 328 companies and 241 institutions in India using some form of biotechnology in agricultural, medical or environmental applications.[18] Although estimates vary, domestic drug molecule production accounts for about 55 per cent of the total health biotechnology market in India. Several multinational pharmaceutical giants, such as Eli Lilly (USA), Glaxo Smith Kline (UK), Novartis (Switzerland), Pfizer (USA) and Astra Zeneca (USA), also carry out manufacturing and clinical trials in India, but they play only a minimal role in developing the local health biotechnology sector. Besides biopharmaceuticals, India is also poised to become a leader in biotechnology services, such as contract research. It has the advantages of lower costs of operations and manufacturing than many nations of the Organisation for Economic Co-operation and Development, a large and relatively inexpensive scientific and technical workforce that speaks English, expertise in software technologies and a well-developed public research and development infrastructure. Successful contract research firms include Biocon subsidiary Syngene (Bangalore) and SIRO Clinpharm (Mumbai).[19]

Public private partnership

The Indian Council of Medical Research (ICMR)[20] has entered into public private partnerships (PPP) with the following pharmaceutical concerns, working on technical collaboration, conducting clinical trials, obtaining patents, transferring technology and evaluating diagnostic kits:

- TDR-Asta Medical, Germany: Phase IV clinical evaluation of Miltefosine for the treatment of visceral leishmaniasis (kala-azar) – a protozoal infection causing fever and enlargement of the spleen – has been completed, and Miltefosine has now been introduced in the national programme for treatment of visceral leishmaniasis.

- OneWorld Health, California: Phase III clinical trial on Paramomycin for visceral leishmaniasis is ongoing.

- E-Merck, (India) Ltd: clinical trial of human papilloma virus (HPV) vaccine is being initiated (infection due to HPV is said to be one of the risk factors for cervical cancer).

- IAVI-Therion: Phase I safety studies with adeno-associated vaccine (AAV) and Modified Vaccinia Ankara (MVA) for prevention of HIV/AIDS has been completed and efficacy trials are ongoing.

- FHI and The Bill & Melinda Gates Foundation: estimation of HIV disease burden is ongoing.

- WHO–SmithKline Beecham: albendazole for co-administration with diethylcarbamazine citrate has been introduced in the country for treatment of filariasis, and now the combination treatment is being evaluated in the national filiaria control programme.

- Shantha Biotech: gamma Interferon as an immuno-modulator for serious illness, such as hepatic failure, and oral cholera vaccine for which fill and finish was done by international action for vaccine initiatives (IAVI).

- Serum Institute of India (SII)–WHO: Phase I clinical trial with aerosol measles vaccine is ongoing as an alternative mode of delivery of vaccine. SII is a large private Indian vaccine manufacturing company.

- Glaxo-Smithkline Beecham: Phase II trial of typhoid and hepatitis vaccine (Phase III).
- Yakult, Honshu, Japan: probiotic field study to investigate its effectiveness as a health drink and to study its role for prevention of diarrhoea in 1–5 year-old children.

The following partnerships are for developing diagnostic kits; for most of the kits, patents have been obtained and there have been technology transfers (or these are under negotiation):

- Zydus Pathline Ltd: for developing MAC-ELISA for JE, DEN and West Nile viruses.
- BBIL, Hyderabad: for Hepatitis A.
- Zydus Cadilla: for diagnosis of infertility.

Screening programmes and registries

There are various screening programmes for early detection and management of illnesses such as cancer, thalassaemia, iron deficiency and sickle-cell anaemia. The ICMR has constructed the *Cancer Registry Atlas*, which provides information on particular cancers in certain states and regions. Based on this information, circumstantially appropriate measures have been implemented to treat problems, such as the ban on *gutka* (a kind of tobacco chewing) because it has been shown to cause oral cancer. India has a major public health problem of thalassaemia, with 25 million carriers and 10,000 children being born each year with thalassaemia major. The cost of treating one 30 kg child per year with transfusions and chelation with desferrioxamine is Rs 200,000 (approximately US$4,500) per year. Realising the importance of this syndrome, the Jai Vigyan Science and Technology Mission mode project on "Community Control of Thalassaemia Syndrome" was initiated in 1999 to educate, screen, counsel and identify couples at risk, and to develop a national referral centre. These screening programmes need to be more broadly available at all facilities if the benefits are to be maximised. Improved awareness through better information could also enable more women to seek such services.

Continuing challenges

Despite these achievements, huge challenges remain.

Health transition

India is currently in demographic and epidemiologic transition. With declining mortality and fertility, it is estimated that by 2020 the proportion of the population aged 15–64 years will increase from 59 per cent to 67 per cent; above 64 years will increase from 7 per cent to 9 per cent; and below 15 years will drop from 35 per cent to 28 per cent. Simultaneously, there is an epidemiological transition, resulting in a "double burden of disease". Many people continue to die from preventable infections such as diarrhoea, pneumonia, under-nutrition, pregnancy complications, TB, malaria and HIV/AIDS, while simultaneously there is a growing incidence of non-communicable diseases such as cardiovascular disease, diabetes, hypertension, cancer and obesity, attributable to changing lifestyles.

Reproductive and child health

Maternal, prenatal and childhood conditions continue to account for a significant percentage of the disease burden.

Infant and child mortality

The infant mortality rate (IMR) is about 58 per 1,000 live births, a substantial improvement over the levels nearly 30 years ago. The under-5 mortality rate (U5MR) was estimated at 74 per 1,000 live births in 2005. Two-thirds of deaths occur within the first week of birth. In India, the ratio of the neo-natal death rate to the 1–5 year death rate is 1.3, compared with 10 in developed countries. The social preference for the male child and the practice of sex-selective abortions and female feticide compound the problem. The causes of infant mortality and under-5 mortality are different, however; the decline in both of these rates has been the result of cost-effective interventions such as encouraging early initiation and exclusive breastfeeding for the first six months and appropriate complementary feeding thereafter, immunisation, use of antibiotics for acute respiratory infections, oral rehydration therapy for diarrhoea and so on. An ICMR study comparing the short-term efficacy of room air versus 100 per cent oxygen in the resuscitation of asphyxiated babies showed that, in resource-poor settings where oxygen cylinders may not be readily available, these babies can be managed at birth just as effectively with room air.[21]

Maternal mortality

A study investigating 4,484 maternal deaths among more than 1.3 million births carried out through the *Sample Registration Survey* indicated that the maternal mortality ratio is still high, at 301 per 100,000 live births. The lifetime risk of maternal death is 1.0 for India as a whole, but in some Indian states is much higher; for example, in Uttar Pradesh it is 2.4 and in Rajasthan 1.9. The main causes of maternal death are haemorrhage, sepsis, anaemia, obstructed labour, hypertensive disorders of pregnancy and unsafe abortions.[22] A high prevalence (70–80 per cent) of anaemia has persisted over the last three decades, and this is both a direct and an indirect cause of mortality. Moreover, in malaria-endemic areas malaria is another cause of mortality, particularly because Quinacrine is the only drug used for cerebral malaria during pregnancy. Viral hepatitis during pregnancy has high fatality rates, and viral hepatitis epidemics are not uncommon. It has also been observed that, although couples are aware of contraceptive options, contraceptive use continues to be low. Permanent methods, particularly female sterilisation, continue to be the preferred choice. Use of spacing methods (about 6 per cent) and male participation in the form of male condom use (7–8 per cent) and vasectomies (1 per cent) are very low. Unmet needs for contraception are very high, particularly among women younger than 20 years (27 per cent), resulting in high rates of unplanned and undesirable pregnancy, and consequent resort to unsafe abortions.

Gender differentials

Gender disparities in India are pronounced. The *2001 Census* shows a sex ratio for children under 6 of 927 females to 945 males in 1991. With technological developments, new forms of discrimination such as sex-selective abortions through prenatal diagnostic techniques have become widespread. Girls have higher levels of malnutrition and poorer access to medical attention and care, thus placing them at higher risk of illness and death. Women, too, have higher morbidity risks, and are also at higher risk of HIV/AIDS infection owing to poor negotiating skills and lack of economic empowerment. In addition, many women are vulnerable to domestic violence.

Nutritional problems

Although severe under-nutrition has decreased over the years, moderate to mild under-nutrition continues to be high, particularly for the rural poor and in states with poor health indicators. Another related issue is the problem of *hidden hunger* – or micronutrient deficiency. It is estimated that the number of people suffering from micronutrient deficiency is as high as 3.5 billion globally; a very high percentage of these are in India. Iron deficiency is perhaps greatest in India, with 70–80 per cent of pregnant women and children having iron deficiency anaemia. This has been persistent for the last three decades owing to the presence of phytates in vegetarian diets (causing poor iron absorption), faulty child feeding practices, repeated infection, worm infestation and so on. Moreover, 10–20 million children suffer from micronutrient vitamin A deficiency (VAD) and 60,000 go blind because of VAD. This leads to impaired physical and cognitive development, disability and mortality.

Problems of health access specific to women

Apart from geographical limitations on access to good-quality medical care, technology advances and rising demand for high-quality, high-cost care have put many medical interventions beyond the reach of ordinary people and are indeed an important cause of indebtedness

Table 8.4   Socio-economic differences in health: Selected
             indicators

Indicators	Lowest quintile	Highest quintile
Total fertility rate	4.1	2.1
Antenatal care (ANC) 3+ visits	21.1%	81.0%
Tetanus toxoid – ANC	56.9%	95.5%
Iron/folic acid – ANC	36.8%	84.9%
Trained attendant at birth	16.4%	84.4%
Home deliveries	88.3%	25.3%
Contraceptive use – women	24.9%	50.6%

Source: Davidson R. Gwatkin, Shea Rutstein, Kiersten Johnson, Eldaw Suliman, Adam Wagstaff, and Agbessi Amouzou, *Socio-Economic Differences in Health, Nutrition, and Population in (Name of Country)*, Washington, DC: World Bank, 2007; available at <http://web.worldbank.org/WBSITE/EXTERNAL/TOPICS/EXTHEALTHNUTRITIONANDPOPULATION/EXTPAH/0,,contentMDK:20216965~menuPK:460195~pagePK:148956~piPK:216618~theSitePK:400476~isCURL:Y,00.html> (accessed 21 June 2009).

in the poor. There is a need to develop a health financing system that will address the shift in disease burden, the increase in health costs and health care management. Income levels are strongly correlated to overall reproductive health outcomes. Although the burden of disease is high among the poorest quintile, access to health services is also poor, as indicated in Table 8.4.

Urban health

India's urban population is 285 million, which amounts to nearly 30 per cent of the total population. By 2030, the urban population is expected to reach 297 million. Slum populations, which constitute the urban poor, will continue to grow. Lack of water and sanitation, poor housing conditions, occupational hazards and environmental conditions are major problems for the urban poor. Vulnerability also results from a lack of back-up savings, food stocks and social support systems to help during times of illness. Thus, even though there is a concentration of health care facilities in urban areas, the urban poor lack access to health care. In addition, there are newer challenges in urbanisation; other agencies involved in non-health activities/programmes, related for example to drinking water, sanitation, housing and environmental pollution, need to join forces with health professionals and programmes in order to form safe and prosperous communities.

Health insurance

There is minimal health insurance available. It is reported that private voluntary insurance schemes constitute less than 1 per cent of the health budget. Social insurance accounts for around 2.36 per cent, and substantial contributions come from Employees' State Insurance Schemes. There is a need to explore alternatives, such as social health insurance, to protect the poor against indebtedness caused by catastrophic illness.

Emerging and re-emerging infections

The ease and rapidity with which people and diseases are able to cross national boundaries make all nations, including India, vulnerable to microbial infections. Some of these are newly emerging infections, whereas other are re-emerging, either as newer variants or in new geographical regions.[23] There is also the threat of terrorist groups using genetically engineered strains of micro-organisms as weapons. This calls for a strengthening of the public health vigilance system and monitoring access to essential drugs and vaccines.

Inter-state differences

Within the country, there is a north/south divide and persistence of extreme inequalities and disparities in terms of access to care as well as in health outcomes. Whereas in Kerala life expectancy at birth is 74 years, in Madhya Pradesh it is 56 years – an 18-year gap. Just a few states and approximately one-quarter of districts account for 40 per cent of the poor, over half of the malnourished and nearly two-thirds of malaria, kala-azar, leprosy, and infant and maternal mortality. All these diseases can be easily averted with access to low-cost public health interventions.

Resource constraints

India is one of the 5 countries in the world where public health spending is less than 0.9 per cent of GDP, and one of the 15 countries where households account for more than 80 per cent of total health spending. The government is committed to raising public spending to 2–3 per cent of GDP in the National Rural Health Mission (NRHM).

Human resource development

There is a need to expand the range and skill base of human resources and public health specialists such as epidemiologists, biostatisticians, entomologists, trained regulators, hospital managers and administrators, health economists and cost accountants, as well as doctors, nurses and other paramedics and technicians, so as to support a more modernised health system.

Governance

Despite states attempting several innovations, the health system continues to be unaccountable, disconnected from public health goals and inadequately equipped to address people's expectations or provide financial risk protection to those unable to afford care. In spite of investments in expanding access, villagers need to travel long distances to receive health care. Other deterrents, such as bad roads, a lack of reliable health providers, no guarantee of sustained care, the high costs of transport and wages forgone, make it cheaper for a person from the village to get treatment from the local unqualified practitioner.

Addressing non-medical issues

Besides ensuring availability of facilities and services, other non-medical factors such as socio-behavioural and cultural issues need to be addressed. It is necessary for people to seek and practice preventive/promotive and curative health care, such as appropriate nutrition during pregnancy, child nutrition, immunisation and sexual behaviour changes for HIV/AIDS, accepting treatment and drug compliance for TB, and leprosy.

Trade-related intellectual property rights, intellectual property rights and drug prices

India was a foundation member of the World Trade Organization (WTO) and when the Trade Related Intellectual Property Rights (TRIPS) Agreement was signed in 1995 India was committed to implementing its obligations from 1 January 2005. To that end, India amended the Indian Patent Act (1970) to regulate pharmaceutical product patents in line with obligations under the WTO and TRIPS. The new patent regime is not expected to affect the prices of medicines dramatically because the government continues to have the power to regulate the prices of medicines and provide safeguards such as compulsory licensing and parallel import exits. Further, at a given time only 5–10 per cent of drugs are under patent protection.[24]

Application of research

Many efforts are being made to implement research outcomes. However, it has been observed that, despite this, there are still gaps between research and action. For example, India is categorised at intermediate endemicity for Hepatitis B, and evidence indicates that infection rates and sequelae are high; yet the Hepatitis B vaccine has not been included in the national vaccination programme (it is available in only a few states). Some progress in bringing research results from bench to bedside has been made by the Department of Biotechnology, which has proposed the establishment of an Institution for Translation Research.

India is therefore currently faced with the problem of addressing the triple burden of communicable diseases, non-communicable diseases and nutritional problems, arising from demographic transitions, lifestyle changes and the continuing problem of the health consequences of the poverty and illness cycle. The Government of India is addressing reproductive and child health issues through the National Rural Health Mission. Alternative finance mechanisms, such as social insurance catering for the health needs of the underprivileged are being piloted for feasibility. The ICMR is undertaking a Risk Factor Surveillance Programme for non-communicable diseases, which is being allied with the national Integrated Disease Surveillance Programme. Intervention studies to improve neo-natal and child survival and for the prevention of sexually transmitted infections including HIV/AIDS are being carried out to identify implementation strategies. Research activities to identify suitable interventions to address these challenges form the thrust of research activities for the ICMR in India's Eleventh Five Year Plan (2007–2012).

Health research systems

Health is multi-dimensional: the health status of a population is an outcome of complex interactions between several sectors. Therefore, health research is not confined to research under various national health programmes or institutions under the Ministry of Health and Family Welfare, but also includes research under a large number of other government ministries/departments such as Science and Technology, Atomic Energy, Human Resource Development, Women and Child Development, and Social Welfare (see Figure 8.4). In addition, research is conducted by academic and research institutions, voluntary agencies and private institutions.

Meeting these challenges and national commitments to achieve goals set in the Health Policy, the Population Policy, the NRHM and the UN Millennium Development Goals requires an active

Figure 8.4   Indian government ministries undertaking research with health components

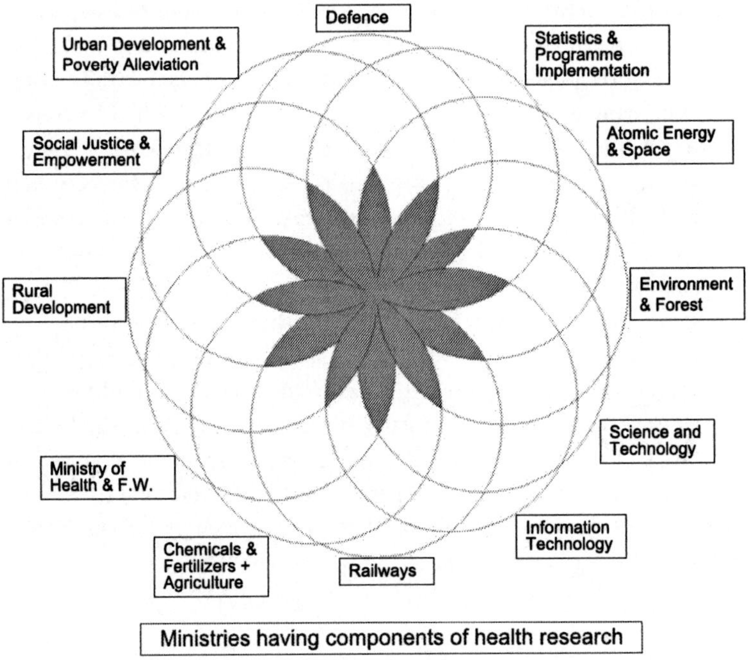

Defence

Urban Development & Poverty Alleviation

Statistics & Programme Implementation

Social Justice & Empowerment

Atomic Energy & Space

Rural Development

Environment & Forest

Science and Technology

Ministry of Health & F.W.

Information Technology

Chemicals & Fertilizers + Agriculture

Railways

Ministries having components of health research

Source: the authors.

health research system providing a scientific evidence base for the optimal delivery of health interventions. The health research system should be the "brains" behind practical health service delivery.

The Indian Council of Medical Research is the peak national bio-medical research institute. ICMR's research findings have found a place globally in the development of the Pulse Polio Control Strategy, establishing domiciliary and short-course chemotherapy for tuberculosis and making multi-drug therapy for leprosy more effective. At the national level, the research conducted has helped in several disease control programmes such as short-course chemotherapy for TB, supervised chemotherapy (now called DOTS) for TB, multi-drug therapy for leprosy, mass drug administration and morbidity management for filariasis, the operationalisation of oral rehydration therapy for diarrhoeal diseases, the development of strategies for the eradication of polio and the elimination of leishmaniasis and filariasis, recommended dietary allowances for Indians, the nutritional value of Indian food, vitamin A prophylaxis for children to prevent nutritional blindness, and iron and folic acid supplementation for pregnant women to address the high prevalence of anaemia.

Many of these research findings have been translated into reproductive health products, which have been introduced in the National Family Welfare Programme. For example, combined oral pills, the Centchroman oral weekly pill, intrauterine contraceptive devices (IUCD), CuT 380 A, Levonorgestrel emergency contraceptive as a back-up method, medical methods of safe abortion and Misoprostol for the prevention of post-partum haemorrhage have all been introduced. Others products have become marketed items, such as the injectable contraceptive NET-EN and the contraceptive TODAY pessary.

A study of the home-based management of newborn care (babies up to 60 days old), including simple interventions such as sepsis management delivered through an appropriately trained village-level worker, has indicated that, in situations where institutional delivery is not sought and the referral of sick babies is not possible, these simple interventions are feasible and acceptable to the community and would decrease the high morbidity and mortality associated with the newborn period.[25] In the long run, this could affect newborn and infant health as well as infant mortality rates.

Health research is carried out by organisations in both the public and the private sectors. In the years to come, prospective health research players must unite under an overarching umbrella representing all key stakeholders through the establishment of a National Health Research Management Forum, enabling India to support and sustain a health system that meets its goals and responds to people's needs.

Notes

1. World Health Organization, *World Health Report 2000: Improving Health Systems: Improving performance*, Geneva: WHO, 2000.

2. Registrar General of India, *Census of India 2001*, Delhi: Government of India, 2001; Registrar General of India, *Sample Registration System Bulletin*, 40(1), Delhi: Government of India, 2006.

3. Government of India, *Report of the Health Survey and Development Committee* (Chairman Sir Joseph Bhore), Delhi: Manager of Publications, 1946.

4. Ministry of Health and Family Welfare, *Report of the National Commission on Macroeconomics and Health*, Delhi: Government of India, 2005.

5. Ministry of Women and Child Development, *Annual Report 2005–06*, Delhi: Government of India, 2006.

6. Ministry of Health and Family Welfare, *Report of the National Commission on Macroeconomics and Health*; Ministry of Health and Family Welfare, *Annual Report 2005–06*.

7. Ministry of Health and Family Welfare, *Initiatives from Nine States*, Delhi: Government of India, 2004.

8. Ministry of Health and Family Welfare, *Report of the National Commission on Macroeconomics and Health*.

9. Registrar General of India, *Census of India 2001*.

10. R. Mishra et al. (eds), *Indian Health Report*, New York: Oxford University Press, 2005.

11. Ibid.

12. Ibid.

13. Ibid. See also Arvind Panagariya, "India: The Crisis in Rural Health Care", *The Economic Times*, 24 January 2008, <http://www.brookings.edu/opinions/2008/0124_health_care_panagariya.aspx> (accessed 21 June 2009).

14. Ministry of Health and Family Welfare, *National Rural Health Mission. Framework for Implementation 2005–12*, Delhi: Government of India, 2005.

15. "National Rural Health Mission(2005–2012): Mission Document", available at <http://mohfw.nic.in/NRHM/Documents/NRHM%20Mission%20 Document.pdf> (accessed 21 June 2009).

16. Registrar General of India, *Census of India 2001*; Registrar General of India, *Sample Registration System Bulletin*, 40(1), Delhi: Government of India, 2006; Ministry of Health and Family Welfare, *National Family Health Survey (NFHS) – III*, Delhi: Government of India, 2006.

17. For further information, see <http://biospectrumindia.ciol.com/> (accessed 24 June 2009).

18. N. K. Kumar et al., "Indian Biotechnology – Rapidly Evolving and Industry Led", *Nature Biotechnology*, 6(22), supplement, 2004, p. 31.

19. Ibid.

20. The Indian Council of Medical Research (ICMR) is one of the oldest research councils in the world. Established in 1911 as the India Research Fund Association it was renamed in 1950. Today it is an autonomous organisation fully funded by the Ministry of Health and Family Welfare, Government of India, and has an active network of 26 disease/discipline-specific Institutes (for example, leprosy, tuberculosis, malaria, pathology, cytology and preventive oncology, desert medicine, reproductive health, nutrition and occupational health) and over 70 field stations

in various parts of the country. For further information, see <http://www.icmr.nic.in/> (accessed 10 June 2009).

21. S. Ramji, R. Rasaily, P. K. Mishra, A. Narang, S. Jayam, A. N. Kapoor et al., "Resuscitation of Asphyxiated Newborns with Room Air or 100% Oxygen at Birth: A Multicentric Clinical Trial", *Indian Paediatrics*, 40, 2003, pp. 510–517.

22. Office of the Registrar General, *Sample Registration System. Maternal Mortality in India, 1997–2003: Trends, Causes and Risk Factors*, Delhi: Government of India, 2003.

23. India had some cases of severe acute respiratory syndrome (SARS), Avian flu and encephalitis resulting from the Chandipura and Nipah virus outbreaks, and diarrhoea cases due to new strains of V.cholerae 0139 Group B adult Rota virus and V.parahaemolyticus 03:K6. Besides emerging infections there is also a change in the spatial distribution of many infections, such as Japanese encephalitis, Chikungunya viral fever spreading from rural to urban areas, and dengue viral fever spreading from urban to rural areas, indicated by the increase in the reported cases and deaths annually.

24. Ministry of Chemicals and Fertilizers, *Annual Report 2005–06*, Department of Chemicals and Petrochemicals, Delhi: Government of India, 2006.

25. Ramji et al., "Resuscitation of Asphyxiated Newborns with Room Air or 100% Oxygen at Birth".

9

Health PPPs in India: Stepping stones for improving women's reproductive health care?

RAMA V. BARU AND MADHURIMA NUNDY

Introduction

A historical overview of the roles of the state and the market in Indian health services describes a mixed economy, with both influencing components such as financing, provisioning, human resources and pharmaceuticals. The financial crisis of the late 1970s resulted in a re-examination of the welfare state, leading to greater market involvement. The characteristics of the state–market mix have varied across regions and over time. Up to the 1970s the influence of markets was relatively small compared with that of the state, and mostly concerned primary-level provisioning. However, there was a shift in this trend through the 1980s and 1990s: market involvement burgeoned in secondary and tertiary levels of care, involving various types of providers ranging from single entrepreneurs to corporate enterprises. During the same period there was an acknowledgement of the crisis in public services and an explicit policy statement on the inability of the state to provide all the required services. The *National*

Partnerships for women's health: Striving for best practice within the UN Global Compact,
Timmermann and Kruesmann (eds),
United Nations University Press, 2009, ISBN 978-92-808-1185-8

Health Policy of 1982 defined roles for the private and voluntary sectors in health services by offering a variety of minor subsidies in the form of free supplies, honorariums and so on.[1]

The entire discourse shifted during the 1990s when the idea of public private partnerships (PPPs) became an important constituent of health policy in India and the rest of the world. The idea of PPPs was informed by new public management practices and techniques that emphasised a shift from traditional administration to public management focused on notions of economic efficiency in markets.[2] PPPs were seen to promote greater efficiency and improve the quality of public services at a time when these were at their lowest ebb.

This chapter seeks to review the experience of PPPs in the Indian health sector generally, with a special emphasis on women's reproductive health. It draws together available evidence on PPPs that captures the variation, both across regions and across levels of care; the interventions for which partnerships have been formed; the design of these partnerships; and the implications for equity, sustainability, replication and comprehensiveness.

Public private partnerships in health: An overview

Globally, PPPs in health are a phenomenon of the 1990s, and arose in the aftermath of market failures in the health sector.[3] The idea of PPPs, encouraged by new public management (NPM) techniques, was promoted across nations. In several developing countries, multilateral agencies such as the World Bank and other bilateral agencies actively promoted PPPs in national health programmes (NHPs) and health sector reforms. As Larbi argues:

A common feature of countries going down the NPM route has been the experience of economic and fiscal crises, which triggered the quest for efficiency and for ways to cut the cost of delivering public services. The crisis of the welfare state led to questions about the role and institutional character of the state. In the case of most developing countries, reforms in public administration and management have been driven more by external pressures and have taken place in the context of structural adjustment programmes.[4]

This kind of trend is clearly visible in the Indian context where the very idea of PPPs enters the health policy discourse as a part of conditionalities of World Bank funding for selected NHPs, which included the Reproductive and Child Health Programme and tuberculosis, leprosy, HIV/AIDS, malaria and blindness control.

A distinction needs to be drawn between the PPPs of the 1990s and earlier forms of non-governmental involvement in the NHPs. The need for non-governmental collaboration with the state in implementing national health programmes was articulated from the first Five Year Plan onwards. Initially, the government mostly sought programmatic support from non-governmental organisations (NGOs), but gradually this collaboration was extended to other primary, secondary and tertiary levels of health services.

A review of committee reports and other policy documents shows that there have been efforts to seek cooperation and enter into collaborative arrangements with the "for-profit" and "non-profit" sectors in health care. Until about the late 1970s most of these collaborations were with the "non-profit" sector, and it is only since the 1980s that one sees the "for-profit" sector gaining prominence in these ventures. The major areas of collaborations were NHPs that included disease control for malaria, tuberculosis and leprosy and the family planning programme. There is plurality in the nature of these collaborations across states but broadly these were restricted to providing curative and preventive services, mostly at the primary and secondary levels of care.

Among the various national programmes it is the family planning programme that has the maximum number of collaborations. Table 9.1 summarises the nature of the collaboration between the government and the private sector in addressing women's reproductive health over the various planning periods. Up to the Fifth Plan, the

Table 9.1   Collaboration between government and the
private sector in family planning and reproductive
and child health programmes in India

Five Year Plans	Components and levels of services rendered
First Plan (1951–1956)	• Establishment of antenatal and post-natal clinics run by NGOs • Licensing of private nursing homes for maternal and child health services
Second and Third Plans (1956–1961) (1961–1966)	• Government subsidies and grants given to states, local authorities, NGOs and scientific institutions for family planning clinics and research relating to demographic issues
Fourth and Fifth Plans (1969–1974) (1975–1977)	• NGOs integrate family planning as part of other health services extended to the community • Distribution of contraceptives and education • Proposal for, in urban areas, private practitioners to provide advice, distribute supplies and undertake sterilisations • Financial support from government to private practitioners and NGOs
Sixth Plan (1980–1984)	• Encouragement of private medical professional and non-governmental agencies to increase investment • Government offers organisational, logistical, financial and technical support to voluntary agencies active in the health field
Seventh Plan (1985–1990)	• NGOs involved in the extension of education about family planning • Continuation of scheme for assisting private nursing homes for family planning work • Increased emphasis on maternal and child health through supporting NGOs, village health committees and women's organisations
Eighth and Ninth Plans (1992–1997) (1997–2002)	• Encouragement of private initiatives and private hospitals • Continuation of NGO role

Table 9.1   (continued)

Five Year Plans	*Components and levels of services rendered*
Tenth Plan (2002–2007)	• Increased involvement of voluntary and private organisations, self-help groups and social marketing organisations in improving access to health care • NGO sector supports government in handling rural child health services, such as transport for emergency obstetric care where funds would be devolved to the village level • Preparation of information, education and communication material • Counselling services for adolescents and parents • Social marketing of contraceptives transferred to NGO sector
Eleventh Plan (2007–2012)	• Enhancing and experimenting with different systems of PPPs • Accreditation of private providers for attaining public health goals • Under the National Rural Health Mission and the National Urban Health Mission (NUHM), PPPs are being promoted to address public health goals. NUHM states that it would ensure partnerships with NGOs, charitable hospitals and other stakeholders • Adoption of PPP at secondary and tertiary levels of care • PPP for setting up diagnostic and radiological services for Central Government Health Services • Critical study of existing PPPs to see whether they fulfil the objective of equity

Source: Government of India, Planning Commission, Five Year Plan documents of various years.

main focus was on NGOs, which, at best, provided supplementary support to the public sector. The role of the for-profit sector was restricted to individual practitioners, mostly in urban areas.

Subsequently, increasing involvement of this sector demonstrates the shift in health policy during the Sixth Plan period, when there was an explicit recognition of the role of the for-profit and non-profit sectors to provide services.[5] For the first time the *National Health Policy* stated that:

> With a view to reducing governmental expenditure and fully utilising untapped resources, planned programmes may be devised, related to local requirements and potentials, to encourage the establishment of practice by non-governmental agencies, establishing curative centres and by offering organised logistical, financial and technical support to voluntary agencies active in the health field.[6]

It further stated that: "Planned efforts should be made to encourage private investments in such fields so that the majority of such centres, within the governmental set-up, can provide adequate care and treatment to those entitled to free care, the affluent sectors being looked after by paying clinics."[7] This legitimised the existence of a dual health service system characterised by private services for the affluent and government services for the poor. It was well recognised that programmes that had a substantial "public good" component required the for-profit and non-profit sectors and the government to enter into partnerships.

By the Seventh Plan, there appears a division of labour and role definition of the non-profit and for-profit organisations in PPPs. The role of the non-profit organisations focused largely on the social mobilisation of communities, the social marketing of devices such as intra-uterine devices (IUDs), providing information on programmes, counselling and ensuring follow-ups. The available evidence suggests that a small proportion of the "non-profit" category provided solely curative interventions in the form of sterilisation, insertion of IUDs and so on. This was essentially the domain of private providers in both rural and urban areas across primary and secondary levels of care.

The role of the for-profit sector gained further momentum in the late 1980s, when the government provided a variety of subsidies in terms of land, water and electricity at lower costs to private entrepreneurs for setting up "super speciality" institutions at the tertiary level. Tax concessions were offered for the import of advanced technology medical equipment, which fuelled the growth of these hospitals at the secondary and tertiary levels of care. This growth opened up opportunities for further public private partnerships at the secondary and tertiary hospitals in the better-developed states of Maharashtra, Gujarat, Tamil Nadu, Andhra Pradesh and Delhi.

Global processes influenced the design of PPPs in the Reproductive and Child Health Programme (RCH). Here, the deliberations of the International Conference on Population and Development (ICPD) in Cairo resulted in a paradigm shift in the approach to population policy in the developing world. There was a shift away from fertility control to the reproductive rights of an individual. Fertility control was to be addressed within the understanding of gender equality, with both men and women taking responsibility.[8] India was a signatory to the Cairo ICPD, and the RCH package was influenced by discussions at the conference. In fact, the ICPD document devotes a substantial section to the importance of PPPs in RCH services.[9] It defines NGOs' role in addressing the needs of marginalised groups, creating awareness, monitoring and advocating for women's reproductive health. The role of the for-profit sector was to include the production and delivery of reproductive health and family-planning commodities and contraceptives.

In order to facilitate implementation of the ICPD agreement, governments were strongly encouraged to set standards for service delivery and to review legal, regulatory and import policies. There was also a suggestion that governments must remove restrictions on the involvement of the private sector. These ideas gained currency in both global and national policies. Multilateral and bilateral agencies endorsed this view and built it into their policy mandates for funding programmes in developing countries. The Ninth and Tenth Plans in India reflect some of these trends, especially with regard to PPPs in the RCH Programme (see Table 9.1).

The National Rural Health Mission was launched in 2005 with the vision of improving public health services through increasing financing and provisioning. The RCH programme is one of the major components of the mission. A separate taskforce was set up under the Mission to examine the possibilities of PPPs. Partnerships have been established with NGOs under the RCH-II programme across 300 districts. The Eleventh Plan is influenced largely by the goals of the NRHM and the newly launched National Urban Health Mission and incorporates PPP in all aspects of health services and across levels. It acknowledges explicitly that partnerships with the private sector – both for-profit and non-profit – are important to attain public health goals and to improve the delivery system.

This review has provided an insight into the extent to which the private and non-profit sectors have always existed within the family planning programme over the past four decades. What started as minor collaborations have now increased in number and complexity; however, there is very little systematic information regarding the design of these collaborations from the plan documents. Based on available studies, we analysed some of the more recent collaborations, which are termed PPPs in RCH programmes. Both the RCH-I and RCH-II documents have defined the role and scope of the private and voluntary sectors in the areas of social marketing, information, education and communication (IEC), monitoring and service provisioning.[10]

Forms of partnership for health in India: A review of the evidence

Designs of PPPs for health care show that they are complex, involving a variety of institutions and actors across different regions, levels of care and socio-economic contexts (Table 9.2 and Figure 9.1). We find that the most prominent forms of PPPs at the primary level are

Figure 9.1   Pathways of partnerships

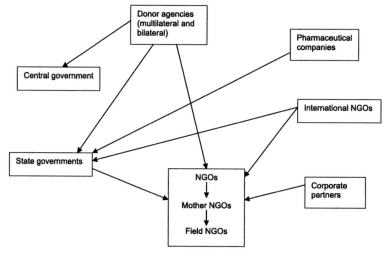

Source: the authors.

social marketing and the contracting-out of services. It is possible to discern some broad prototypes:

- contracting-out of facilities by the government to NGOs for either fully managing public institutions or partially managing a few services (normally non-clinical services);
- contracting-in of health professionals from the private sector to provide clinical services;
- social marketing that involves advocacy, providing information and marketing of products for prevention and curative purposes;
- social franchising.

Contracting

Both contracting-in and contracting-out operate at all levels of care, whereas social marketing and franchising are largely restricted to the primary level of provisioning. There are a few examples of primary health centres being contracted out to NGOs where the government

Table 9.2 Forms and designs of health PPPs in India

Type	States	Type of institution giving contracts	Services included under PPP	Design of PPP
1 Contracting-in and -out	Rajasthan, Jaipur	Tertiary teaching hospital	Drugstore	Hospital provides physical space, electricity, water and computers for the drugstore to the private operator
			CT scan/MRI services	Services given to a private agency. Agency is given a monthly rent, and must provide 20 per cent of services free
	Himachal Pradesh, Karnataka, Orissa, Punjab, Uttaranchal and Tripura, Maharashtra	Hospitals at secondary and tertiary level	Cleaning and maintenance of building, security, waste management, scavenging, laundry, dietary services, etc.	Cleaning and maintenance of hospitals contracted to Sulabh International in some states; dietary services in Bombay municipal hospitals and some government hospitals either contracted in or out
	Gujarat	National Disease Control Programme (State Malaria Control Society)	IEC services for malaria control	IEC budget from various pharmaceutical companies is pooled on a common basis and agencies hired by the private sector are allocated money for the development of IEC material through special sanction

| Tamil Nadu, Theni District | Non-governmental organisation (NGO) | Emergency ambulance services | This scheme is self-supporting through the collection of user charges. Government supports the scheme only by supplying the vehicles. The NGO recruits drivers, trains staff, maintains the vehicles, operates the programme and reports to the government. It bears the entire operating costs of the project, including communications, equipment and medicine, and publicising the service in the villages, particularly the telephone number of the ambulance service. However, the project is not self-sustaining in the longer term because revenue collection is less than anticipated. |
| Widespread in 439 districts | NGOs | Various rural child health services, capacity-building of field NGOs (FNGOs), conducting Community Needs Assessment, liaison, networking and coordination with state and district health services, *Panchayati Raj* institutions (PRIs) and other NGOs; monitoring performance and progress of FNGOs and documentation of best practices, advocacy and awareness generation. SNGOs provide an integrated package of clinical and non-clinical services directly to the community | The mother NGO (MNGO) and service NGO (SNGO) schemes are implemented by NGOs for population stabilisation and RCH. The MNGOs involve smaller FNGOs in the allocated districts. |

Table 9.2 (continued)

Type	States	Type of institution giving contracts	Services included under PPP	Design of PPP
	Gujarat, Karnataka	NGOs	Management of primary health centres (PHCs) in rural areas and urban health services	The government of Gujarat provided grants to an NGO to manage one PHC and three child health centres. The NGO provides rural health and medical services and manages the public health institutions. The NGO can accept employees from the district *panchayat* on deputation. It can also employ its own personnel by following the recruitment decision of either the government or the district *panchayat*.
				Management of PHCs in two districts contracted out by the government of Karnataka to an NGO in 1996 to serve the tribal community in the hilly areas. The costs are borne 90 per cent by the government and 10 per cent by the trust. It has full responsibility for providing all personnel at the PHC and the health sub-centres within its jurisdiction and for the maintenance of all assets at the PHC. The agency ensures adequate stocks of essential drugs at all times and supplies them free of cost to patients.

Delhi	NGO	Management of urban health services	As contractual partners, an NGO and the Municipal Corporation of Delhi (MCD) each have fixed responsibilities and provide a share of resources as agreed in a partnership contract. The NGO is responsible for organising and implementing services in the project area, while the MCD is responsible for monitoring the project. The MCD provides the building, furniture, medicines and equipment, while the NGO maintains the building and provides for water and electricity charges and the management of staff and medicines.
Andhra Pradesh	NGO	Urban Slum Health Centre Project	The Andhra Pradesh Ministry of Health and Family Welfare contracts NGOs to manage health centres in the slums of Adilabad. The basic objectives of the project are to increase the availability and utilisation of health and family welfare services, build an effective referral system, implement national health programmes and increase health awareness and better health-seeking behaviour among slum dwellers, thus reducing morbidity and mortality among women and children.

Table 9.2 (continued)

Type	States	Type of institution giving contracts	Services included under PPP	Design of PPP
	Gujarat (Chiranjivi experiment in five selected districts)	Private providers	Emergency obstetric care, transport, caesarean section, forceps delivery, ultrasonography, anaesthesia, blood, education to popularise the scheme	Federation of Gynaecologists and Obstetricians, empanelled private providers
	Andhra Pradesh	Charitable trust	Tuberculosis (TB)	The Trust Hospital acts as a coordinator, intermediary and supervisor between the government and private medical practitioners (PMPs). PMPs refer patients suspected of having TB to the hospital or to any of 30 specified neighbourhood Directly Observed Treatment (DOTS) centres operated by PMPs. The patients pay the fees to the PMPs.
	Rural Uttar Pradesh	Private sector	Sterilisation and IUD services, pre- and postoperative medicines, follow-up, transportation and reporting to district society	Government reimburses and district societies implement the programme through private institutions

	Madhya Pradesh, Bhopal	*Rogi Kalyan Samiti* (RKS) or patient welfare committee formed as a society. Its members are from local PRIs, NGOs, local elected representatives and government officials.	Secondary level hospital	RKS to manage a secondary level government hospital	RKS functions as an NGO and not a government agency. It may impose user charges. It may raise funds additionally through donations, loans from financial institutions and grants from government as well as other donor agencies. The funds received are available to be spent by the executive committee, constituted by the RKS or the Hospital Management Society. Private organisations could be contracted for the provision of super specialty care at a rate fixed by RKS. Through RKS, the hospital has also been able to provide free services to patients living below the poverty line.
	Bihar			Immunisation, managing HIV/AIDS, voluntary counselling, testing, DOTS, leprosy, RCH services	State, district hospital and charitable trust (part of London-based organisation)
II Social franchising	Bihar		Primary level (preventive and curative)	Janani scheme (mostly contraceptives and basic health services)	Mix of social franchising, marketing, outsourcing and external funding
III Social marketing	Several states		NGOs	Promotion and sale of contraceptives with subsidies for the products	SIFPSA, HLL, PSI, Hindustan Latex Family Planning Promotion Trust

Sources: V. B. Annigeri et al., *An Assessment of Public–Private Partnership Opportunities in India*, United States Agency for International Development/India, November 2004; Futures Group, "Contracting out Health Facilities in India", prepared for Policy Division of the Ministry of Health and Family Welfare, GOI, ITAP, IFPS II Technical Assistance Project, 2005; Government of India, "Draft Report on Recommendation of Task Force on Public Private Partnership for the 11th Plan", New Delhi: Planning Commission, GOI, 2006.

provides infrastructure, equipment and medicine and meets recurring expenses in varying proportions across states. Although some of these have been cited as example of "best practices", they have not been replicated in any significant way. This is because the necessary and sufficient conditions required for making these partnerships work are often lacking in other socio-economic and institutional contexts. There have been efforts to contract out primary-level facilities in both rural and urban areas to NGOs for the delivery of RCH services, as seen in the case of the Urban Slum Health Centre project in Vishakapatnam and Hyderabad, Andhra Pradesh.[11]

Another model of contracting is seen in parts of rural Uttar Pradesh between district societies,[12] the state Department of Health and Family Welfare, and private hospitals and nursing homes. The government reimburses private hospitals and nursing homes that provide sterilisation and IUD services. District societies implement the programme through funds allocated to them. The target group is the rural poor. Interested private providers sign a memorandum of understanding with the district societies covering service protocols, quality standards, roles and responsibilities. Once providers are selected, if training is needed it is provided by the district societies. The private providers provide free sterilisation and IUD services, including pre-operative investigations, postoperative medicines, follow-up visits and transportation, and they send periodic reports to the district society. Upon verification, the district society reimburses the provider the fixed amount depending on the service provided.

Gujarat has initiated PPPs through the Chiranjivi scheme, which covers services at the secondary level for deliveries. The scheme also provides emergency obstetric care and emergency transportation for poor pregnant women. The state government has entered into a partnership with selected private hospitals and also supports the hiring of private practitioners for government hospitals. The private provider submits an application that is forwarded to the health officer at the district level. A memorandum of understanding (MOU) and appointment letter are sent to the private provider. The beneficiary is registered with the auxiliary nurse midwife (ANM) from the relevant area for antenatal checks. The ANM informs the beneficiary of the papers required and prepares beforehand for transportation by alerting the local transport operator of the tentative date of delivery. The private providers are initially given a fee as soon as they are registered by the state. They are further reimbursed for their services on a monthly or fortnightly basis. The officers at the block and district level conduct monitoring of the private providers. The ANM receives feedback on the services delivered by the private provider to the beneficiary, and if there are discrepancies she has to report it to the officials. A modified version of this scheme has been implemented in one district of Tamil Nadu (for details see Table 9.2).

There are also several examples of contracting-out at the secondary and tertiary levels of care in terms of non-clinical services such as laundry, catering and cleaning. One such PPP involves the contracting-out of catering services by public hospitals in Mumbai.[13] The rationale for contracting-out was to minimise wastage and promote cost-effectiveness. The contractors for two hospitals were provided with space, water and electricity at fixed monthly charges, whereas the third contractor brought the prepared food in containers to the hospital. Two of the contractors employed their own staff, but the third had to use the hospital canteen staff. Another form of simple contracting that is evident at the tertiary level is the contracting-out of diagnostic services such as computed tomography (CT) scanning and magnetic resonance imaging (MRI) to a private agency.

Social marketing

Social marketing has been included in the RCH and malaria programmes. This includes the marketing of a variety of related products such as contraceptives (condoms, oral pills, injectables and IUDs), oral rehydration salts, safe delivery kits and mosquito nets for the malaria programme.[14] A specific case of social marketing has been implemented in rural Uttar Pradesh by the State Innovations in Family Planning Services Agency (SIFPSA), which is involved in the social marketing of contraceptives. SIFPSA has awarded performance-based contracts to several organisations for communications support and distribution of contraceptives. The Government of India provides contraceptives at a subsidised rate to SIFPSA's partners for distribution and sale. The private partners, such as Hindustan Latex Limited (HLL), Population Services International (PSI) and Hindustan Latex Family Planning Promotion Trust, have created standard sales distribution systems in their assigned areas. A distributor–retailer chain has been established and field personnel are employed to maintain this chain.[15]

Social franchising

Although social franchising is not widely prevalent, it has been tried in selected districts of Bihar, Uttar Pradesh and Andhra Pradesh under the RCH programme. There are a great many different models and we present some of these initiatives in order to capture the variations in design.

One of the frequently cited cases of franchising is that of Janani in Bihar.[16] Janani adopted a strategy of social franchising and social marketing of subsidised products to reach out to a wider population. It operates through a network of shops and other retail outlets (mainly in the urban area), rural health practitioners (RHPs) and health centres run by private medical practitioners. The rural health centres of the trained RHPs are called Titli (butterfly) Centres. Janani provides the centres with the logo of the butterfly and supplies them with its brand of contraceptives. It franchises selected RHPs, who provide a primary-level service, at an annual fee of Rs 300. At the secondary level there are well-equipped medical centres with medical personnel that serve as training centres for private medical practitioners and establish benchmarks for the standardisation of services. They provide clinical contraceptive services, abortion services up to 10 weeks and the treatment of reproductive tract infections and sexually transmitted infections. This model symbolises a mix of franchising, marketing, subsidies from international funders and the Indian government contracting-in and -out.

The major models of PPPs that have been reviewed show diversity in design scope and content. In India, the older and more complex of these partnerships occur mainly in states such as Andhra Pradesh, Bihar, Chattisgarh, Jharkhand, Uttaranchal, Uttar Pradesh, Gujarat, Madhya Pradesh and Rajasthan.

The scope of PPPs in women's reproductive health

The major objective behind PPPs is to increase efficiency and equity and to reduce bureaucratic interference in services, but there is insufficient evidence to assess whether this objective has been fulfilled. The parameters used for assessing these partnerships are diverse and often it is not possible to judge their effectiveness because of the varied contexts in which the partnerships occur. Thus, there is variation in terms of strengths, weaknesses, costs and the extent to which they address issues of equity, sustainability, scalability, coverage, equality of partnership and their impact on health outcomes. Based on an extensive review of PPPs in health, Annigeri et al. conclude that there are "strengths and weaknesses in each implementation intervention reviewed. These strengths and weaknesses vary from intervention to intervention based on the unique design of each."[17] Since these partnerships are so varied, it is difficult to draw firm conclusions about replication and scalability.

On the issue of equity, one finds that whereas services under some partnerships are able to reach out effectively to target groups such as the poor, in other cases the poorest may get left out because the services must still be paid for partially by the patient. This would certainly have negative consequences for equity, as social franchising experience has shown; the really poor are excluded from accessing services. Similarly, when services are contracted out there is typically a user fee instituted to recover costs. This, once again, could lead to the exclusion of the poorest, and these are concerns that the design of PPPs needs to examine and address. In our view, equity concerns in stratified societies and representation of the "voice" of the poor need to be kept in mind while evaluating and monitoring PPPs.[18] If the main objective of PPPs is improving "efficiency" and "equity"[19] then there is very limited evidence to point to the fulfilment of these objectives.

It is fallacious to assume that PPPs contribute to reducing bureaucratisation, which is a common criticism of the public system. In fact, studies on PPPs show that multifaceted capacities relating to technical and administrative inputs are necessary for selecting partners, formulating MOUs and monitoring these partnerships.

PPPs vary from simple to complex, depending on the interventions and the levels at which they operate. The important issues for design are: what services are rendered through the partnership, and how is the arrangement or memorandum of agreement spelled out and defined so as to make it transparent, accountable, equitable and scalable? The success of any PPP will depend on how well it has set up proper regulation and accreditation of the heterogeneous private providers (from a private medical practitioner to a hospital). Experience has shown that developing MOUs is extremely technical and may require legal expertise. This would require a much more systematic enquiry into the suitability of institutions and their adherence to treatment protocols and ethical guidelines. In most developing countries there are no overarching regulatory frameworks for the private sector and definitely none for PPPs. As a result, most partnerships are developed in an ad hoc manner. In the Indian context, the heterogeneity of the private sector, in terms of both regional variations and institutional forms, is a potential impediment to creating and sustaining partnerships.

All of this falls into the domain of additional and specialised technical inputs on the part of government that are not adequately accounted for when assessing financial and administrative efficiency. Prakash and Singh's study observes that:

> contracting out of healthcare services entails high transaction costs as it includes the costs of writing, negotiating and enforcing the agreement, information asymmetry, difficulty in defining and pricing the "product", opportunism, reduced flexibility of re-allocating resources, and limited entry and exit of providers.... Contracting distributes risk

and responsibility between the purchaser and the provider. Thus, it follows that high risk for the provider translates into higher price. Pricing is, therefore, a difficult decision in contracts.[20]

All these factors both directly and indirectly influence the budgets of PPPs, which may also be affected by the available levels of government subsidy, foreign funding to NGOs and the administrative costs incurred to initiate, sustain and monitor these partnerships.

The nature of the contractual arrangements and the number of players who can even qualify for selection to these partnerships are of serious concern. Given the unequal distribution of for-profit and non-profit organisations across the country, questions of with whom to partner and the duration of these contracts become debatable. These have further consequences for replication and scalability. As stated by Prakash and Singh: "Due to fragmented adoption of the approach, difficulties in measurement, market imperfections and the nascence of the private sector in many areas of healthcare, the experience of contracting-out health services is limited, ambiguous and more rhetorical than substantive."[21]

Although the best practices of PPPs are worthy in and of themselves, they cannot be replicated without considering whether the necessary and sufficient conditions are available to ensure success. In this regard, the variations in socio-economic and institutional contexts where the partnerships are formed have not received sufficient analysis. Best practices invariably focus on the technical details of the design rather than raising questions about the capacity and capabilities of the institution that is implementing the partnership or the socio-economic context in which the institution is situated.[22]

Ethical concerns for PPPs

Monitoring, accountability and transparency of partnerships are important issues for success. Since partnerships are built on notions of equality, associations between agencies with different values can

Box 9.1   Some ethical concerns

Global norms and principles: "there are no global norms and principals [*sic*], to set a framework within which global public health goals can be pursued in a partnership arrangement."

Legislative frameworks, policies and operational strategies: "many developed countries have legislation to interface with the private sector. However in the developing world, there is a general lack of overarching legislation relating to public-private partnerships. As a result, such arrangements develop on an *ad hoc* and opportunistic basis and may have questionable credibility; as a result of this failure, polices [*sic*] and specific operational strategies fail to develop."

Governance structures: "workable partnerships require a well-defined governance structure ... to allow for distribution of responsibilities to all the stakeholders. Public-private partnerships may run into problems because of ill-defined governance mechanisms."

Power relationships: "skewed power relationships are a major impediment to the development of successful relationships. Governments in developing countries usually tend to assume core responsibility of the joint initiative and take charge of the weaker partner. In case of NGOs with outreach-related strengths, this usually takes the form of a 'contractual relationship' without much regard to the participatory processes, which should be key to a public-private partnership arrangement. In case of relationships with NGOs with technical strength, there are issues relating to power relationships of a more serious nature with regard to who assumes the leadership role."

Criteria for selection: "the criteria for selection are an important issue both from an ethical and process-related perspective as it raises the questions of competence and appropriateness. In many instances the public sector is vague about important issues related to screening potential corporate partners and those in the non-profit sector."

Source: S. Nishtar, "Public–Private 'Partnerships' In Health – A Global Call to Action", *Health Research Policy and Systems*, 2(5), 2004; available at <http://www.health-policy-systems.com/content/2/1/5> (accessed 18 June 2009).

raise ethical dilemmas. Very often the partners are not held accountable for the quality of the services delivered, sometimes because the MOU does not detail the required parameters or because monitoring is inadequate. In addition, even when services are not up to the mark, there is a lack of clarity as to how they can be rectified and made accountable. We agree with Nishtar that "[t]o hold partners accountable for their actions, it is imperative to have clear governance mechanisms and clarify partner's rights and obligations. Clarity in such relationships is needed in order to avoid ambiguities that lead to break up of partnerships."[23]

There is serious concern regarding monitoring and ensuring accountability because, technically, a partnership is meant to be between two equals, yet there is tension between the government and the private players. The latter often sense that they are mistrusted by the former, resulting in a situation in which they feel "policed". Some NGOs that have entered into partnerships in health have commented that the government wants them to motivate communities to accept programmatic interventions but, when shortcomings of the programme are pointed out, the government tends to play the role of "big brother". This is extremely frustrating because there is no semblance of equality or trust in these partnerships.[24]

It is well acknowledged in the literature on PPPs that there is tension in opposing values:

> Many partnerships are initiated on the premise that they fulfill a social obligation, and can involve good intentions on the part of individuals and organisations. However the basic motive that drives the "for-profit" sector *demands* that these involve a financial pay-off in the long term. In such cases, the difference between corporate sponsorships and philanthropic donations with long-term visible public health goals needs to be clearly separated. This issue has been further complicated in recent years as many global health initiatives funded by endowments generated by foundations have partnerships with the private sector as a key feature ... Such donor-recipient relationships ... include concerns relating to such arrangements providing the "for profit" private sector an opportunity to improve their organisational image by engaging in cause-related marketing and concerns relating to these engagements

facilitating access of the commercial sector to policy makers. On the other hand, many NGOs even in the developing countries are little more than lobby groups with a particular interest, which may or may not be aligned to public good.[25]

Therefore, keeping the heterogeneity of the private, non-profit sector in mind, motivations and objectives may vary across these two sets of institutions. There are inherent tensions characterised by opposing values in these partnerships. This needs to be kept in mind when defining the choice of institutions and reducing these tensions by ensuring that they are explicitly addressed in MOUs.

Fragmentation of national health policies

There are also concerns that partnerships redirect national and international health policies and priorities. PPPs tend to aim for short-term high-profile goals and focus on a set of specific interventions. As a result, they may be seen to obstruct a comprehensive approach to health service development.

> If public-private partnerships are not carefully designed, there is a danger that they may reorient the mission of the public sector, interfere with organizational priorities, and weaken their capacity to uphold norms and regulations. Such a shift is likely to displace the focus from the marginalized and may therefore be in conflict with the fundamental concept of equity in health.[26]

This has been further exemplified by the global PPPs for disease control in the World Health Organization (WHO), where there is concern that the global agenda influences funding to national governments, which in turn disrupts a comprehensive approach to planning. The recent debates on the Polio Eradication Programme in India are a case in point.[27]

Based on the available evidence, there are obvious drawbacks for sustainability, replication and equity. First, despite the attention that PPPs have received, the administrative and technical inputs required for initiating, sustaining and monitoring these initiatives are still embryonic. Secondly, criteria for the registration and regulation of private and voluntary players are a necessary precondition for initiating a partnership. Thirdly, there is a need to assess the socio-economic and institutional prerequisites for the partnership to succeed. Lastly, the most important aspect is the monitoring of these partnerships to ensure that equity is not compromised and that the MOU addresses this aspect adequately. Our analysis shows that the process of forming and sustaining a partnership requires various forms and levels of preparedness, including the societal, institutional, administrative and technical. Therefore PPPs can, at best, play only a supplementary role to government in women's reproductive health services.

Acknowledgements

We are grateful to Ranjana Kumar, J. P. Mishra, K. B. Singh, Ellora Guhathakurtha and Sangeeta Singh for helping us gain access to documents and papers.

Notes

1. Government of India (GOI), *National Health Policy*, New Delhi: Ministry of Health and Family Welfare, 1982.
2. G. A. Larbi, "The New Public Management Approach and Crisis States", Discussion Paper No. 112, United Nations Research Institute for Social Development, New York, 1999.
3. Market failures in health were widely debated during the 1980s when policies of blanket privatisation proved to have negative consequences for health outcomes, access and utilisation of health services across developed and developing countries. For example, see Giovanni Cornia, Richard Jolly and Frances Stewart, *Adjustment with a Human Face. Volume 1: Protecting the Vulnerable and Promoting Growth*, Oxford: Clarendon Press, 1987. As a response to these various debates, there was a redefinition of the role of

markets and states in policy discourses. It was argued that states must play an important role in providing preventive services, while markets would provide the curative component. The World Bank's *World Development Report 1993: Investing in Health* (New York: Oxford University Press, 1993) articulates this position clearly, providing the conceptual framework for PPPs.

4. Larbi, "The New Public Management Approach and Crisis States", p. iv.

5. Government policy sought to encourage private practitioners to settle in rural areas, so their services could supplement government efforts in rural health. The Andhra Pradesh government, for example, initiated a scheme under which some allowance was provided to medical practitioners who settled in a village where there was no doctor and where they provided a part-time service at the nearest sub-centre. The Tamil Nadu government adopted the Mini Health Centre Scheme under which financial assistance was supplied to NGOs providing medical care facilities at the village level through doctors employed on a part-time basis. These experiences were seen as steps to promote the settling of doctors in rural areas (GOI, *Sixth Five Year Plan*, New Delhi: Planning Commission, 1980).

6. Government of India (GOI), *National Health Policy*, New Delhi: Ministry of Health and Family Welfare, 1982, p. 8.

7. Ibid.

8. For further elaboration, see the "Introduction" in M. Rao (ed.), *The Unheard Scream: Reproductive Health and Women's Health in India*, New Delhi: Zubaan and Panos Institute, 2004.

9. For more details, see United Nations, *Report of the International Conference on Population and Development, Plan of Action*, Chapter XV, New York: United Nations Population Information Network, 1994; available at <http://www.un.org/popin/icpd2.htm> (accessed 18 June 2009).

10. RCH-I and RCH-II have been supported by "soft loans" from the World Bank and also bilateral agencies. For details regarding the role of PPPs, see GOI, *RCH Phase II: National Program Implementation Plan*, New Delhi: Ministry of Health and Family Welfare, 2005.

11. The Urban Slum Health Centre Project in Andhra Pradesh was started in 2001 as an extension of the Indian Population Project and is funded by the World Bank. Under PPP, 192 urban health centres (UHCs) have been set up in 72 urban municipalities to provide primary-level curative, preventive and promotive services to the urban poor. The focus is on providing proper referrals when required and on maternal and child health by providing comprehensive antenatal care, institutionalised deliveries and immunisation for children. Community participation and social mobilisation are two other activities taken up by the UHCs. To manage the UHCs, 192 NGOs have been hired across the state. The UHCs are either rented or owned by the Andhra Pradesh government. NGOs were chosen by a selection committee at the district level and a UHC was contracted to an NGO for a year. Staffing norms are set by the government so the number of employees and their salaries are fixed. Hiring of staff is on a contract basis. NGOs retain the power to ensure good-quality health care provision from employees and

to not renew the contracts of those performing poorly. UHC doctors are hired on a part-time basis. The major cost of running the UHC is directly borne by the government in the form of the building, furniture, equipment, drugs and supplies. It provides each NGO with an annual budget of Rs 280,000 for salaries and other operational costs. For each UHC, a 15-member women's group from the community is to be formed to mobilise the community and create awareness about maternal and child health. The major concern regarding this model was salaries, which were lower than regular government scales. Other than this project, there has also been contracting-out of rural primary health centres to NGOs in several states. World Bank, *Project Appraisal Document: Reproductive and Child Health II*, Vol. 1, Report No. 28237-IN, Human Development Sector Unit South Asia Region, 2006.

12. District-level societies in national programmes have been constituted primarily to ensure the smooth flow of funds to the local level, monitoring, and accountability and transparency.

13. M. Bhatia and A. Mills, "Contracting out of Dietary Services by Public Hospitals in Bombay", in S. Bennett et al. (eds), *Private Health Providers in Developing Countries: Serving the Public Interest?*, London and New Jersey: Zed Books, 1997, pp. 250–263.

14. V. B. Annigeri et al., *An Assessment of Public–Private Partnership Opportunities in India*, United States Agency for International Development/India, November 2004, <http://pdf.usaid.gov/pdf_docs/PNADC694.pdf> (accessed 18 June 2009).

15. Ibid.

16. Janani was registered as a non-profit organisation in 1995 and started working in Bihar in 1996. It operates in the field of family planning by providing contraceptives and sexual and reproductive health services, such as counselling (including HIV/AIDS prevention); educational packages on relevant issues of reproductive health; pregnancy testing; treatment of reproductive tract infections and sexually transmitted infections.

17. Annigeri et al., *An Assessment of Public-Private Opportunities in India*, p. 42.

18. District societies in RCH and TB programmes are seen as effective mechanisms for ensuring people's voices are adequately represented. However, studies tend to show that the membership composition of district societies reflects the social, economic and political hierarchies of the community and results in the exclusion of the voices of the poor. The very definition of "poor" is complex. Sociologically, caste, class and gender are heterogeneous. Other studies use differentials to identify groups as "not so poor", "poor" or "very poor".

19. Mills and Broomberg review the contracting of health services in developing countries and find very little data on the impact of these contracts on efficiency and equity. See A. Mills and J. Broomberg, "Experiences of Contracting Health Services: An Overview of Literature", Working Paper 01, Health Economics and Financing Programme, LSHTM, London, 1998.

20. G. Prakash and A. Singh, "Outsourcing of Healthcare Services in Rajasthan: An Exploratory Study", paper presented at the conference on Global

Competitiveness through Outsourcing: Implications for Services and Manufacturing, Indian Institute of Management Bangalore, India, 13–15 July 2006.

21. Ibid.

22. David Mosse discusses how project designs tend to focus much more on technical aspects than on acknowledging the political and institutional contexts. D. Mosse, *Cultivating Development: An Ethnography of Aid Policy and Practice*, New Delhi: Vistaar Publications, 2005.

23. S. Nishtar, "Public–Private 'Partnerships' in Health – A Global Call to Action", *Health Research Policy and Systems*, 2(5), 2004, p. 5; available at <http://www.health-policy-systems.com/content/2/1/5> (accessed 18 June 2009).

24. Based on discussions with the Mahila Samakhya Programme, National Resource Group Meeting, New Delhi, 2005.

25. Nishtar, "Public–Private 'Partnerships' in Health", p. 3; M.R. Reich, "Introduction: Public-Private Partnerships for Public Health", in M. R. Reich (ed.), *Public-Private Partnerships for Public Health*, Cambridge, MA: Harvard University Press, 2002. Also see Martina Timmermann, "Meeting the MDG Challenges of Women's Health, Human Rights and Health Care Politics: The 'Women's Health Initiative (WHI) for Improving Women's and Girls' Reproductive and Maternal Health in India'", in C. Raj Kumar and D. K. Srivastava (eds), *Human Rights and Development: Law, Policy and Governance*, Hong Kong: LexisNexis, 2006, pp. 475–493.

26. Nishtar, "Public–Private 'Partnerships' in Health", p. 3.

27. See P. Yash, "Polio Eradication Programme: A Failure", *Economic and Political Weekly*, 41(43 and 44), 2006, pp. 4538–4540.

Bibliography

Allison, C. J. and V. R. Muraleedharan (2004) *Reproductive and Child Health (Phase 2) Programme India: Towards a Comprehensive Sector (Private-Public) Approach*, London: DFID Health Systems Resource Centre.

Annigeri, V. B., et al. (2004) *An Assessment of Public–Private Partnership Opportunities in India*, United States Agency for International Development/India, November.

Baru, R. V. (1998) *Private Health Care in India: Social Characteristics and Trends*, New Delhi: Sage Publications.

Bhat, R. (2000) "Issues in Health: Public-Private Partnership", *Economic and Political Weekly*, 35(52), pp. 4705–4716.

Baru, R. V. (2005) "The National Rural Health Mission and Public-Private Partnerships", *Journal of Health and Development*, 1(4), pp. 19–22.

Bennett, S. et al., eds (1997) *Private Health Providers in Developing Countries: Serving the Public Interest?*, London and New Jersey: Zed Books.

Bhatia, M. and A. Mills, (1997) "Contracting out of Dietary Services by Public Hospitals in Bombay", in S. Bennett, et al. (eds), *Private Health Providers in Developing Countries: Serving the Public Interest?*, London and New Jersey: Zed Books, pp. 250–263.

Caldwell, J. and P. Caldwell, (1986) *Limiting Population Growth and the Ford Foundation Contribution*, London: Frances Pinter.

Cornia, G., et al., eds (1987) *Adjustment with a Human Face. Volume 1: Protecting the Vulnerable and Promoting Growth*, Oxford: Clarendon Press.

Futures Group (2005) "Contracting out Health Facilities in India", prepared for Policy Division of the Ministry of Health and Family Welfare, GOI, ITAP, IFPS II Technical Assistance Project.

Government of Gujarat (2006) "Chiranjivi Yojna", unpublished document.

Government of India (1951, 1956, 1961, 1966, 1980, 1985, 1992, 1997, 2002) *Five Year Plan*, New Delhi: Planning Commission, GOI.

Government of India (1982) *National Health Policy*, New Delhi: Ministry of Health and Family Welfare.

Government of India (2005) *RCH Phase II: National Program Implementation Plan*, New Delhi: Ministry of Health and Family Welfare.

Government of India (2006) "Draft Report on Recommendation of Task force on Public Private Partnership for the 11th Plan", New Delhi: Planning Commission, GOI.

Government of India and European Commission (1999), "Situational Analysis of District Level Management Societies", ECTA Situational Analysis 1999/14, New Delhi.

Kanjilal, B. (2004) "Private-Public Collaboration in Providing Reproductive and Child Health Care in India", in N. S. Badri et al. (eds), *Population Policy of India: Implementation Strategies at National and State Levels*, New Delhi: Sterling Publishers.

Kavadi, S. N. (1999) *The Rockefeller Foundation and Public Health in Colonial India 1916–1945: A Narrative History*, Pune/Mumbai: Foundation for Research in Community Health.

Larbi, G. A. (1999) "The New Public Management Approach and Crisis States", Discussion Paper No. 112, United Nations Research Institute for Social Development, New York.

Mills, A. and J. Broomberg (1998) "Experiences of Contracting Health Services: An Overview of Literature", Working Paper 01, Health Economics and Financing Programme, LSHTM, London.

Nishtar, S. (2004) "Public–Private 'Partnerships' in Health – A Global Call to Action", *Health Research Policy and Systems*, 2(5); available at <http://www.health-policy-systems.com/content/2/1/5> (accessed 18 June 2009).

Prakash, G. and A. Singh (2006) "Outsourcing of Healthcare Services in Rajasthan: An Exploratory Study", paper presented at the conference on Global Competitiveness through Outsourcing: Implications for Services and Manufacturing, Indian Institute of Management Bangalore, India, 13–15 July.

Reich, M. R. (2002) *Public-Private Partnerships for Public Health*, Cambridge, MA: Harvard Series on Population and International Health, Harvard Center for Population and Development Studies.

Sathyamala, C., et al. (2005) "Polio Eradication: Some Concerns", *Economic and Political Weekly*.

Smith, E., et al. (2001), *Working with Private Sector Providers for Better Health Care: An Introductory Guide*, London: London School of Hygiene and Tropical Medicine and Options.

Timmermann, M. (2006) "Meeting the MDG Challenges of Women's Health, Human Rights and Health Care Politics: The 'Women's Health Initiative (WHI) for Improving Women's and Girls' Reproductive and Maternal Health in India'", in C. R. Kumar and D. K. Srivastava (eds), *Human Rights and Development: Law, Policy and Governance*, Hong Kong: LexisNexis.

United Nations (1994) *Report of the International Conference on Population and Development, Plan of Action*, Chapter XV, New York: United Nations Population Information Network; available at <http://www.un.org/popin/icpd2.htm> (accessed 18 June 2009).

World Bank (2006) "Project Appraisal Document: Reproductive and Child Health II", vol. 1, Report No. 28237-IN, Human Development Sector Unit South Asia Region.

10

Pro-poor capacity-building in India's women's health sector

ARABINDA GHOSH

Introduction

Reducing poverty is the fundamental objective of economic development. In 2001, more than 1 billion people in the developing world
lived in poverty. Poverty has many faces, changing from place to
place and across time, and has been described in many ways. The
World Health Organization (WHO) stated in 1999 that poverty
must be addressed in all its dimensions, not income alone, because
the resulting inequalities in health outcomes are stark. For example,
the under-five mortality rate is five times higher for people who are
living in absolute poverty than for those in higher income groups.
Further, those living in absolute poverty are two-and-a-half times
more likely to die between the ages of 15 and 59, and in parts of
sub-Saharan Africa, where almost 50 per cent of the population live
in absolute poverty, the lifetime risk of dying in pregnancy is 1 in 12,
compared with 1 in 4,000 in Europe.[1]

Among the poor, women are more vulnerable in terms of access to
resources. The present scenario of women in most of the developing
countries corroborates the collective household model,[2] which helps

Partnerships for women's health: Striving for best practice within the UN Global Compact,
Timmermann and Kruesmann (eds),
United Nations University Press, 2009, ISBN 978-92-808-1185-8

to explain why gender inequalities persist even though household income increases over time. Under this model, the welfare of individual household members is not synonymous with overall welfare, but depends on their relative bargaining power for resources within the collective. Bargaining power is determined not only by social and cultural norms but also by such external factors as opportunities for paid work, laws governing inheritance and control over productive assets and property rights.[3]

This chapter examines the multidirectional relationship between poverty, poor health and illiteracy and attempts to formulate a strategy to build capacity for improving the reproductive health status of women. The reproductive health status of Indian women provides a particular focus for this study. The chapter identifies factors influencing safe delivery and ranks these according to their relative importance.

The discussion is arranged in four sections. The first section provides a background to the study and a brief review of existing relevant studies in this area, along with a snapshot of the relationship between economic growth and human development and the multidirectional relationships between poverty, poor health, illiteracy, women and reproductive health. The second section explains the data and methodology adopted in the construction of a model to examine factors influencing safe child delivery. The third section highlights the results, and conclusions are drawn in the final section, highlighting possible areas for intervention.

Background

There is a close relationship between poverty and poor health. The poorest people in every society usually experience higher levels of child and maternal mortality. The low capabilities of the poor individuals (low nutritional status, marginal living and hazardous working conditions), coupled with poor access to health services, mean that poor health shocks are experienced more often.[4] Owing to inadequate social security provisions, poor people are vulnerable to these shocks and tend to experience temporary welfare losses.[5]

Inequality and powerlessness are increasingly seen as being important root causes of poor health. This has gender implications because women are commonly less powerful than men in their societies and communities. Lack of self-esteem and poor education may lead to women being unaware that they are suffering from a health condition that could successfully be treated, particularly with reproductive health problems.[6] In India, the perceived need for medical help is determined partly by socio-cultural factors governing how pain and discomfort are expressed, how symptoms of illness are recognised; and which symptoms are perceived to warrant medical care. Women typically have little autonomy, living under the control of first their fathers, then their husbands and finally their sons.[7]

Economic growth and human development

The purpose of development is to improve the quality of life. An improved quality of life in the world's poor countries generally calls for higher incomes – not as ends in themselves but as a means for acquiring human well-being. However, development requires other things as well, such as higher standards of health and nutrition, better education, more equality of opportunity, political freedom, personal security, community participation and guaranteed human rights.

Although economic growth fulfils the necessary condition for human development, if the distribution of income is unequal and if social expenditures are low or distributed unevenly, quality of life may not improve much, despite rapid growth of gross national product (GNP). There is no automatic mechanism linking economic growth and human development. Some developing countries have been very successful in managing growth to improve human conditions, others less so. The exact process through which growth translates, or fails to translate, into human development under different developmental conditions is a matter of great concern in development economics.

The human development experience in various countries during the past three decades reveals three broad categories of performance. First are countries that sustained their success in human development, sometimes achieved very rapidly, sometimes more gradually, as in Botswana, Costa Rica, the Republic of Korea, Malaysia and Sri

Figure 10.1   Similar income, different Human Development Index (HDI)

| GDP per capita (US$) | HDI | Life expectancy | Adult literacy (%) |

Venezuela values: 3,489; 0.772; 72.9; 93.0
South Africa values: 3,326; 0.658; 48.4; 82.4

--•-- Venezuela   --*-- South Africa

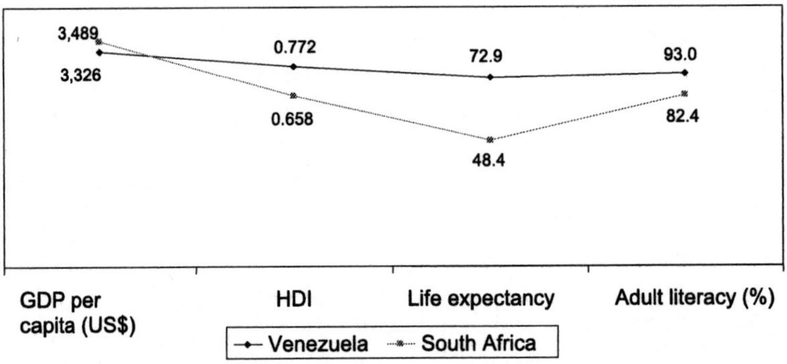

Source: Developed from data available in United Nations Development Programme, *Human Development Report, 2006: Beyond Scarcity: Power, Poverty and the Global Water Crisis*, New York: Palgrave Macmillan, 2006.

Lanka. Second are countries where initial success slowed down significantly or sometimes even reversed, as in Chile, China, Colombia, Jamaica, Kenya and Zimbabwe. Third are countries that had good economic growth but did not translate it into human development, as in Brazil, Nigeria and Pakistan.

For example, Figure 10.1 shows that Venezuela and South Africa have similar incomes but a different Human Development Index (HDI). GDP per capita for Venezuela and South Africa is similar, but life expectancy in Venezuela is 72.9 years, compared with 48.4 years in South Africa. The adult literacy rate is also higher in Venezuela. As a result, the HDI in Venezuela is much higher than that in South Africa, though they have similar per capita income.

Poverty and health

Table 10A.1 (in the appendix to this chapter) indicates the number of people living on less than US$1 a day. Of the world's total poor, 39.5 per cent live in South Asia and 32.8 per cent live in India, which makes that country a focus of major international concern. Interna-

Figure 10.2   Multidirectional relationships between poverty, ill health and illiteracy

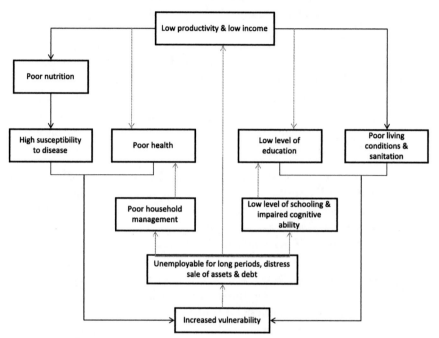

Source: the author.

tional concern is also reflected in the first UN Millennium Development Goal (MDG), which calls for the development community to reduce the global rate of extreme income poverty, measured by the share of the population living on less than US$1 per day, by half between 1990 and 2015.

Still, the relationship between poverty and poor health is not a simple one. It is multifaceted and bi-directional. Poor health can be a catalyst for poverty spirals and, in turn, poverty can create and perpetuate poor health status. The relationships work in both directions. As with poverty, poor health has an effect on both the individual and the household, and may have repercussions for the wider community, too.[8] Figure 10.2 illustrates these complex relationships.

Low productivity and low income lead to low nutrition. Low nutrition makes the poor highly susceptible to disease. In addition, low income leads to poor living conditions and sanitation facilities. These in turn increase the vulnerability of the household. The wage earner in the family remains unemployable for longer periods owing to frequent and prolonged illness. Increased vulnerability to disease may also compel a distress sale of assets, leading to indebtedness. As a result, productivity and income are further reduced. "The capabilities of poor individuals (low nutritional status, hazardous living and working conditions, inability to afford to adequately treat illness) mean that ill-health shocks are more often repeated for poor individuals."[9]

By illustrating how poverty, health and education are interlinked, the model in Figure 10.2 allows us to identify appropriate entry points to break the spiral. Improved health contributes to economic growth in various ways: it reduces production losses caused by prolonged illness; it not only enhances the enrolment of children in school but also makes them better able to learn; and it provides the opportunity for alternative uses of resources that would otherwise have to be spent on treating illness.[10] Households with more education enjoy better health, both for adults and for children. This result is strikingly consistent in a large number of studies, despite differences in research methods, time periods and population samples.[11]

Literacy and health

In most households, women have the main responsibility for a broad range of activities that affect health. They manage household chores, keep the house clean, process foods and prepare meals, feed and care for young children, and look after the sick. Education greatly strengthens women's ability to perform their vital role in creating healthy households. It increases their ability to benefit from health care access and to make good use of health services. The strength of this observed association has led to the suggestion that even the direct effect on mortality rates of doubling everyone's income, providing every household with a flush lavatory and piped water, and turning every agricultural labourer into a professional or white-collar worker would be less than the direct effect of providing 10 years of schooling for each woman.[12]

Health status is a very important part of human well-being. Several studies have shown that literacy and other measures of education are more closely correlated than per capita income with life expectancy.[13] In order to identify the importance of GDP per capita and female literacy in explaining variations in life expectancy at birth, a regression model was developed. The latest data relating to 166 countries as available in the *Human Development Report 2007/08* were used.[14] It was found that the standardised β values for GDP per capita and female literacy are 0.336 and 0.528, respectively. Standardised β values provide a better insight into the importance of a predictor of a model. The larger standardised β value of female literacy indicates the higher degree of importance of this variable.

Further, the t-test indicates whether the predictor is making a significant contribution to the model. The larger the value of t, the greater the contribution of that predictor. The regression model shows that GDP per capita [$t(160) = 5.680$, $p < .001$] and female literacy [$t(160) = 8.917$, $p < .001$] are both significant predictors of life expectancy at birth, but female literacy has more impact than GDP. An explanation for this relationship may be that education helps determine both the level of knowledge about how to combat disease and the instances in which this knowledge is transmitted and utilised.

From childhood, poor health and nutrition impair access to the benefits of education, particularly in three key areas: enrolment, ability to learn and participation by girls. Children who enjoy better health and nutrition during early childhood are more ready for school and more likely to enrol. Health and nutrition problems affect a child's ability to learn. Girls are particularly liable to suffer from iodine or iron deficiency – reasons why fewer girls complete primary school. Other health-related reasons for dropping out of school include pregnancy and parental concern about sexual violence. In societies where girls' education is given lower priority than boys', girls miss school because they have to stay at home to look after sick relatives.

Health, poverty and gender

According to WHO, there is no direct correlation between poverty and poor health for women. Until the benefits of economic growth are equally distributed, economic growth does not necessarily guarantee better health or higher status for all women.[15] Human development is a process of expanding the choices available to people. It is not limited to a section of the society. Economic growth can, in fact, become an unjust and discriminatory process in itself if most women are excluded from its benefits. Progress in literacy in India in the twentieth century suggests an illustration of this problem. In India, the literacy rate has increased since 1901, but the male–female gap in literacy also increased considerably until 1981.

It is now widely accepted that poverty elimination cannot be based on a narrow approach that relies solely on rising incomes or macro-economic growth. As the benefits of growth do not trickle down automatically to all households and to all household members, we need to address the gender differences and incidence of poverty in a contextualised way.

In less developed countries (LDCs), there is a preponderance of surviving men over surviving women, despite the biological advantages that women seem to have over men in survival and longevity. This is happening because of unequal treatment in the allocation of survival-related goods, such as nutrition, health care and medical attention. In developed countries, the situation is in sharp contrast. Whereas there are about 106 women per 100 men in Europe and North America, there are only 97 women per 100 men in the LDCs as a whole. Since mortality and survival are dependent on care and neglect and are influenced by social action and public policy, even this extremely crude perspective cannot fail to isolate gender as an important parameter in development studies.[16] In India, census data show that the trend in the sex ratio (the number of women per thousand men) since 1901 has also been one of decline.

Much of this discrepancy can be understood in the context of women's powerlessness and inequality, which are increasingly seen as important root causes of ill health. Gender inequity is the archetypal "inequality trap". The interaction of political, economic and socio-cultural inequalities shapes the institutions and rules in all societies. Therefore, inequality prevails everywhere – in income, in education and in health. Inequalities in health often translate to inequalities in other dimensions of welfare. The combined effects of gender inequality and poverty on nutrition lead to poor health for women and girls. Intergenerational transmission of poverty may occur through the under-nourishment/overwork of pregnant or lactating women. Furthermore, certain conditions of poor health may lead to women's social exclusion, incapacity and subsequent poverty, highlighting the importance of recognising cycles of poor health and poverty. It is important to recognise that women's health problems and access to health care are affected not only by poverty but also by gender inequality.[17]

Gender equality and reproductive health

Gender equality is a human right, one of the eight MDGs, and key to achieving the other seven. The UN Millennium Project concluded that reproductive health is essential to achieving the MDGs, including the goal of gender equality.[18] The leading cause of women's poor health and death worldwide is associated with reproductive health problems. When both women and men are taken into account, reproductive health conditions are the second-highest cause of ill health globally, after communicable diseases.[19] Reproductive health services enable individuals to decide freely and responsibly the number, spacing and timing of their children, and consequently to have greater control over their own destinies, including better opportunities to overcome poverty. Despite this, millions of people around the world are deprived of exercising their reproductive rights and safeguarding their reproductive health because of poverty and gender discrimination.

A survey on "Morbidity and Health Care" in India was undertaken by the National Sample Survey Organisation (NSSO) during the National Sample Survey (NSS) 60th Round (January–June 2004). This survey produced estimates of the prevalence of morbidity, termed Proportion of Ailing Persons (PAP) and measured as the number of persons reporting an ailment during a 15-day period per thousand persons within broad age groups. These are not strictly prevalence rates as recommended by the Expert Committee on Health Statistics of the WHO. The WHO defines a prevalence rate as the ratio between the number of spells of ailments suffered at any time during the reference period. The survey revealed that females suffered more than males, particularly in the reproductive age groups, though less in their childhood. This corroborates the statement of the UN Millennium project.

Every minute one woman dies needlessly of pregnancy-related causes. This adds up to more than half a million mothers lost each year – a figure that has hardly improved over the past few decades. Another 8 million or more suffer life-long health consequences from the complications of pregnancy. Every woman, rich or poor, faces a 15 per cent risk of complications around the time of delivery, but maternal death is practically nonexistent in developed regions. The lack of progress in reducing maternal mortality in many countries highlights the low value placed on the lives of women and testifies to their limited voice in setting public priorities. The lives of many women in developing countries could be saved with reproductive health interventions that people in rich countries take for granted.[20] Safe delivery plays the most significant role in ensuring women's health.

In India, the District Level Household Survey under the Reproductive and Child Health Project was conducted during 2002–2004 in 593 districts in accordance with 2001 census practice. Figure 10A.1 in the appendix to this chapter highlights the percentage of pregnant women having delivery complications in Indian states. It shows that 40.8 per cent of pregnant women in India had delivery complications, with the highest figures recorded in Bihar, followed by Maharashtra. The survey further revealed that only 18.7 per cent of childbirths took place in government hospitals and 21.8 per cent of childbirths took place in private hospitals. Therefore, the remaining 59.5 per cent of childbirths took place in the home. There is also a significant negative correlation between safe delivery and women having post-delivery complications. The correlation is −.398 (significant at the .01 level). Therefore, it is vital to ensure 100 per cent safe delivery.

However, this will be very difficult to achieve in the near future if we depend only on government hospitals. A study on the availability of primary health centres in the villages of West Bengal, an Indian state with a population over 80 million and reasonably good economic progress, shows that 30.4 per cent of the villages have no primary health centre within 10 km.[21] This varies from 10.2 per cent to 45.9 per cent between districts. In many situations, rural road conditions are poor. The lack of infrastructure restricts poor people's access to government hospitals. On the other hand, the cost of delivery of a baby in a private hospital can be as high as Rs 4,692, compared with Rs 1,111 in government hospitals.[22] Therefore, the high costs of childbirth in private hospitals renders this option unaffordable to the underprivileged. In the present circumstances, it is difficult to enhance government health infrastructure in a way that would increase considerably the number of childbirths in government hospitals, and it is a big challenge to achieve 80 per cent institutional deliveries and 100 per cent deliveries by trained persons, as envisioned in the National Population Policy 2000.

Methodology and database

Data

The present chapter uses the data set of the District Level Household Survey (DLHS) under the Reproductive and Child Health (RCH) interventions that are being implemented by the Government of India.[23] In Round 2, a survey was completed during 2002–2004 in 593 districts, in accordance with 2001 Census practice, and those data are used in this chapter. A systematic multistage stratified sample design was used for collecting data. A total of 620,107 households were interviewed, of which 415,135 households were in rural areas and 204,972 households were in urban areas. The overall household response rate was 99 per cent. In the interviewed households, interviews were completed with 507,622 currently married women (aged

15–44 years) who were a usual member of the household or had stayed the night before the household interview. 330,820 husbands were also interviewed. There were five questionnaires: (i) household questionnaire; (ii) women's questionnaire covering background characteristics, antenatal, natal and post-natal care, immunisation and child care, contraception, assessment of quality of government health services and client satisfaction, and awareness of reproductive tract infections (RTI) and sexually transmitted infections (STI) and of HIV/AIDS; (iii) husbands' questionnaire; (iv) health questionnaire; and (v) village questionnaire.

The main focus of the DLHS was on the following aspects: coverage of antenatal care (ANC) and immunisation services, proportion of safe deliveries, contraceptive prevalence rates, unmet need for family planning, awareness about RTI/STI and HIV/AIDS, utilisation of government health services, and users' satisfaction. District-wide data have been used for developing the model.

In this DLHS, every woman who delivered at least one child in the preceding three years of the survey was asked about the type of antenatal care and place of delivery. The full ANC comprises at least one tetanus toxoide (TT) injection, more than 100 iron and folic acid (IFA) tablets/syrup and at least 3 antenatal care visits. Safe delivery is defined as either institutional delivery at government or private hospitals, or home delivery assisted by a doctor, nurse or trained birth attendant. Data on the mean marriage age for girls, girls married below the legal age of 18 years, knowledge of any modern family planning methods and institutional delivery at government or private hospitals are also included. Data on women who had pregnancy complications, women who had delivery complications, women who had post-delivery complications, women visited by health workers, women who utilised government health facilities for antenatal care and women who utilised government health facilities for treatment of pregnancy complications have also been used.

In addition, the percentages of urban population, sex ratio, child sex ratio (0–6), percentage of scheduled caste and percentage of scheduled tribe, literacy rate, and female literacy rate have been gathered from the 2001 census report.[24]

Model

Each year about 430,000 women in developing countries die from complications associated with childbearing. In the absence of obstetric care, women who give birth before the age of 18 are three times as likely to die in childbirth as those who give birth between the ages of 20 and 29. India has set the legal age of marriage for girls at 18 years. Age of marriage has a strong influence on safe delivery outcomes.

The use of family planning services by couples is an effective means of avoiding many of the fertility-related health risks, and can enable families to achieve their fertility goals. Government can do much to help couples by promoting family planning as a socially acceptable practice, by providing information on the health effects of fertility regulation, by teaching couples about effective methods of contraception and by removing restrictions on the marketing of contraceptives.[25]

Maternal health care services utilised in reducing maternal morbidity and mortality have gained prominence in India since the Safe Motherhood Initiative of 1987 and following the 1994 International Conference on Population and Development (ICPD). The Safe Motherhood Initiative proclaims that all pregnant women must receive basic, professional antenatal care.

Ideally, antenatal care should monitor a pregnancy for signs of complications, detect and treat pre-existing and concurrent problems of pregnancy, and provide advice and counselling on preventive care, diet during pregnancy, delivery, post-natal care and related issues. In spite of these efforts and programmes, maternal and child health situations in the country have not improved to the desired level.

Therefore, in the present study, I have used a multilinear regression model to identify the social and other non-medical factors responsible for improving safe delivery. Data relating to 593 Indian districts have been used to explain the variations in the safe delivery resulting from changes in female literacy, the marriage age of girls, the number of eligible women with knowledge of all modern family planning methods and the number of eligible women who have received full antenatal care.

$$Y_i = \beta + \beta_1 X_{1i} + \beta_2 X_{2i} + \beta_3 X_{3i} + \beta_4 X_{4i} + u_i,$$

where

Y_i = percentage of safe deliveries (either institutional delivery or home delivery attended by doctor, nurse or trained birth attendant) in district i in the period 2002–2004.

X_{1i} = percentage of literate females in district i in the period 2002–2004.

X_{2i} = percentage of girls married below the legal marriage age of 18 years in district i in the period 2002–2004.

X_{3i} = percentage of eligible women with knowledge of all modern family planning methods in district i in the period 2002–2004.

X_{4i} = percentage of eligible women who have received full antenatal care (at least 3 visits for antenatal care + at least one TT injection + 100 or more IFA tablets/syrup) in district i in the period 2002–2004.

Results

The estimated model has the following values:[26]

$$Y = 21.881 + 0.461^{**} X_{1i} - 0.147^{**} X_{2i} + 0.064^* X_{3i} + 0.668^{**} X_{4i}.$$
$$\quad\;\; (8.057) \qquad (3.352) \qquad (2.357) \qquad\quad (4.797)$$

The model reveals that 59.5 per cent of the variation in safe delivery is accounted for by the estimated sample regression plane (SRP), which uses female literacy rate, percentage of girls married below the legal marriage age of 18 years, full antenatal care and knowledge of all modern family planning methods. It is found that safe delivery would increase by 4.61 percentage points for every 10 percentage point increase in female literacy. This is true only if the effects of girls married below the legal marriage age, knowledge of all modern family planning methods and full antenatal care are held constant. Similarly, every 10 percentage point fall in the proportion of girls married below the legal age of marriage would increase safe delivery by 1.47 percentage points, if other variables are held constant; and safe delivery would increase by 6.68 percentage points for every 10 percentage point increase in full antenatal care where the other variables are held constant.

To have better insight into the importance of a predictor in the model, the standardised β values are measured. This will help in formulating a strategy for pro-poor capacity-building in India's women's health sector. The standardised β values of female literacy rates, percentage of girls married below the legal marriage age, full antenatal care and knowledge of all modern family planning methods are 0.303, –0.119, 0.470 and 0.063, respectively. So the ranking of these predictors according to their relative importance in explaining safe delivery would be as follows: (1) for full antenatal care, (2) for female literacy, (3) for percentage of girls married below the legal marriage age of 18, and (4) for knowledge of all modern family planning methods.

The box plots based on these data (see Figure 10.3) illustrate the present scenario of women's reproductive health and selected predictors in the 593 districts of India. The box plot is a summary based on the median, quartile and extreme values, and represents the inter-quartile range, which contains the middle 50 per cent of the values.

The box plots show us the lowest value (the bottom horizontal line on each plot) and the highest value (the top horizontal line of each plot). Safe delivery is as low as 9.0 per cent in Phek district, Nagaland, and as high as 100 per cent in five districts of Kerala. The distance between the lowest horizontal line and the lowest edge of the tinted box is the range in which the values of the lowest 25 per cent of districts fall. In safe delivery, it is between 9.0 per cent and 37.2 per cent. The box (the tinted area) shows the percentage of safe deliveries in the middle 50 per cent of districts. The slightly thicker horizontal line in the tinted box represents the value of the median. The median value for safe delivery is 54.5 per cent. The distance between the top edge of the tinted box and the top horizontal line shows the range in which the values of the top 25 per cent of districts

**Figure 10.3   Present scenario of selected RCH programmes'
performance and female literacy**

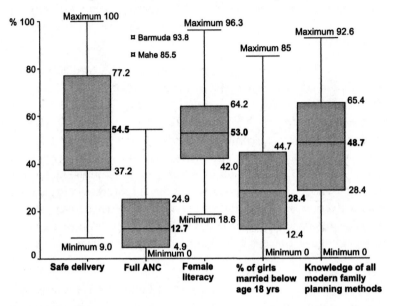

Source: the author.

fall. The range is 77.2 per cent to 100 per cent. In full antenatal care,
the distribution is skewed. Some circles above the box plot relating
to full antenatal care indicate outliers. It is evident that a minimal
number of women receive full antenatal care.

Conclusions

This discussion has focused primarily on capacity-building for improving the socio-economic conditions of poor women in India.
Reproductive child health plays an important role in the overall
improvement in women's health. Safe delivery reduces many post-
delivery complications, and in order to ensure safe delivery it is necessary to have significant improvement in the areas of full antenatal care,
female literacy, the percentage of girls married below the legal marriage age, and knowledge of all modern family planning methods.

It is now widely felt that, in the short term, it is quite impossible for the government alone to improve women's health in this way. In India, provincial governments have primary responsibility for population health, but most of these governments are currently undergoing serious financial crises.

In this context, the Planning Commission in India established a working group on public private partnerships to seek to improve health care delivery from the *Eleventh Five Year Plan* (2007–2012). In the working group's draft report, it is noted that the success of health care systems in Tamil Nadu and Kerala is not only a result of success in the public sector; the private sector, too, has made a useful contribution. However, because there is wide disparity in the availability of quality care at a reasonable cost from the private sector, the expansion of health care provision by non-profit sectors is necessary. For example, in designing and implementing innovative approaches to RCH services, collaborating with community-based organisations and non-governmental organisations (NGOs) is a significant step. These organisations often work in remote rural areas where access to RCH services is difficult.[27] Recent NGO policy development at the Ministry of Health and Family Welfare envisages a scheme where each district would have a "mother" NGO, linked to several more autonomous and decentralised field NGOs within the district.

Constructing an index for development

In general terms, however, progress in the social sector in India continues to be slow, and an urgent need remains to improve living standards, health, education, gender justice, welfare and the development of downtrodden people.[28] This is a key task for regional administrations and institutions, noting that decentralisation of governance processes in India has been strengthened by the 73rd amendment to the Indian Constitution. Here, three-tier *Panchayati Raj* institutions (PRIs)[29] have been revitalised as units of local self-government at district level and below. PRIs now have responsibility for framing policy and implementing socio-economic improvement programmes. One-third of the seats of office bearers in the PRIs have been reserved for women, and it is hoped that women's development in particular, and social development in general, will therefore get priority in the activities of the PRIs. However, various studies have shown that the presence of women alone has not always led to actual improvements, and, further, it has been revealed that, even at the grassroots level, market forces are influential in the success of development activities.[30] Making markets more people-friendly will require a strategy that maintains their dynamism but supplements this with other measures to allow many more people to capitalise on the advantages they offer. Further, to ensure human well-being, particularly of downtrodden peoples, special initiatives are required, and policy-makers at the grassroots level must recognise this.

The Human Development Index (HDI), developed by the United Nations Development Programme (UNDP), has made a significant contribution in drawing the attention of national leaders towards human well-being since 1990. The HDI measures average achievements in a country on three basic dimensions of human development: a long and healthy life; knowledge; and a decent standard of living. Subsequently, many countries have drawn on this to prepare national human development reports aimed at influencing policy-makers at sub-national level. It is now widely felt that India needs a development indicator for grassroots level organisations. This development indicator should be simple and easy to calculate, and be able to sensitise people to gender discrimination within the priority of meeting basic human needs. UNDP/India has begun to develop district-level human development reports but when the author took an effort, there had not been development of an index for Maternal and Child Health Care. To construct an index, to popularise and update it on a regular basis can assist in utilizing local resources in improving health in general, and women's health in particular.

Developing a model for convergence

Health infrastructure in poor countries is often limited in its ability to reach highly dispersed populations in rural areas. Although it is preferred that government systems play the major role in reproductive health service provision, there are limits to public sector outreach. At the margins of this outreach, increasing community and NGO involvement can be effective. Reproductive services provided through community-based distribution are a highly cost-effective means of improving maternal and child health.[31]

However, although community and NGO involvement in reproductive health service provision has proved to be successful in many cases,[32] there is wide disparity in their success and sustainability. Monitoring the performance is a major issue. A model is needed whereby government, community and NGO activities may converge and be coordinated to sustainably improve women's reproductive health care. Such a model will serve as a framework of reference for the monitoring, sustainability and replicability of the programme.

Capacity-building through women's self-help groups

Capacity-building amongst women themselves is also essential. Women's self-help groups now constitute a strong and vibrant institutional network in India. The strength of these groups is increasing day by day, and such groups may be utilised within organisational and administrative frameworks in creating awareness, providing support and disseminating required knowledge and skills – for example, as grassroots-level knowledge and skill hubs for RCH. Self-help groups may play a key role in developing the capacity of the rural poor to take care of their health properly; and, in this context, literacy is an essential asset in order for members of women's self-help groups to be able to provide, disseminate and understand information.

This study shows that female literacy has a significant influence on ensuring safe birth delivery. Female literacy enhances women's ability to convert available resources into practical capabilities. Figure 10A.2 shows that the total fertility rate (TFR) decreases as female literacy increases, corroborating the fact that female literacy empowers women to control fertility using available modern family planning methods. It is further demonstrated in Figure 10A.3 that the TFR influences the maternal mortality rate.

In order to examine the relevance of this finding, the correlation between female literacy and the maternal mortality rate (MMR) has been calculated for 79 countries of medium and low human development. The correlation is −.673 (significant at the .01 level).[33] An urgent effort is needed to improve female literacy in India. Further, it has been noted that improving the female literacy rate enhances other well-being variables, including the mean age of marriage of girls (Figure 10A.4), which in turn promotes a decline in the maternal mortality rate (Figure 10A.5). Women's self-help groups can play a key role in building rural women's capacity to make good uses of health services. To realise these possibilities for improved women's health, it is necessary to develop an institutional mechanism at grassroots level for ensuring better coordination between government, *Panchayati Raj* institutions, NGOs and women's self-help groups in providing health services in general and reproductive health services in particular.

Appendix

Table 10A.1   Poverty measured by people living on less than US$1 a day (2001)

| Region | People living on less than US$1 per day | | Head count indices: percentage of population living on less than US$1 per day |
	No. (million)	Per cent	
East Asia	271.3	24.8	14.9
Eastern Europe & Central Asia	17.6	1.6	3.7
Latin America & Caribbean	49.8	4.6	9.5
Middle East & North Africa	7.1	0.6	2.4
South Asia	431.1	39.5	31.3
India	358.6	32.8	34.7
Sub-Saharan Africa	315.8	28.9	46.9

Source: S. Chen and M. Ravallion, "How Have the World's Poorest Fared since the Early 1980s", Development Research Group, *World Bank Research Observer*, 19(2), 2004, pp. 141–170.

**Figure 10A.1   Women experiencing delivery complications
(per cent)**

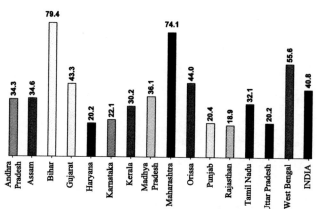

Source: Data from the District Level Household Survey under the Reproductive
and Child Health project conducted in India during 2002–2004.

**Figure 10A.2   Female literacy rate (FLR) and total fertility
rate (TFR)**

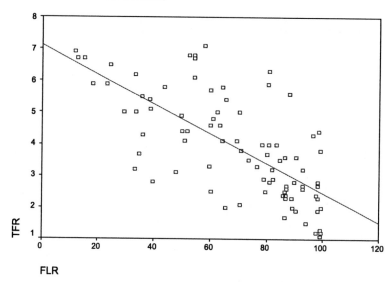

Data source: Data available from United Nations Development Programme, *Human Development Report 2006. Beyond Scarcity: Power, Poverty and the Global Water
Crisis*, New York: Palgrave Macmillan, 2006.

Figure 10A.3   Total fertility rate and maternal mortality rate

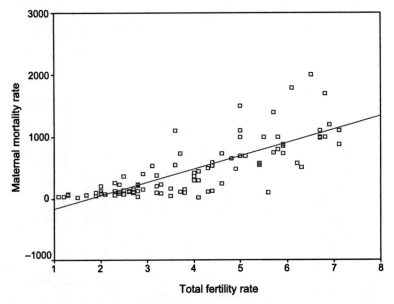

Data source: Data available from United Nations Development Programme, *Human Development Report, 2006. Beyond Scarcity: Power, Poverty and the Global Water Crisis*, New York: Palgrave Macmillan, 2006.

Figure 10A.4   Female literacy rate (per cent) and mean age at marriage for girls (years)

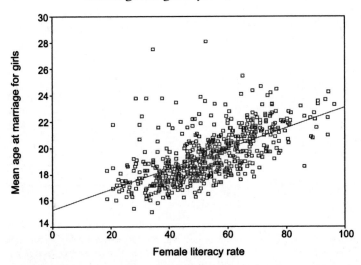

Source: Data from the District Level Household Survey under the Reproductive and Child Health project conducted in India during 2002–2004.

Figure 10A.5   Mean age at marriage for girls (years) and safe delivery (either institutional delivery or home delivery)

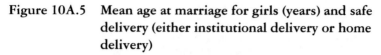
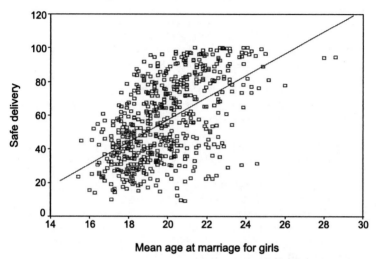

Mean age at marriage for girls

Source: Data from the District Level Household Survey under the Reproductive and Child Health project conducted in India during 2002–2004.

Notes

1. World Health Organization, "Provisional Agenda Item 2", Executive Board 105th Session, EB 105/5, 14 December 1999.
2. M. Maser and M. Brown, "Marriage and Household Decision-Making: A Bargaining Analysis", *International Economic Review*, 21, 1980, pp. 31–44; and M. McElroy and M. J. Horney, "Nash-bargained Household Decisions: A Bargaining Analysis", *International Economic Review*, 22, 1981, pp. 33–49.
3. World Bank, *Towards Gender Equality: The Role of Public Policy*, Washington, DC: World Bank, 1997.
4. J. Goudge and V. Govender, *A Review of Experience Concerning Household Ability to Cope with Resource Demands of Ill Health and Health Care Utilisation*, EquiNet Policy Series No 3, Centre for Health Policy, University of Cape Town, 2000.
5. J. Pryer, S. Rogers and A. Rahman, "Work Disabling Illness, and Coping Strategies in Dhaka Slums, Bangladesh", paper presented at "Staying Poor: Chronic Poverty and Development Policy" conference, University of Manchester, 7–9 April 2003, <http://www.cprc.abrc.co.uk/pubfiles/Pryer.pdf> (accessed 26 June 2009).

6. Z. Oxaal and S. Cook, "Health and Poverty Gender Analysis", briefing prepared for the Swedish International Development Co-operation Agency, Bridge, Institute of Development Studies, University of Sussex, 1998.

7. Victoria A. Velkoff and Arjun Adlakha, "Women of the World: Women's Health in India", WID/98-3, US Bureau of the Census Population Division, International Programs Center, December 1998, <http://www.census. gov/ipc/prod/wid-9803.pdf> (accessed 26 June 2009).

8. U. Grant, *Health and Poverty Linkages: Perspectives of the Chronically Poor*, DFID Health System Resource Centre, 1995.

9. Goudge and Govender, *A Review of Experience Concerning Household Ability to Cope with Resource Demands of Ill Health and Health Care Utilisation.*

10. World Bank, *World Development Report 1993: Investing in Health*, Oxford: Oxford University Press, 1993.

11. Ibid., p. 42.

12. P. Sandiford et al., "The Impact of Women's Literacy on Child Health and Its Interaction with Access to Health Services", *Population Studies*, 49, 1995, pp. 5–17.

13. S. H. Cochrane et al., "The Effects of Education on Health", Staff Working Paper 405, World Bank, Washington DC, 1980.

14. United Nations Development Programme, *Human Development Report, 2007/08. Fighting Climate Change: Human Solidarity in a Divided World*, New York: Palgrave Macmillan, 2007. In the model, adjusted R^2 = .540; Durbin–Watson Statistic = 1.777; N = 166.

15. World Health Organization, "Women's Health: Improve Our Health, Improve the World", WHO Position Paper, Geneva 1995.

16. A. Sen, "Gender and Co-operative Conflicts", in Irene Tinker (ed.), *Persistent Inequalities: Women and World Development*, New York: Oxford University Press, 1990, pp. 123–149.

17. Oxaal and Cook, "Health and Poverty Gender Analysis".

18. United Nations Population Fund (UNFPA), *State of the World Population 2005. The Promise of Equality: Gender Equity, Reproductive Health and the Millennium Development Goals*, New York: UNFPA, 2005; available at <http:// www.unfpa.org/swp/2005/pdf/en_swp05.pdf> (accessed 18 June 2009).

19. Ibid.

20. Ibid.

21. Directorate of Census Operations, West Bengal, *Census of India*, <http://web. cmc.net.in/wbcensus/DataTables/08/FrameTables-h_1.htm> (accessed 26 June 2009).

22. Government of India, *Morbidity, Health Care and the Condition of the Aged*, NSS 60th Round (January–June 2004), National Sample Survey Organisation, New Delhi: Ministry of Statistics and Programme Implementation, 2006.

23. See Ministry of Health and Family Welfare, Government of India, District Level Household Survey Reproductive and Child Health (RCH) Project, <http://www.rchiips.org/> (accessed 26 June 2009).

24. See Office of the Registrar General & Census Commissioner, *Census of India*, <http://censusindia.gov.in> (accessed 18 June 2009).

25. World Bank, *World Development Report 1993*, pp. 82–83.
26. The figures in parentheses are *t*-values; ** indicates significance at the .01 level (2-tailed); * indicates significance at the .05 level (2-tailed); adjusted R^2 = .595; Durbin–Watson statistic = 1.122; N = 593.
27. Management of primary health centres in Gumballi and Sugganhalli was contracted out by the government of Karnataka to Karuna Trust to serve the tribal community in the hilly areas. See Government of India, *Draft Report on Recommendation of Task Force on Public Private Partnership for the 11th Plan*, New Delhi: Ministry of Health and Family Welfare; available at <http://www.mohfw.nic.in/NRHM/Documents/Draft_report_task_grp.pdf> (accessed 18 June 2009).
28. Government of India, *Economic Survey 2006–07*, New Delhi: Ministry of Finance, Economic Division, 2007, p. 205; available at <http://indiabudget.nic.in/es2006-07/esmain.htm> (accessed 18 June 2009).
29. *Panchayati Raj* institutions are grassroots units of self-government, and have been proclaimed as vehicles of socio-economic transformation in rural India.
30. J. Devaki, "Panchayati Raj: Women Changing Governance", Gender in Development Monograph Series, New York: UNDP, 1996; A. Thomas, "Women's Participation in the Panchayati Raj: A Case Study of Maharashtra, India", PhD dissertation, Western Michigan University, 2004; and A. Ghosh, "Operational Strategy for Development of Rural Women in Amdanga Block, West Bengal", unpublished Management Research Report, Asian Institute of Management, Manila, 2003.
31. World Bank, *World Development Report: Investing in Health*, New York: Oxford University Press, 1993, pp. 82–83.
32. Planning Commission (1973) *Report of the Taskforce on Agrarian Relations*, New Delhi: Government of India; K. Gill, "If We Walk Together: Communities, NGOs and Government in Partnership for Health – The IPP VIII Hyderabad Experience", World Bank, Washington DC, 1998.
33. Standard error and *t*-value are 1.387 and –7.989, respectively (UNDP, *Human Development Report 2006. Beyond Scarcity: Power, Poverty and the Global Water Crisis*, New York: Palgrave Macmillan, 2006). In India, there is wide variation in the MMR. It is as low as 87 in Kerala, where female literacy is 87.7 per cent. On the other hand, the MMR is as high as 707 in Uttar Pradesh, where female literacy is as low as 42.2 per cent. See National Population Policy, Appendix III, at <http://www.unescap.org/esid/psis/population/database/poplaws/law_india/indiaappend3.htm> (accessed 18 June 2009).

PART B

A CASE STUDY IN INDIA

11

Introduction to the case study: The Women's Health Initiative – A trilateral partnership within the framework of the UN Global Compact

MARTINA TIMMERMANN

The main goal of the Women's Health Initiative (WHI) for Improving Women's and Girls' Maternal and Reproductive Health in India was to contribute to the improvement of women's and girls' reproductive and maternal health care in India.

The project idea

The major underlying idea of the public private partnership (PPP) project was that treating women with a new technology, such as endoscopy, which guarantees excellent medical care, also implies that patients will recover more speedily. And this, in turn, should mean that women who benefit from minimally invasive surgery can return to work and their families much faster. A reduction in the length of

Partnerships for women's health: Striving for best practice within the UN Global Compact,
Timmermann and Kruesmann (eds),
United Nations University Press, 2009, ISBN 978-92-808-1185-8

hospital stay benefits both the patient and the hospital – and, when applied to public hospitals, should also benefit the public health system.

Six training centres in six different states of India were to be equipped with state-of-the-art technical equipment for endoscopic surgery. The corporate partner, KARL STORZ, donated the technology in its effort to make a particular contribution to improving women's health care in India. However, this was only the first step. From its inception the project had as its second major goal to go beyond charity and become a viable and lasting initiative after the two years of the initial project period. It aimed at realizing the highest efficiency based on mutual cooperation and commitment to achieving a sustainable impact.

The approach followed the train-the-trainer principle. Endoscopic expert surgeons from six well-known training hospitals were to train medical doctors in endoscopic surgery. The trainers alone decided on the contents of the training courses, complemented by a module related to the United Nations Global Compact (UN GC). Such module was provided by the second public partner, Deutsche Gesellschaft für Technische Zusammenarbeit (GTZ), an international cooperation enterprise for sustainable development with worldwide operationss who operated on behalf of the German Federal Ministry for Economic Cooperation and Development (BMZ).

The doctors who wanted to participate in the training programme were required to pay a (reduced) fee to ensure that the training centres could generate enough income to keep them viable and independent in the long run. The doctors were picked with particular regard to their background, that is, they were to come from rural areas to ensure that patients living in such areas would profit from better diagnosis and treatment on the doctors' return from training. Furthermore, the participating doctors were requested to commit themselves to using the methods they learned for treating underprivileged women and girls in addition to their other patients. The integration of the training centres within existing hospitals was intended to create a self-supporting structure of training centres with a high multiplier impact.

Though initially operating only in India, the project was thought to have the potential for subsequent extension to other countries in Asia, Africa and other regions of the world.

The project structure

The project idea was originally developed in August and September 2004 between, on the one hand, KARL STORZ (KS) and TIMA[1] and, on the other, the United Nations University (UNU). It comprised a business model[2] and an assessment approach that aimed at responding to the several challenges outlined above.

In consideration of the UN GC principle of transparency, UNU was to function as an independent international assessment agency. It therefore could not be systematically involved in the implementation or monitoring of the project on the ground; thus, GTZ was approached as an experienced third partner for cooperation and monitoring in the field.

The first exploratory meetings between KS, UNU and GTZ were held in Berlin in October and in Geneva in November 2004. In March 2005, right before the official launch of the project, a planning meeting was conducted where roles and responsibilities were defined and the criteria for choosing the hospitals discussed.[3]

On 2 April 2005, in a ceremony at the headquarters of the KARL STORZ in Tuttlingen, Germany, KARL STORZ, the Gesellschaft für Technische Zusammenarbeit and the United Nations University formally launched the project "Women's Health Initiative (WHI) for Improving Women's and Girls' Reproductive and Maternal Health in India: A PPP within the Framework of the Global Compact".

On 29 June 2007, the PPP project between KARL STORZ and GTZ officially ended. UNU received the final field monitoring report from GTZ India on 2 June 2008 and finalised its assessment by the end of July 2008.

The trilateral partnership between two UN GC members and UNU

An important feature of the project structure is its three partners (see Figure 11.1). Two partners, KARL STORZ GmbH & Co. KG and the GTZ as technical arm of the German Federal Ministry for Economic Cooperation and Development (BMZ), formed the actual PPP in India. Both parties are members of the UN Global Compact.

In accordance with their Global Compact commitments, KARL STORZ and GTZ agreed to have their PPP assessed by a third

Figure 11.1   WHI partnership structure

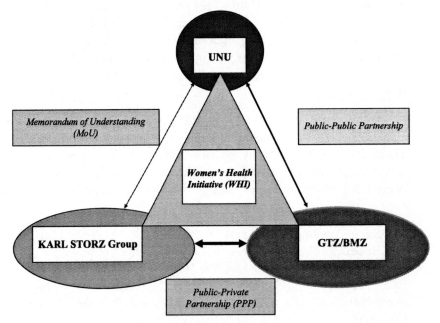

Source: Martina Timmermann, "Meeting the MDG challenges of women's health, human rights and health care politics: The Women's Health Initiative (WHI) for improving women's and girls' reproductive and maternal health in India", in Raj Kumar, C. and Srivastava, D. K., (2006) *Human Rights and Development: Law, Policy and Governance*, (City University of Hong Kong, LexisNexis) pp. 475–493, here p. 480

international partner, the United Nations University. Learning from studies of global health PPPs,[4] and especially noting the problem of institutional loyalties and interests, UNU, as the academic representative without any particular business- or policy-related stake in this undertaking, came on board to ensure objective academic observation and evaluation. It formed a public–public partnership with GTZ, which pledged €50,000 for organizing two workshops and the publishing costs. The funds for the honoraria for the expert authors were raised by UNU from an independent outside source to ensure their independence.

WHI partner profiles

KARL STORZ GmbH & Co. KG

KARL STORZ Company was founded in Tuttlingen, Germany, in 1945.[5] Since then, it has produced instruments and developed technological solutions for endoscopic diagnosis and therapy. Beyond the production and marketing of endoscopy instruments, a core element of the activities of KARL STORZ is the provision of comprehensive technical support with regard to diagnosis and therapy and setting up and supporting state-of-the-art training centres.[6]

In November 2004, the KARL STORZ Group joined the UN Global Compact and thereby made the ethical GC framework a part of the company's strategy, culture and day-to-day operations. KARL STORZ committed itself to publicly advocate the Global Compact and its principles via communications vehicles (press releases, speeches, annual reports and other documents) and to support and provide links to relevant medical doctors so as to facilitate the implementation of the GC principles in submitting medical solutions for health and by offering training tools and equipment. KARL STORZ also committed itself to contribute to the Global Compact at the global and local levels through dialogue, learning and partnership projects in health, and especially in women's health as manifested in Millennium Development Goal (MDG) 5.

GTZ[7]/BMZ[8]

For the past 30 years, GTZ has worked to provide viable and sustainable solutions for political, social, economic and ecological development in a globalizing world. GTZ's corporate objective is to improve people's living conditions on a sustainable basis. An active supporter of the UN Global Compact Initiative, the GTZ Office for Cooperation with the Private Sector also hosts a German Global Compact Focal Point.

The German Federal Ministry for Economic Cooperation and Development (BMZ) is GTZ's main client. In 1999, BMZ launched a Public Private Partnership programme to find and coordinate new opportunities for cooperation with the private sector. BMZ understands that a PPP is generally characterised by the private partner assuming its own risks. To qualify for support by the PPP programme, projects have to be compatible with the German government's development policy principles. The contributions of the partners must be complementary, the private partner must make a significant contribution and the scope of the project must clearly go beyond the limits of normal commercial activity. Support activities by BMZ/GTZ, therefore, start by assessing each company's contribution towards social and economic development, as well as the general environment of the partner country. "It is of crucial importance to BMZ/GTZ that PPPs in the health sector develop a broad impact and reach out to the poor, the main target group of development cooperation. PPPs shall therefore be integrated into the bilateral cooperation under official agreements."[9] Beyond that, various stakeholders such as nongovernmental organisations (NGOs), unions and scientific institutions should participate in PPP projects to broaden the projects' impacts.

United Nations University (UNU)

The United Nations University (UNU) is an international community of scholars engaged in research, postgraduate training and the dissemination of knowledge in furtherance of the purposes and principles of the Charter of the United Nations. The idea for this type of international organisation was originally proposed in 1969 by then United Nations Secretary-General U Thant, who suggested the creation of "a United Nations university, truly international in character and devoted to the Charter's objectives of peace and progress".

The overarching goal of UNU is the advancement of knowledge in areas relevant to addressing global issues of human security and development. As an international community of scholars, UNU serves as a think-tank for the UN system, a bridge between the United Nations and the international scientific community, a builder of capacities (particularly in developing countries), and a platform of excellence for the dialogue on new and creative ideas. The special nature of UNU is that it not only combines research, policy studies and teaching, but that it also brings to this work a global perspective that incorporates both theoretical and practical approaches.

Institutional roles and responsibilities

Learning from the lessons of other global health PPPs, the three partners' roles and responsibilities were clearly defined in contracts taking into consideration the nature and goals of each partner. The three partners were interlinked, however, through their shared goal, namely to improve women's maternal and reproductive health in India.

KARL STORZ delivered the equipment and training materials, and took over the maintenance of the state-of-the art technology and instruments. The company provided technical equipment for six Endoscopy Training Centres (ETCs) in India (for details, see Chapters 12, 15 and 17 in this volume, and the GTZ final monitoring report 2008[10]); offered the opportunity for expert counselling via videoconferences using IT communication networks; and supported capacity-building of medical doctors in up-scaling courses which were designed and conducted by especially qualified medical experts of the project.

GTZ accepted responsibility for managing the government funds and for reporting on progress in the field. Its particular task was to monitor the project at the local level in India to ensure that the social goals were reached. In compliance with its Global Compact activities and goals, GTZ also informed the ETCs and trainees about the UN Global Compact and the objective of the project.

KARL STORZ and BMZ/GTZ shared the costs of the project as a way to combine private resources with those of governmental development cooperation policy. On behalf of KARL STORZ, a project coordinator from the corporate sector (TIMA GmbH) who had also been one of the project designers was installed (until December 2006). He was responsible for inter-partner coordination and mediation to consolidate partnership-wide planning, manage conflicts and foster communication and transparency, and thereby help push things forward.

Finally, UNU as the international observing partner was assigned to evaluate the outcome of the German–German PPP health initiative in India and discuss its impact and its potential for up-scaling and/or replication in other countries. In line with its mandate to contribute to debates of global concern and provide new ideas and approaches to the global public, UNU accepted responsibility for organizing two workshops and making the outcome evaluation accessible to the public in the form of a printed publication (for the differences on monitoring, reporting and evaluation see Figure 11.2).

Setting up a steering committee

During the preparatory meeting in April 2005, a steering committee was formed comprising representatives of KARL STORZ, GTZ and UNU, with project management by KARL STORZ/TIMA. It was the committee's particular task to ensure transparency of communication, procedures and results. There was to be continuous open mutual exchange of information. Part of this involved a clear understanding of the role of individuals within the project team (see Figure 11.3).

Clarifying individual responsibilities

Dr Achim Deja (CEO of TIMA GmbH) was chosen to function as KARL STORZ's GC coordinator, with all partners still taking and

Figure 11.2   Monitoring, reporting and evaluation

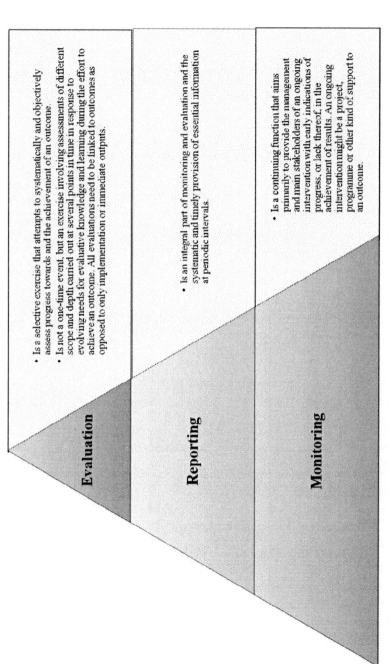

Evaluation

- Is a selective exercise that attempts to systematically and objectively assess progress towards and the achievement of an outcome.
- Is not a one-time event, but an exercise involving assessments of different scope and depth carried out at several points in time in response to evolving needs for evaluative knowledge and learning during the effort to achieve an outcome. All evaluations need to be linked to outcomes as opposed to only implementation or immediate outputs.

Reporting

- Is an integral part of monitoring and evaluation and the systematic and timely provision of essential information at periodic intervals.

Monitoring

- Is a continuing function that aims primarily to provide the management and main stakeholders of an ongoing intervention with early indications of progress, or lack thereof, in the achievement of results. An ongoing intervention might be a project, programme or other kind of support to an outcome.

Source: Based on UNDP Evaluation Office, *Handbook on Monitoring and Evaluating for Results*, New York: Evaluation Office, 2002, pp. 6–7.

Figure 11.3   WHI internal structure

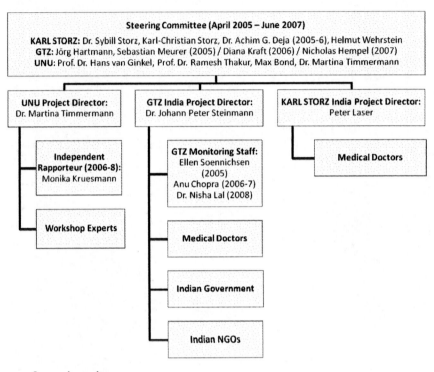

Source: the author.

exercising their individual responsibilities in this project. Dr. Martina Timmermann from UNU was responsible for the organisation of the two workshops, inviting the outside experts and providing a final outcome report based on the monitoring data from GTZ, the experts' observations and recommendations, and the rapporteur's report.

The actual implementation was delegated to the directors in the field, that is, the KS Project-Director in India, Mr. Peter Laser, and the programme head of health projects at GTZ India, Dr. Johann P. Steinmann. It was the KS director's task to contact the chosen hospitals and organise the technical set-up of the six ETCs. Within his realm of activity also lay the negotiation of subsequent contracts as necessary, for example on maintenance issues. He was also to take care of providing the necessary technical information for the trainers and training participants. GTZ India was responsible for liaising and coordinating the initiative with the Indian government and for organizing the monitoring team of the initiative, as well as for making sure that the information on the UN GC was provided to the training participants.

The UNU outcome assessment model

UNU's methodological design rested on the experiences, definitions and recommendations of the United Nations Development Programme (UNDP), the United Nations Children's Fund (UNICEF) and the World Bank. Taking into consideration the lessons learnt from other health PPPs, however, the model had as an additional particular feature a self-learning structure with two workshops. In this way, the requested external sources and evaluations (see Table 11.1) were systematically embedded in the project design from the start.

GTZ was to monitor the output and outcome on the ground. UNU was to provide the outcome assessment/evaluation based on the outcome monitoring data from GTZ, the corporate data from KARL STORZ, a UNU mission report and, most important of all, the insights and advice from external invited experts. UNU's final outcome assessment approach therefore had three complementary parts: organizing two workshops for a self-learning process; ensuring impartial reporting through an independent outside rapporteur; and organizing a platform for transparency and comprehensive documentation.

Organizing two workshops for a self-learning process

For assessing the project and in compliance with its mandate, UNU decided to assemble teams of scientific experts who, in two academic workshops, were to discuss the context-related issues in greater detail and critically apply their expert experience to the PPP itself.

To enable the project partners to learn from this exchange and thereby motivate their self-learning processes, the first workshop was held at the very beginning of the project, in October 2005. The second workshop was to focus on the achievements of the project and to discuss its impact, effectiveness, up-scalability and replicability.[11]

Table 11.1 The difference between outcome monitoring and outcome evaluation

	Outcome monitoring (GTZ/KS and UNU)	Outcome evaluation (UNU Final Report)
Objective	To track changes from baseline conditions to desired outcomes. (GTZ)	To validate what results were achieved, and how and why they were or were not achieved.
Focus	Focuses on the output of projects, programmes, partnerships and soft assistance activities and their contribution to outcomes. (GTZ and KS)	Compares planned with intended outcome achievement. Focuses on how and why outputs and strategies contribute to achievement of outcomes. Focuses on questions of relevance, effectiveness, sustainability and change.
Methodology	Tracks and assesses performance (progress towards outcomes) through analysis and comparison of indicators over time. (GTZ)	Evaluates achievements of outcomes by comparing indicators before and after the intervention. Relies on monitoring data on information from external sources.
Conduct	Continuous and systematic by Programme Managers and key partners. (GTZ/medical doctors/KS)	Time-bound, periodic, in-depth. External evaluations and partners.
Use	Alerts managers to problems in performance, provides options for corrective actions and helps demonstrate accountability. (GTZ/KS Interim reports; UNU Mission Report, April 2007; GTZ Final Monitoring Report, May 2008)	Provides managers with strategy and policy options; provides basis for learning and demonstrates accountability.

Source: Based on UNDP Evaluation Office, *Handbook on Monitoring and Evaluating for Results*, New York: Evaluation Office, 2002, p. 12, <http://www.undp.org/eo/documents/HandBook/ME-HandBook.pdf> (accessed 16 June 2009).

It was therefore organised close to the official end of the project in December 2006.[12]

Workshop I

The first WHI project workshop took place in Chennai, India, during 1–4 October 2005, with 23 expert participants from international institutions, various UN organisations present in India, and Indian and international academia.[13]

Since the project was designed to be a self-learning process, the first workshop had as its major objective the creation of a platform for exchange and learning with experts from academia and different organisations working in the field of women's health in India. Business, academia and international organisations were invited to meet in a constructive atmosphere to discuss their opinions and experiences with health PPPs in India. The two implementing project partners thereby had the opportunity to learn proactively from others in and for the process of their new PPP project and – if necessary – modify its approach.

The concept paper delineating the workshop content was sent out to the participants on 19 September 2005. Every presenter was asked to provide his or her specific angle of expertise. The workshop started with a reception on 1 October 2005. The following day was reserved for the exchange of expertise on important factors framing the PPP, namely: MDGs and Women's Reproductive and Maternal Health; Human Rights and Women's Rights and Needs; Human Rights and the Private Sector; Financing Health Care via Public Private Partnerships; India's Health Politics. The third day started with a presentation on the German government perspective on the role and value of PPPs. The representative from the Indian government had to cancel, but arranged that his points were incorporated into the presentation by the representative from the World Health Organization (WHO) and made sure they were considered by the workshop participants. Since hands-on experience is preferable to mere paper-based discussion, the workshop members were offered the chance to take a look at the first of the six ETCs – Joseph's Nursing Home in Chennai, a private hospital. The presentations by KARL STORZ and GTZ, questions and answers, and the discussion on the PPP therefore took place at that hospital.[14] In the morning of the fourth day, the results of the discussions and suggestions were summarised, synthesised and then further elaborated into concrete steps of project improvement during a concluding meeting of the project partners only.

Workshop II

The second workshop was held at the UN Campus in Bonn, Germany, during 3–5 December 2006. In compliance with its goal to serve as a stocktaking workshop, it was entitled "Aspirations, Actions and Achievements: Which Lessons Learnt? Where to Go from Now?"

The workshop was opened with an overview presentation on the goals and structure of the project and workshop. Since there were new experts (who were not all from the medical field) attending, a keynote lecture on endoscopy and laparoscopy for women's health aimed at broadening the participants' understanding of the options of endoscopy and laparoscopy prior to the following workshop days.

The second day started with a stocktaking session by the project partners. In session I, the partners presented their individual project reports, experiences and perspectives. Session II focused on the issue: "Improving Women's Health Care in India?" Three expert presentations were followed by a discussion of the WHI's contribution to women's sexual health care in India. In session III, the participants discussed the WHI's original aspirations, actions and final achievements, with particular regard to sustainable development. Finally, session IV tackled the question of whether or not the WHI could and should be replicated beyond India.

Day three was open to the public under the title: "WHI's Future Perspectives: The Challenges of Business, Ethics and the Right to Health". Here, three high-level speakers from business and politics provided the contextual framework for the WHI with regard to health care ethics, the UN Global Compact, corporate social responsibility and the right to the best attainable health care. The final speaker linked the WHI with the needs and challenges in Africa, thereby taking up the vital issue of WHI's potential for replication.

Ensuring impartial reporting through an independent outside rapporteur

To ensure impartiality, a workshop rapporteur from Australia, Monika Kruesmann, who had not been involved in the design process or project implementation on the ground, was invited to the second workshop on stocktaking. It was of particular benefit that the rapporteur was able to both understand and speak the working languages of German and English. In addition, Monika Kruesmann worked in the Australian government sector in the field of education, which gave her some additional understanding with regard to the capacity-building part of this project.

The reports on both the workshops were sent to the participants for their comments before incorporating them into UNU's final report. This was to ensure that the comments and recommendations made by the experts during the workshops were adequately understood and reported and as objectively as possible considered and incorporated.

Organizing a platform for transparency and comprehensive documentation

A comprehensive outcome assessment needs to take into consideration the various national and global challenges outlined above. In addition, it needs to build on outside expert resources. But it is also vital to consult with the shareholders in this process.

In order to provide the partners as well as the experts with more scope for their arguments, UNU invited the partners to each contribute a chapter wherein they could present their particular positions and perceptions from the management side in Germany and the implementing side in India. By offering such a publication platform to all stakeholders in this project, UNU aimed to create additional opportunity for transparency and information-sharing as well as constructive further debate on the issues that formed the starting point of this endeavour. When looking at the results and impact of this project, the following contributions shall also serve as a frame of reference to all those who need to prepare and learn on the needs and measures of PPPs (not only) for women's health within the framework of the UN Global Compact.

Notes

1. TIMA (Transition Integration Management Agency) GmbH was established in 1996 by Achim G. Deja, who instigated KARL STORZ's joining the UN Global Compact. He was responsible for developing the business model and overall GC strategy while serving as interim manager and UN GC representative for KARL STORZ until the end of 2006.
2. For the business model, see Achim G. Deja, TIMA GmbH, 2004 (internal document).
3. The criteria for selection were: 1. ownership: private/public; 2. location: north/eastern states were chosen because they have the least developed health care system/catchment areas; 3. institutions that were financially sound and could be sustained; 4. hospitals that had gynaecologists who are experienced trainers; 5. institutions KS had previous experience with; 6. hospitals where KS had previous experience with the medical personnel; 7. integrity of leaders. See Anu Chopra, GTZ Monitoring Plan, Appendix, ES 29.6.2005.
4. See, for instance, the study on PPP and international health policy-making by Judith Richter ("Public–Private Partnerships and International Health Policy-Making: How Can Public Interests Be Safeguarded?", Development Policy Information Unit, Ministry for Foreign Affairs of Finland, Helsinki, 2004), and the studies by Kent Buse from the Overseas Development Institute (ODI). Kent Buse was invited to the first UNU project workshop (WS I) in Chennai in October 2005, where he presented his ideas for discussion. He published his findings (together with Andrew Harmer) as "Global Health: Making Partnerships Work. Seven Recommendations for Building Effective Global Public–Private Health Partnerships", ODI Briefing Paper No. 15, London, January 2007; also published in *Social Science and Medicine*, 64(2), 2007, pp. 259–271.
5. Apart from the headquarters in Tuttlingen, Germany, there are production facilities in Munich (Germany), Tallin (Estonia), Dundee (UK), Schaffhausen and Widnau (Switzerland), and Charlton and Goleta (USA). Marketing facilities or distribution partners can be found in 26 countries in four continents. In 2008, KARL STORZ Group had about 4000 employees worldwide, and an annual turnover of about €700 million.
6. See Chapter 12 in this volume.
7. See Chapter 14 in this volume.
8. See Chapter 13 in this volume.

9. Nicolaus von der Goltz, "Abstract for UNU Project Workshop in Chennai", 1–4 October 2005.
10. "Reaching beyond Boundaries. Women's Health Initiative: A Public–Private Partnership. GTZ Monitoring Report", by Dr Nisha Lal and Dr J. P. Steinmann, GTZ, New Delhi, 28 May 2008 (unpublished manuscript).
11. Effectiveness is a measure of quality and goodness. Effectiveness says that getting it right is more important than cost or time, in contrast to efficiency, which is a mere measure of speed and cost. See Neil Kendrick, *The Reporting Skills and Professional Writing Handbook*, <http://www.reportingskills.org/secure/5_moreaboutreporting.htm> (accessed 11 June 2009).
12. For a detailed discussion of the workshops, see the report by Monika Kruesmann, "UNU Report of the Women's Health Initiative Workshop Bonn, Germany, 3–5 December 2006" (unpublished manuscript).
13. For the programme and participants, see Appendix A.
14. For a report with photos, see "KARL STORZ: Women's Health Initiative in India. Public–Private Partnership Hopes to Prompt Global Replication", *Compact Quarterly*, 2006(1), <http://www.enewsbuilder.net/globalcompact/e_article000513981.cfm> (accessed 14 June 2009).

12

KARL STORZ's WHI goals and expectations

Sybill Storz

Introduction

KARL STORZ, a family company founded in 1945 by Dr. Karl Storz, is a leading global producer of endoscopes and endoscopic instruments and equipment. The company employs 3,800 people worldwide, with 1,500 employees at its head offices in Tuttlingen, Germany. KARL STORZ has maintained trading relations with India since the 1960s, and in 1998 set up its own marketing subsidiary in New Delhi. In November 2004, KARL STORZ became a signatory to the Ten Principles of the United Nations Global Compact.

Corporate responsibility

KARL STORZ remains a family-run company, with a proven tradition of social awareness, both in responsibility towards its employees and in the long-term sustainability of its business activities. Many years of doing business all over the world have engendered a strong

Partnerships for women's health: Striving for best practice within the UN Global Compact,
Timmermann and Kruesmann (eds),
United Nations University Press, 2009, ISBN 978-92-808-1185-8

sense of ethics and global responsibility within the company. A fundamental principle of KARL STORZ's entrepreneurial activities is the balancing of economic interests with sustainable use of resources for the benefit of society. Sustainable management and taking the interests of society into consideration do not stop at the door of the factory in Tuttlingen or even at the state or national borders; it is a concern that applies internationally.

However, a company cannot and should not overestimate its individual ability to solve social injustices. Companies are, after all, dependent on a high level of political and legal stability in their operational environments. It is clearly in the best interests of industrialised nations to reduce inequity in wealth distribution – one of the major sources of conflict in the world. There is no doubt that economic success can be achieved only in a stable world economy. This also relates to companies' need for certain levels of basic infrastructural development. Most companies seeking involvement in health care, in particular, require a certain level of infrastructure to be in place before engaging in a project or investment activity so appropriate improvements can be added to existing structures.

From a company's standpoint, real success and sustainable measures are achieved when it operates within its core competencies. Corporate responsibility can be applied and sustained in the longer term only where a company is economically successful. A family-run company with a strong history of economic success such as KARL STORZ is not under any short-term pressure to succeed – unlike many publicly listed companies – and consequently has the capability to develop sustainable measures and thus future markets. Combining sustainable economic interests with the social goals of development policy is an approach KARL STORZ recognises as being the rationale behind the private public partnership (PPP) projects it wishes to support.

Endoscopic training: Significance and benefits

Endoscopy is a medical procedure that offers benefits that can be summarised as follows:

- minimal discomfort for the patient and less trauma;
- shorter operation times;
- increased operating theatre capacities;
- less postoperative pain;
- faster convalescence for patients resulting in shorter absences from work.

Between the 1930s and 1980s, endoscopy was used in isolated fields such as bronchoscopy, urology and gynaecology, and was utilised primarily in diagnostic cases and only rarely in therapeutic cases. The effectiveness of endoscopy subsequently meant it began spreading to other fields, in particular laparoscopy, and increasingly it began to be used therapeutically. This led to the term "minimally invasive surgery" becoming widely used at the end of the 1980s and in the early 1990s, and familiarity helped the procedure to gain broad acceptance in many disciplines.

In India, diagnostic endoscopy has been available since the 1960s and 1970s, mainly in the field of gynaecology. In addition, therapeutic endoscopy has been practised there since the 1980s.[1]

Endoscopic operations are characterised by the following specific aspects, which increase the need for specialised training:

- working with a video camera and monitor without tactile feedback or three-dimensional vision;
- coping with miniaturised, remotely controlled instrumentation;
- limited space and reciprocal sequences of movements.

To ensure that the benefits of endoscopy can be used for the patient's full advantage, doctors must complete special training and gain experience in using this technique.

KARL STORZ recognised many years ago that support for endoscopic training is a fundamental element in sustainable market development. As a producer of medical technological products, the

company is confined to providing logistics and infrastructure support for training activities. Medical training should be performed
exclusively by medical specialists. This ensures that competency remains in the hands of the medical experts and that the role of KARL
STORZ is primarily to provide support in the form of appropriate
equipment. Over the past decade, the company has supported training activities along these lines within the framework of many individual projects around the world.

The Women's Health Initiative:
Training for better health care

What makes the Women's Health Initiative (WHI) special is the
impetus it has achieved through the company's cooperation with its
partners the Gesellschaft für Technische Zusammenarbeit (GTZ) and
the United Nations University (UNU). Thanks to the training support already provided by KARL STORZ in many individual projects
and the experience gained as a result, it was possible to establish
this PPP project on a broader basis: not just one, but six Endoscopy
Training Centres (ETCs) were set up in parallel. Furthermore, approaches that were both social in nature and desirable for development aid policy were specifically included for the first time. This is
demonstrated, for example, in the methods for implementing project
aspects such as the selection of trainees, the voluntary commitment
by trainees to devote some of their time to disadvantaged regions
and/or sectors of the population and an assessment of whether the
model is suitable for use in other regions of the world.

Women in India

The decisive reasoning for conducting this project in India – the first
of its kind for KARL STORZ – involved, first, the fact that India
already has a fairly well-developed health system compared with
other emerging and developing countries. This means, for example,
that the necessary basic infrastructure is available. Furthermore, India

has outstanding endoscopy specialists with many years of experience in the field. This met KARL STORZ's condition that the project should achieve a "multiplier" effect, by ensuring that trained doctors would be available to pass on their experience of using the technology to other colleagues, thus undergirding the longer-term sustainability of the project. These aspects were regarded as key factors for the project's success.

Over the course of many trips throughout India, one comes into close contact with the proverbial "Indian paradox" – the country's transformation into an affluent economic power for an aspiring upper class in stark contrast to the unbelievable poverty suffered by the majority of the population. Such key in-country experiences highlight the need to contribute to the improvement of living conditions via the implementation of programmes and projects that are specifically adapted to the local environment. A functioning health care system is certainly a major factor influencing the improvement in people's living conditions and standard of living.

In addition to using these parameters to select a suitable national setting for the project, careful consideration was given to which medical field was most suitable for this project. The central issue, in this case, was a woman's place and role within a society or cultural environment. In almost all cultures, women play a vital role in the continuing development of a society, because they are often primarily responsible for the rearing of its children. Most people receive their environmental conditioning, values and skills from their mothers. This perception suggests that progress in a developing society can be effectively fostered in the long term by improving women's living conditions. Women thus take on a multiplier role by passing on the improved living standards directly to the next generation through childrearing.

A further consideration as to why the project should focus on supporting women is the discrimination they still suffer in various areas of life and the multiple burdens they have to bear in bringing up children, caring for their families and contributing to their livelihoods. This also reinforced the view that improving women's medical care is a key objective. Women's health builds a foundation for a better future for society as a whole.

Project focus: Using endoscopy to improve women's health

The project focus incorporated the desired aims for the project in a working model.

The WHI aims to spread medical know-how in the use of endoscopic techniques in India. The ongoing commitment of the trainees, on completion of their training, will – to some extent at least – expand patients' access to this type of medical care to areas currently lacking these services. In India, in particular, this means rolling out endoscopy to rural areas. According to current figures, around 70 per cent of Indians live in the countryside. By setting up Endoscopy Training Centres in several states the objective is to achieve optimal regional coverage. The project definition stresses, in particular, the creation of a self-supporting methodology structure to make long-term sustainability possible after the PPP contract comes to an end. This self-supporting structure would also benefit from the integration of the training centres into existing hospitals and from a fee paid by all trainees.

Expectations and success factors

An interim review, conducted in 2006 by GTZ, provided the following results. Six Endoscopy Training Centres had been set up with the help of Indian endoscopy specialists. Training courses in the centres began in November 2005 and at the start of 2006, a delay of about six months. Because of this delay, the intended annual target of 240 doctors trained in all six centres had not yet been reached. The trend, however, is considered to be positive. By January 2007, some 200 doctors had been trained and about 130 registrations were pending. Monitoring data relating to 2,000 treated patients had also been collected by January 2007. Up until then, the majority of patients had been treated within the training centres. However, the fundamental intention of the project has always been that increasing numbers of women will be treated using endoscopic methods in rural areas, as trained doctors return to their "home" health centres, sharing and transferring their new knowledge and skills. The effect is expected to be incremental because the trained doctors only gradually begin to practise new forms of treatment following their return to their institutions or practices.

Although the stated expectations had already been achieved to a large extent, the delay led to an extension of the project from May 2006 to June 2007. This extension was agreed to by GTZ, so as to better assess the effects of the project.

The project's self-learning structure, involving collaboration between the project partners, enabled a considered and detailed assessment to be made of the project's feasibility, project effects and success rate. This provides useful indications as to the future capacity and transferability of the model.

Mechanisms must be established to monitor the project's long-term effects, possibly over a number of years. From an entrepreneurial perspective, measures need to be found to prove the economic viability of such long-term investments in order to win new companies over to the principles of responsible management.

In summary, three key factors that have contributed to the project's success are:

1. cooperation with strong partners that are independent, well known and accepted locally;
2. unequivocal validation of the project content by the doctors involved;
3. the careful selection of doctors as trainers and trainees.

In addition to the structural organisation of the training units, the practical project implementation and the monitoring of the project, it must be emphasised that only the protagonists themselves – that is, the doctors on-site – can successfully pass on this model and its goals to the target groups. With this in mind, the staffing of the training centres and the selection of trainees are certainly crucial factors in a successful outcome. It is only by involving the trainees in the voluntary commitment that the social goals can be achieved in tandem with the transfer of medical knowledge.

From KARL STORZ's viewpoint, we can draw a positive conclusion from the results and trends achieved by the WHI. In addition, we consider the trilateral cooperation with our partners GTZ and UNU to be an important exemplar of the vital partnerships between industry, government and non-governmental organisations which need to be reinforced to foster responsible management.

Note

1. On the development of endoscopy in India, see Tehemton E. Udwadia, "Laparoscopy in India – A Personal Perspective", *Journal of Minimal Access Surgery*, 1(2), 2005, pp. 51–52.

13

The German PPP Programme: A viable way to improve women's health in India?

NICOLAUS VON DER GOLTZ

Introduction

Over the past decade, the business sector has taken an increasingly important role in development cooperation. Today, several major donors have special business partnership programmes. Examples include Germany's "PPP Facility", the United States Agency for International Development's "Global Development Alliance", the UK Department for International Development's "Business Linkages Challenge Fund", the United Nations Development Programme's "Growing Sustainable Business" and the United Nations Industrial Development Organization's "Business Partnership Programme". At the same time, a variety of international public private health programmes or funds have been launched: for example, the Global Alliance for Vaccines and Immunizations (GAVI), the Global Alliance for Improved Nutrition (GAIN) and the Global Fund to Fight AIDS, Tuberculosis and Malaria (GFATM).[1]

Several trends underlie the growing importance of partnerships with the business sector in development cooperation. In particular,

Partnerships for women's health: Striving for best practice within the UN Global Compact,
Timmermann and Kruesmann (eds),
United Nations University Press, 2009, ISBN 978-92-808-1185-8

foreign direct investment (FDI) flows into developing countries have increased remarkably in the past 15 years. According to the United Nations Conference on Trade and Development (UNCTAD), FDI into developing countries amounted to more than US$334 billion in 2005.[2] Thus, FDI surpassed official development assistance (ODA) in 2005 by more than a factor of three and became the most important source of capital inflow into developing countries.[3]

However, even though public and private capital inflows into developing countries have recently increased, more resources are still necessary to attain the Millennium Development Goals (MDGs). The UN Millennium Project, for example, calculated that annual ODA must increase to US$195 billion until 2015 in order to achieve the MDGs.[4] Partnerships with the private sector promise to generate additional resources for development purposes. In addition, cooperation between private and public partners aims to increase the effectiveness of aid. The private sector often contributes specific sector knowledge and efficient management systems, as well as the necessary financial and human resources.[5] The general assumption is that partnerships yield better results because they build on the complementary competencies of corporations, government and civil society. Thus, it is no surprise that most of the recent development policy framework agreements such as the *United Nations Millennium Declaration*, the *Johannesburg Plan of Implementation* or the "Monterrey Consensus" refer to closer collaboration with the private sector.

At the same time, both private and public actors have recognised that they can benefit each other. Supporting the MDGs is not primarily a question of selfless charity, but also offers the opportunity to develop new areas of business.[6] Furthermore, environmental degradation, climate change, the HIV/AIDS pandemic, violent conflict and inadequate health and education systems not only cause great human suffering but also increase the costs and risks involved in economic activity. Most analysts agree that the markets of the future are not in Europe or North America but in Asia, Africa and Latin America.[7] Companies, however, need conducive legal, economic and political environments as well as a well-trained and healthy workforce. The achievement of the MDGs would help to create the right conditions for economic activity.

Finally, consumers are more and more interested in the conditions under which products have been manufactured (for example, whether companies abstain from the use of child and forced labour, pay fair wages and meet environmental standards). Therefore, many enterprises increasingly understand the voluntary acceptance of social and ecological responsibility, often labelled corporate social responsibility (CSR), as part of their corporate strategy.[8]

Against this general background, this chapter introduces the German Public Private Partnership (PPP) Programme. The chapter is based on a paper presented at a United Nations University (UNU) workshop in Chennai in October 2005 that focused on a PPP between the German medical equipment retailer KARL STORZ GmBH, the German development agency Gesellschaft für Technische Zusammenarbeit (GTZ), the German Federal Ministry for Economic Cooperation and Development (BMZ) and the UNU. This project is supported by the German PPP Programme and aims to introduce endoscopic gynaecology procedures in India. Therefore, this chapter concludes by briefly addressing health PPPs and perspectives for future cooperation with India.

Germany's PPP programme

Just like the world in which it operates, German development policy has been evolving over the past few years. A decisive change of course occurred in January 1999 when BMZ launched its PPP Programme. For the first time ever, German development agencies were encouraged to seek opportunities actively to work with the private sector in developing countries.[9]

With its PPP strategy, BMZ intends to strengthen the coordinated action of development cooperation and private business activity. Instead of having a clear division of roles – with commercial projects by the private sector on one side and development measures by the public sector on the other – BMZ is looking at a whole spectrum of activity between these two extremes. The strategy focuses on covering special risks and/or costs that would otherwise prevent the realisation of projects that make sense in development policy terms and that are economically viable. Support activities start not by looking at the companies' need for support but by assessing their contribution to social and economic development, as well as to the general environment of the partner country.[10]

How does BMZ define PPPs?

A remarkable confusion about the nature of PPPs in development cooperation still exists. So far, no common definition of PPPs in development cooperation has evolved.[11] Development cooperation has worked with the private sector for a long time, and development cooperation has frequently delegated tasks to the private sector. Not all forms of collaboration between development cooperation and the private sector, however, should be labelled public private partnerships. Eeva Ollila therefore suggests distinguishing between public private interactions (PPI) and public private partnerships (PPP), the latter referring to "interactions in which the private sector is included in the agenda setting, policy-making and priority setting exercise."[12]

The definition of partnerships according to the BMZ's PPP Programme is as follows:

> PPPs are voluntary and collaborative relationships between the State and for-profit organizations. Participants agree to work together to achieve a common purpose and to share risks, responsibilities, resources, and benefits. Partnerships should serve a business purpose, but at the same time go beyond the core business activities of the private partners.

In many respects, this definition is closely aligned with the United Nations (UN) definitions of PPP.[13] It differs in two ways, however. First, this definition focuses on for-profit organisations. This does not mean that civil society, academia or international organisations should not be included in partnerships, but cooperation between the public and the corporate sector is at the core of the partnership. Second, the definition highlights the business interests of private partners explicitly, while at the same time emphasising efforts going beyond the core business activities of the partners in question. In this regard, PPPs differ from private sector participation (PSP), which is what the World Bank and other development banks often call the participation of the private sector (for example, in management contracts). In such forms of collaboration, the private partners bring in their own capital and therefore share risks, but they typically engage only within their core business areas (for example, water companies supply water). At the same time, PPPs differ from sole charity, since PPPs must be related to a specific business purpose of the private partners in question.

The three pillars of the German PPP Programme

The German PPP Programme is based on three pillars. These are the PPP Facility, so-called "Integrated PPPs", which are an aspect of bilateral cooperation arrangements, and support for multi-stakeholder forums.[14]

The PPP Facility

The PPP Facility is a separate fund of €20–25 million allocated annually for development partnerships with the private sector. This fund is particularly flexible and available to projects that could otherwise not be supported as part of the usual procedures because of their short duration or their small scale or because they cover more than one country. The PPP Facility targets projects of European enterprises that are engaged in investments, joint ventures, or export or import relations with partner countries and that aim to contribute to the development of the country in question. The Facility's operation is demand orientated, given that most projects are proposed by the private partners themselves. The projects are implemented jointly by the enterprise concerned and by one of the German implementing agencies (GTZ, the Deutsche Investitions- und Entwicklungsgesellschaft and SEQUA). The average financial value of partnership projects is €500,000 each[15] and project duration varies from one to three years.

Projects financed by the PPP Facility are generally intended to serve as pilot projects, which provide examples for private partners to replicate such projects in other regions or for other companies to carry out similar measures. Based on these experiences we are now witnessing both an increasingly intense dialogue with industry associations and top-ranking companies with the aim of extending the use of PPP tools at the transnational level and growing participation of other actors, such as trade unions, non-governmental organisations and UN organisations.[16] Well-known examples of such strategic alliances are the "Common Code for the Coffee Community", which aims to develop and implement an industry-wide code of conduct for the production, processing and trade of coffee, and the implementation of social standards in the textile industry in South East Asia together with the European Foreign Trade Association.

Integrated PPPs

Private enterprises are increasingly contributing resources of their own to bilateral financial and technical cooperation projects, for instance in developing economic and social infrastructure, improving professional education, introducing model solutions for (industrial) environmental protection and certifying local products and production methods. In the health sector, for example, the private sector participates in areas such as health infrastructure, insurance, social franchising or subcontracting.[17] However, most of these types of public private collaboration more properly fall into the category of PSPs.

German development cooperation also increasingly aims to mainstream PPPs in the sense of the BMZ's definition given above. There is already a routine check during the planning stage of bilateral development projects and programmes to assess whether cooperation with the private sector might translate development challenges into business opportunities. In contrast to the PPP Facility, PPP activities carried out under bilateral official agreements are not limited to European enterprises. They also often have a higher financial value and the public financial contribution might exceed the private one.

Mainstreaming, however, has proved to be a daunting task. It is particularly difficult to adjust development cooperation procedures to the needs and planning intervals of the private sector. In addition, the character and management requirements of partnership projects are usually much more complex than traditional development projects and project managers often lack strong incentives to pursue partnership models.[18]

Support for multi-stakeholder forums

In addition to these two kinds of PPPs, BMZ supports multi-stakeholder forums such as the United Nations Global Compact or the German Round Table Codes of Conduct.[19] By supporting such initiatives, BMZ aims to increase private sector awareness of development-related concerns. The rise of CSR and its connection with developing country problems could be a cornerstone of the solution to some development obstacles.

The Global Compact is an important instrument in this regard. This global alliance between the United Nations and private enterprise comprises 10 principles, which are derived from the Universal Declaration of Human Rights, the International Labour Organization's "Declaration on Fundamental Principles and Rights at Work", the UN Convention Against Corruption and the "Rio Declaration on Environment and Development". By November 2006, more than 3,900 companies had joined the initiative. They have each declared their support for the 10 principles and promised to implement them in their own enterprises, while being accountable for their actions.

Participation in the Global Compact has often led to the launch of partnership projects. The PPP with KARL STORZ is merely one of numerous examples in this regard.[20]

On behalf of BMZ, GTZ established a contact office for the German Global Compact Network. The network has established itself as an important platform for joint learning processes and sharing experiences in implementing the 10 principles. A steadily growing number of corporate global players and representatives from civil society, politics and academia actively participate in the German network. In November 2006 the German network had more than 75 corporate members – among them 17 of the 30 largest German stock corporations.

Criteria for PPPs and mutual benefits

In order to gain support from BMZ, PPP projects must meet various requirements:

(1) contributions by both the public and the private partner must complement each other in such a way that both partners achieve their objectives better, faster and at lower cost;

(2) the partner companies must provide a significant proportion of the project costs (in the Facility, at least 50 per cent);

(3) partnerships must be in line with German development policy guidelines and with the cooperation priorities that have been negotiated with the partner countries in question;

(4) the support of BMZ must be subsidiary and the scope of the project must clearly go beyond the limits of the partner company's normal commercial activity, because PPPs are not subsidies.

The mutual benefits for both the private partners and development cooperation are multifaceted. Private corporations benefit from additional financial as well as personnel resources. They also gain access to local networks of the implementing agencies and benefit from their specific country and sector know-how. Finally, PPPs often also facilitate market entry and provide new marketing possibilities for corporations. Development cooperation, on the other hand, benefits from the mobilisation of additional resources, the utilisation of private management know-how with a view to more efficient service delivery, and the promotion of private-sector investment as a growth engine for Germany's partner countries' development processes. In addition, the involvement of private partners often increases the sustainability of projects due to the companies' vested interest in the projects' long-term success. Thus, the limited ODA funding available can be used as a catalyst to create new structures needed for development. Finally, partnerships raise corporate awareness of global problems such as poverty, pandemics and environmental degradation.

The record

Between 1999 and 2005, 833 PPP projects were supported under the PPP Facility, with an overall value of nearly €330 million, of which the public sector contributed €126 million and the private sector invested €203 million. Thus, for every €1 of public money that has gone into these projects, around €2 of private funding has been attracted. Under bilateral cooperation agreements, 916 partnership projects were initiated in this period with an overall value of €1.7 billion. However, many of these projects are PSPs rather than PPPs.

The projects were carried out in more than 70 countries, most of them in Asia and Africa. These countries included emerging economies, such as India and China, but also poorer countries such as Nicaragua, Ethiopia and Bangladesh. Although it is often claimed that PPPs mainly target transnational corporations, about 70 per cent of the corporate partners in the German PPP Programme are small and medium-sized enterprises. PPPs have been undertaken in nearly all areas of relevance to development policy. In concrete terms, that includes training specialist staff on the ground, improving water supplies and sanitation, promoting renewable energies, introducing environmental and social standards and implementing projects to combat HIV/AIDS.[21]

PPPs in the area of health

Until 2005, roughly 6 per cent of all PPPs (or 108 in total) were carried out in the health sector. These projects had a financial value of some €170 million, and most of them dealt with HIV/AIDS. This is a result partly of the enormous spread of the HIV/AIDS problem in many developing countries but also of the exceptional public and corporate awareness of this issue.

Many HIV/AIDS partnerships are implemented as private sector workplace programmes. Prime examples are BMZ's HIV/AIDS Workplace Programmes with Private Companies in South Africa, which are carried out with companies such as DaimlerChrysler, Volkswagen, Roche, Robert Bosch and T-Systems. Through employee education, prevention and treatment programmes, workplace projects aim to prevent further HIV infection among employees and their families and to support HIV-positive employees and employees living with AIDS in a fair and appropriate manner.

Together with the pharmaceutical producer Pharmakina, the German PPP Programme also supports the production and gradual distribution of antiretroviral drugs as well as accompanying therapies for HIV-infected persons in the Democratic Republic of Congo. For that purpose, production facilities were built, an HIV diagnosis and treatment centre was equipped and medical staff were trained for the treatment of HIV/AIDS patients. BMZ currently plans to undertake similar projects in other least developed countries.

PPPs that exclusively address women's health are relatively rare. Up to now, women's health has often been a cross-cutting issue. Individual components of HIV/AIDS-related projects, for instance, specifically address women (particularly in the wake of information campaigns). Projects in the realm of family planning and reproductive health usually address women first and foremost. One example was a project with Schering in Bolivia, which aimed to increase the knowledge of the population about modern high-quality family planning methods. Schering set up a contact office and a free hotline to provide information and personal advice with regard to family planning methods. A similar project was implemented with Beiersdorf. This PPP aimed at improving sexual education for adolescents to prevent HIV/AIDS infection as well as unintentional pregnancies. Selected adolescents were trained to disseminate knowledge further by conducting small information events and workshops in schools and youth prisons.

In sum, PPP projects in the health sector with women as the main target group have been the exception rather than the rule thus far. In the eyes of BMZ, PPPs addressing women's health nevertheless have great potential. Possible areas of cooperation include medication and reproductive health supplies and materials, as well as social insurance.[22]

German development cooperation with India

Germany considers India an "anchor" country.[23] In both economic and political terms, the further development of anchor countries is of great importance. According to a study conducted by Goldman Sachs, by 2050 the four countries Brazil, Russia, India and the People's Republic of China – known as the BRICs – can be expected to generate a higher gross national product than the industrialised countries of the Group of Six.[24] This means that the global demand structure will also shift more towards these countries. Germany cooperates with these countries as equal partners and is endeavouring to establish strategic alliances with politics, business and science in order to ensure that their development is socially and economically sustainable. Ultimately, the economic success of the anchor countries has an enormous knock-on effect in neighbouring countries.

In the last bilateral government negotiations in December 2005, India and Germany agreed on energy, environmental policy and economic reform as priority areas of Indo-German development cooperation. Health, which had been a priority area of Indo-German cooperation until then, will in future not form a priority area, although activities will continue in the realm of health care financing, social health insurance, prevention of pandemic contagious diseases (HIV/AIDS, polio) and support to related health sector reforms.

There is, however, remarkable potential to expand cooperation with private companies in the Indian health sector. First, the Indian government considers health to be one of the main deficit sectors in relation to the MDGs. Therefore, the Indian government recently issued plans for new and far-reaching health initiatives. Second, the private sector is already a big player in the Indian health sector. Some 80 per cent of all health services are already supplied by the private sector.[25] Finally, the health sector is seen as a key future market in India. This could provide strong incentives for enterprises to engage in health PPPs in India.

Conclusion

PPPs are a comparatively new instrument and there are still many areas of development cooperation where state interventions are first and foremost needed. In addition, development cooperation has to tackle major challenges with regard to PPPs, such as improved project monitoring and impact assessments, as well as the mainstreaming of partnership projects.[26] However, PPPs are instruments that have given new impetus to cooperation between development policy and the private sector. Used properly, public private partnerships offer many advantages over traditional means of state-centred development cooperation.

The success of future health PPPs in India depends on a variety of factors. First, it should be noted that development cooperation projects and programmes are implemented according to the policy priorities of the partner countries. This is particularly true in India's case, where the German contribution is only marginal compared with the dedication of the Indian government's own resources. Ultimately, therefore, the Indian government itself determines whether health PPPs are promoted or not. Second, the private sector has to be interested in carrying out health PPPs. Successful PPPs depend primarily on the interest and innovative capacity of the private sector itself. Finally, the main target group of development cooperation are the poor. Therefore it is of crucial importance that health PPPs are designed with their needs in mind.

Notes

1. See World Economic Forum, *Building on the Monterrey Consensus: The Growing Role of Public–Private Partnerships in Mobilizing Resources for Development*, Geneva: WEF, 2005, pp. 60–79.
2. See UNCTAD, "FDI from Developing and Transition Economies: Implications for Development", *World Investment Report 2006*, Geneva: UNCTAD, 2006, p. 299.
3. According to preliminary figures, ODA amounted to US$106 billion in 2005. This would represent a 31.4 per cent increase compared with 2004. This increase can mainly be accounted for by debt relief to Iraq and Nigeria, as well as tsunami aid. ODA was expected to reduce slightly over 2006 and 2007 as debt relief declines. See OECD Development Cooperation Directorate, "Aid Flows Top USD 100 billion in 2005", Press Release, 4 April 2006, <http://www.oecd.org/document/40/0,2340, en_2649_33721_36418344_1_1_1,00.html> (accessed 12 June 2009).
4. See UN Millennium Project, *Investing in Development: A Practical Plan to Achieve the Millennium Development Goals*, London: Earthscan, 2005.
5. For a similar assessment, see World Commission on the Social Dimension of Globalization, *A Fair Globalization: Creating Opportunities for All*, Geneva: ILO, 2004, p. 128.
6. See C. K. Prahalad, *The Fortune at the Bottom of the Pyramid: Eradicating Poverty Through Profits*, Philadelphia: Wharton School Publishing, 2004.
7. See Goldmann Sachs, "Dreaming with BRICs: The Path to 2050", Global Economics Paper No. 99, 2003.
8. See D. Vogel, *The Market for Virtue: The Potential and Limits of Corporate Social Responsibility*, Washington DC: Brookings Institution Press, 2005; and "CSR Supplement" in *Financial Times Deutschland*, 7 December 2005.
9. See T. Altenburg and T. Chahoud, "Public–Private Partnerships – Assessment of the First Years", *Development and Cooperation (D+C)*, No. 4, 2003, pp. 144–147.
10. See Nicolaus von der N. Goltz, "Public Private Partnerships in der Entwicklungszusammenarbeit: Partnerschaften für eine nachhaltige Entwicklung", *Forum Wirtschaftsethik*, No. 3, 2005, pp. 33–43.
11. See J. Richter, *Public Private Partnerships and International Health Policymaking: How Can Public Interests Be Safeguarded?*, Helsinki: Hakapaino Oy,

2004, pp. 5ff; and A. Zammit, "Development at Risk: Rethinking UN–Business Partnerships", South Centre and United Nations *Research Institute for Social Development*, 2003, pp. 51ff.

12. See E. Ollila, "Global-Health Related Public–Private Partnerships and the United Nations", Policy Brief No. 2, GASPP, Helsinki, 2003, p. 2. Jane Nelson suggests distinguishing partnerships from other forms of interactions by means of a shared decision-making process. See J. Nelson, *Building Partnerships: Cooperation between the United Nations System and the Private Sector*, Report commissioned by the United Nations Global Compact, New York: United Nations Department of Public Information, 2002.

13. The UN General Assembly characterises partnerships as "voluntary and collaborative relationships between various parties, both public and non-public, in which all participants agree to work together to achieve a common purpose or undertake a specific task and, as mutually agreed, to share risks and responsibilities, resources and benefits". United Nations General Assembly, *Towards Global Partnerships*, UN Document A/RES/60/215, 14 December 2005.

14. Besides such development partnerships, various other forms of cooperation with the business sector exist in German development cooperation. For example, BMZ also aims to attract private equity for its bilateral financial cooperation in order to realise development projects – typically in the infrastructure sector. These forms of cooperation are labelled PSP. In addition, the Deutsche Investitions- und Entwicklungsgesellschaft provides long-term finance and advice to German and international private enterprises as well as enterprises from partner countries with a view to investment in places where no such services are available in the local market. To that end, it offers equity capital, mezzanine finance, loans and guarantees, and provides advice on the design of investments. For a detailed categorisation of cooperation projects with the private sector, see BMZ, "Entwicklungspartnerschaften mit der Wirtschaft – Public Private Partnership (PPP)", *Jahresbericht 2005*, Bonn: BMZ, 2006, pp. 6f.

15. The public contribution usually amounts to €200,000.

16. See E. Demtschück, *Von PPP zu strategischen Allianzen. Ansätze zur Weiterentwicklung im Lichte nationaler und internationaler Erfahrungen*, Bonn; German Development Institute, 2004.

17. See Kreditanstalt für Wiederaufbau (KfW), "Private Sector Participation (PSP) in der FZ", Position Paper, KfW, Frankfurt am Main, 2004.

18. On the problems of mainstreaming PPPs in bilateral development cooperation, see also United States Agency for International Development, *The Global Development Alliance: Public Private Alliances for Transformational Development*, Washington DC: USAID, 2006.

19. On the German Round Table Codes of Conduct, see *Codes of Conduct on Social Standards*, Eschborn: Secretariat of the Round Table Codes of Conduct, 2004.

20. For further examples, see German Global Compact Network, *Global Compact Yearbook 2005*, Berlin: Macondo, 2006.

21. For an in-depth statistical analysis of Germany's PPP Programme, see BMZ, "Entwicklungspartnerschaften mit der Wirtschaft, pp. 1–5.
22. See BMZ, "Sexual and Reproductive Health (SRH)", Policy Paper No. 90, Bonn: BMZ, 2003, p. 16.
23. On the concept of anchor countries, see A. Stamm, "Schwellen- und Ankerländer als Akteure einer globalen Partnerschaft – Überlegungen zu einer Positionsbestimmung aus deutscher entwicklungspolitischer Sicht", DIE Discussion Papers No. 1/2004, Bonn: German Development Institute, 2004.
24. See Goldman Sachs, "Dreaming with BRICs: The Path to 2050".
25. See Martina Timmermann, "Meeting the MDG Challenges for Women's Health, Human Rights and Health Care Politics: The Women's Health Initiative (WHI) for Improving Women's and Girls' Reproductive and Maternal Health", in C. Raj Kumar and D. K. Srivastava (eds), *Human Rights and Development: Law, Policy and Governance*, Hong Kong: City University, 2006, pp. 475–493, at p. 491.
26. On similar challenges for partnership projects within the UN system, see Global Public Policy Institute, *Business UNusual. Facilitating United Nations Reform through Partnerships*, New York: UN Global Compact Office, 2005.

14

GTZ's goals and expectations for the WHI public private partnership from a development cooperation point of view

DIANA KRAFT AND JÖRG HARTMANN

Introduction

The Women's Health Initative (WHI) was founded in 2004 as a public private partnership (PPP) between three project partners: the company KARL STORZ GmbH, the United Nations University (UNU) and the Deutsche Gesellschaft für Technische Zusammenarbeit (GTZ), which implements the PPP Programme of the German Development Cooperation on behalf of the German Federal Ministry for Economic Cooperation and Development (BMZ). As a trilateral development partnership, the WHI was given a very specific framework of action.[1]

The project goals are framed by the basic philosophy behind a public private development partnership (PPP), which is to combine each partner's technical, subject-specific and regional know-how in the best possible way and to create a mutually advantageous situation for all participants. The core project objective of the WHI is to

Partnerships for women's health: Striving for best practice within the UN Global Compact,
Timmermann and Kruesmann (eds),
United Nations University Press, 2009, ISBN 978-92-808-1185-8

optimise disadvantaged Indian women's and girls' access to high-quality health services, particularly gynaecological treatment involving endoscopic diagnostics and therapy (minimally invasive surgery). In more global terms, the WHI hence also contributes to the achievement of the fifth Millennium Development Goal (MDG) for the improvement of maternal health, as well as to MDG 9, strengthening global partnerships for development.

In its country-specific operation, the project addresses a weakness of the Indian health system – its current inability to ensure sufficient access to good-quality, adequate and affordable health services for the rural population. Because diseases are not diagnosed early enough and the quality of health services is poor, in many cases there is a need for more expensive treatment at a later stage, many patients are incapacitated and some are unable to continue earning a living. An overall improvement in the population's health would therefore make a crucial contribution to alleviating poverty and promoting the country's economy.

Against this background, the PPP project contributes to two focus areas of German development policy. The first is promoting women's and girls' health in a development policy context. This issue has a high priority on the German development policy agenda and at the project implementation level. However, it is also a cross-sectoral issue that runs "horizontal" to the classic main areas of bilateral development cooperation in India, namely energy, environmental and resource management, and sustainable economic development. Health as a main topic of bilateral cooperation is in danger of becoming marginalised and being perceived merely as a peripheral issue. The WHI's particular character as a PPP project focused on disadvantaged women in India who still do not have sufficient access to good-quality, adequate and affordable health services – despite some forthcoming positive development effects in this field – serves to give a stronger impetus to women's health. In this way, it gives health a clear priority status for project implementation, rather than treating it as a peripheral matter as is happening in other projects.

The second objective of the WHI PPP is close involvement of the private sector – in case of the WHI, the medical technology company KARL STORZ, an actor with specific know-how and important structural contributions to the project's sustainability and the local impacts of the project results. The close involvement of a private partner also aims at transforming the private partner's commitment at the project level into a longer-term business case for entrepreneurial engagement in the partner country's markets – based on mutual advantages for all project partners. In this way it would be possible to develop a *model* for a sustainable improvement in health services for disadvantaged parts of the population that can be transferred to projects in other regions.

Development policy impacts of the WHI: Evaluation methodology

Whereas KARL STORZ's project input is predominantly of a technical nature[2] and the UNU's contributions focus on the final overall scientific evaluation of the project, GTZ's contribution to implementing the WHI measures is that of a *facilitator* which co-monitors the PPP's intended impacts at the development policy level. This involves ensuring well-founded, continuous monitoring and documentation of progress on-site and evaluating all activities in connection with the setting up of Endoscopy Training Centres in the selected Indian project hospitals. GTZ also offers training for local hospital personnel (Indian gynaecologists and relevant medical staff). To achieve this, GTZ mainly uses the computer-based evaluation programme e-VAL, which is used more widely by GTZ as a proprietary instrument for evaluating its development cooperation projects around the world.[3]

The use of e-VAL in the evaluation process makes sense in the case of the WHI because the evaluation is not based on predetermined or pre-developed questionnaires, but rather enables the project partners and target groups to individually determine the evaluation criteria they consider most crucial. These relate mainly to the time-frame, an assessment of the successful implementation concepts or measures used by the various partners and the inputs and contributions of each partner. In addition, e-VAL employs various evaluation filters and allows for different modes for presenting the evaluation outcomes (consensus vs. disagreement within the interviewed group, factors in success or failure, and so on).[4] For the WHI, a highly complex and participatory PPP that is to be replicated in other contexts for improving the health situation for disadvantaged women, the use of e-VAL will produce a robust basis for sustainable project management and possibly a future roll-out of the project.

In addition to qualitative interviews with trained doctors, medical personnel and other project participants using e-VAL, there are evaluation tools based on different methodological approaches. These include the collection and analysis of quantitative patient treatment data based on socio-demographic criteria and exit interviews with patients undergoing endoscopic treatment.

GTZ's detailed project monitoring, based on the above instruments, delivers valuable information on the effectiveness and scope of impact of the implemented project activities.

Evaluation outcome levels

The expected development policy results and effects, defined in the preparation of the WHI, were designed to form a coherent functional impact chain. The project partners are assigned specific roles and tasks in accordance with their core competences. In the case of public private development partnerships within the BMZ's PPP Programme, a project's impact chain is composed of different outcome levels. Figure 14.1 shows the outcome levels of the WHI.

The very bottom of the impact chain is represented by the predetermined project output to be performed by the project partners in the course of the project. For the WHI, this means that Endoscopy Training Centres (ETCs) in selected health institutions in medium-sized and small Indian cities have been set up and that KARL

Figure 14.1   WHI – functional impact chain

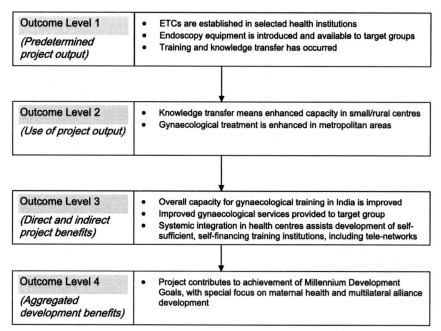

Outcome Level 1 (Predetermined project output)	• ETCs are established in selected health institutions • Endoscopy equipment is introduced and available to target groups • Training and knowledge transfer has occurred
Outcome Level 2 (Use of project output)	• Knowledge transfer means enhanced capacity in small/rural centres • Gynaecological treatment is enhanced in metropolitan areas
Outcome Level 3 (Direct and indirect project benefits)	• Overall capacity for gynaecological training in India is improved • Improved gynaecological services provided to target group • Systemic integration in health centres assists development of self-sufficient, self-financing training institutions, including tele-networks
Outcome Level 4 (Aggregated development benefits)	• Project contributes to achievement of Millennium Development Goals, with special focus on maternal health and multilateral alliance development

Source: the authors.

STORZ's endoscopic diagnosis, treatment and surgical methods in the field of gynaecology have been introduced for disadvantaged women and are offered to the target group. In addition, knowledge will have been transferred by means of training for doctors and operational personnel, long-term training concepts and material are prepared, and treatment is put in place in coordination with identified gynaecological areas of concern. This level of WHI project outputs also includes ongoing monitoring of activities in relation to the ETCs, scientific and academic support, plus a final project evaluation by the UNU.

The second level in the WHI's impact chain focuses on the use of these outputs. The main question at this level is: who actually uses the project outputs and in what way? In terms of the WHI, output use consists largely of the broad transfer of medical and technical knowledge to other regions in India. The surgeons, doctors and operational personnel who undergo the training come from various parts of the country and it is intended that the knowledge they acquire of endoscopic operation and treatment methods will be passed on to previously under-served areas of India. In turn, it will be possible to further develop the capacity of even smaller health centres, particularly in rural locations, at a later stage. On that basis it is assumed that, in the rapidly growing metropolitan areas and urban centres as well as in rural locations, modern medical and health-related services will be offered, enhancing the quality of gynaecological treatment. This impact level also includes the output use achieved for the indirect target group – the female patients – among whom the WHI measures are intended to create higher demand, especially from women from rural areas, for minimally invasive endoscopic treatment.

The third impact level focuses on the direct and indirect benefits of the WHI. Thanks to improved training capacity, more Indian doctors than before are able to receive low-cost training in minimally invasive surgery in their own country, especially in the field of gynaecological treatment. In addition, past experience has shown that the introduction of endoscopy in hospitals and surgeries can create additional jobs because more qualified medical personnel become necessary.

At this impact level, access to treatment for disadvantaged women and children is also clearly improved. Following the project, the broad use of modern endoscopic surgery will enable more disadvantaged women to receive an early diagnosis and have their gynaecological complaints treated sooner.[5] Besides improved access, the use of endoscopic technologies can also enable surgeries in rural areas, away from the urban, metropolitan centres and major hospitals, to diagnose diseases faster and more conclusively.

Another benefit is that minimally invasive surgery reduces the duration of hospital stays and postoperative recovery periods, thus enabling female patients to return to their families sooner. For patients this results in an earlier return to work, meaning also less income loss and a reduction in transactional costs in general. Hence, working women in India have a better choice in terms of planning surgery. In addition, provided the new surgical methods continue to be applied in the long term, they will result in a fall in the cost of treatment, for example for painkillers and dressing materials. The range of family planning measures in India – based on principles of good governance – is also assumed to be extended thanks to endoscopy, accompanied by improved medical consulting services.

At the technical and organisational level of providing endoscopic health services, the integration of ETCs into existing hospitals and health centres can also be seen as promoting the rapid development of a self-sufficient, self-financing system for the training centres, with fee-paying training courses, a strong multiplier function and the potential in the long term to establish additional training centres. In the medium to long term, the range of medical services offered by Indian hospitals in the field of gynaecology could be fundamentally improved.

Besides the direct benefits, the WHI impact chain includes an indirect benefit level. This comprises the overarching effect of the use of tele-medicine, a system that enables the fast and efficient electronic exchange of information on patients and their treatment, promotes the exchange of knowledge and experience between doctors and improves their skills in this area. A worldwide "tele-network" for endoscopic medicine could – as a long-term effect of the project – ultimately lead to new working methods and the holistic, cross-regional, cross-cultural treatment of gynaecological complaints. It could also mean that medical performance records in the field of gynaecology in India will be improved in general. Moreover, it is likely that the relationship between patients and doctors will be optimised and the medical outcome of a successful course of treatment improved.

In a longer-term perspective on the indirect benefits resulting from the WHI, good practice and governance policy employed by doctors in relation to the appropriate use of endoscopic technology could be strengthened. For instance, the doctors involved provide evidence of having treated disadvantaged women and girls with the new technology. Finally, it is assumed that the indirect benefits include a greater spread of the use of endoscopic devices among medical personnel, thanks to better and more readily available training, which will help to consolidate the Indian market for endoscopic technologies.

These positive effects on the local market for health services and health technologies hence imply the potential for a stronger commitment by the private partner KARL STORZ to the WHI project and its future development. This would create more "private ownership" within the project, even beyond the official project phase. In turn, such strong private involvement will give rise to greater entrepreneurial commitment to generally supporting capacity-building in the field of endoscopic diagnosis and treatment among local technical personnel. Another indirect benefit is that UNU's academic support and overall assessment of the project create a robust foundation for developing follow-up projects and rolling out the WHI concept to other areas in the long term. The outcomes of the evaluation elaborated by UNU will provide insights into the potential for KARL STORZ and other companies in the health sector to help to improve medical care for disadvantaged population groups in other parts of the world. In general, UNU functions within the project as a provider of academic input: it delivers a basis for comprehensive PPP project assessment and through that for an objective observation of the WHI, and it embeds the project in a contextual framework of relevant development cooperation topics.

The WHI PPP is a prime example of the implementation of corporate social responsibility in a real-life setting and of an entrepreneurial commitment to the UN Global Compact and its 10 principles (including, for example, human rights, environmental protection and the fight against corruption). In that respect, KARL STORZ, a UN Global Compact member since 2004, demonstrates how corporate responsibility can be realised in close connection with a company's core business and how a sustainable business case for alleviating poverty can lead to better health services in developing countries. It also demonstrates a new dimension of corporate citizenship: companies as political, and at the same time moral, actors invest in better local and global institutional conditions for their own commercial action and thereby transcend the trade-off between economic self-interest and societal benefits such as improvements in the health sector related to development policy.[6]

At the fourth and highest level of the impact chain, defined as highly aggregated development policy benefits, the WHI contributes – as mentioned at the very beginning – to the achievement of the Millennium Development Goals, in particular the improvement of women's health around the world and the establishment of long-term multilateral alliances to facilitate development.[7]

Outlook

Thanks to its multi-level approach and self-learning process structure, the WHI, being a trilateral development partnership, may be a pioneering example of effective interaction between development policy benefits (improving health services for disadvantaged Indian women) and business benefits (the positioning of KARL STORZ in the Indian market). The project's special concept promises the potential of being transferred to other countries and companies and hence makes an important contribution to putting health, as well as gender issues, into a stronger position within development cooperation by means of collaboration with the private sector.

Notes

1. Public private partnerships, also known as development partnerships with the private sector, generally aim to combine the strengths of public and private partners and employ these in order to achieve a common goal. PPP projects reconcile companies' business interests with the German Federal Government's development policy objectives. For further information on the PPP concept, please refer to N. von der Goltz, "Public Private Partnerships in der Entwicklungszusammenarbeit. Partnerschaften für eine nachhaltige Entwicklung", *Forum Wirtschaftsethik*, No. 3, 2005, pp. 33–34; and T. Altenburg and T. Chahoud, "Public–Private Partnerships – Assessment of the First Years", *Development and Cooperation (D+C)*, No. 4, 2003, pp. 144–147.
2. KARL STORZ, a manufacturer of endoscopic devices, provides the technical equipment for the project, installs it in the Endoscopy Training Centres at selected health centres, trains gynaecologists to apply endoscopic diagnoses,

therapies and surgical methods and rolls out the technical aspects of tele-medicine in India.

3. For more information on e-VAL, see GTZ, Gruppe Evaluierung, *e-Val Manual – Methodik-Handhabung-Interpretation, Kap. 2*, January 2005.

4. See also GTZ, Stabsstelle Evaluierung, *Kurzinformation e-Val*, June 2006; and A. Chopra, "GTZ – Health Sector Support India. Assessment of the Women's Health Initiative", Private Public Partnership GTZ, KARL STORZ and UNU, November 2006, p. 19.

5. See also Chopra, "GTZ – Health Sector Support India. Assessment of the Women's Health Initiative", p. 21.

6. For a detailed description of the concept of corporate citizenship, see I. Pies, *Ordnungspolitik in der Demokratie. Ein ökonomischer Ansatz diskursiver Politik-beratung*, Tübingen: J. C. B. Mohr (Paul Siebeck), 2000; and M. Beckmann and I. Pies, "Sustainability by Corporate Citizenship – The Moral Dimension of Sustainability", Discussion Paper No. 04-12, Research Institute of the Wittenberg Center for Global Ethics in collaboration with the Chair of Economic Ethics, Martin Luther University Halle-Wittenberg, 2005.

7. See also World Health Organization, *Health and the Millennium Development Goals*, Geneva: WHO, 2005.

15

The WHI: Management perspectives from the private and the public partners in the field

The trilateral partnership structure of the Women's Health Initiative (WHI) is one of its most innovative features. Taking a collaborative approach to developing, implementing and monitoring the project encourages both continuity of planning and coordination of action. Nevertheless, the geographical dispersal of the partners across continents and time zones, as well as their nuanced interests and objectives, does present challenges. Consequently, the role of on-the-ground project managers from the main implementation partners – KARL STORZ (KS) and the Gesellschaft für Technische Zusammenarbeit (GTZ) – remains critical to maintaining links between the partners, as well as between the officers of GTZ and KS at the project sites and the officers situated at company and agency headquarters.

Peter Laser (KS) and Anu Chopra (GTZ, 2006–7) filled these roles in India for the WHI, and their comments and reflections on the experience provide an engaging personal insight into the challenges and considerations that a project manager may confront in such an undertaking. Their comments also demonstrate how lessons for future action can be derived within a self-learning project.

Partnerships for women's health: Striving for best practice within the UN Global Compact,
Timmermann and Kruesmann (eds),
United Nations University Press, 2009, ISBN 978-92-808-1185-8

Management perspectives:
KARL STORZ GmbH

Peter Laser

Introduction

KARL STORZ has maintained close relations with the medical fraternity in India since the early 1960s. It has contributed significantly to the development of minimally invasive surgery (MIS) in that country, and is currently the unchallenged market leader in the field. Nevertheless, there is more to be done; all major efforts to bring modern health care to India have, thus far, been limited to metropolitan areas, owing to the absence of adequate facilities in the rural areas. This has led to the phenomenon of patients travelling great distances, often for several days, with an average of three accompanying family members.

The objective for KARL STORZ's activity in India became quite clear following the establishment of its own subsidiary in 1998: health care had to expand to rural areas rather than requiring patients in need to travel to urban centres. Coinciding with KARL STORZ's participation in the UN Global Compact in 2004, the idea of the Women's Health Initiative was created. The concept was unique but simple: create centres of training expertise, staffed by experienced doctors with mastery of laparoscopic techniques; provide them with the necessary equipment to deliver ongoing training; and, most essentially, ensure that those trained return to the rural areas where health care is scarce.

Establishing the Endoscopy Training Centres

When the Women's Health Initiative was formally launched by Sybill Storz in April 2005, it was not completely clear how the major focus of our company's work in India would be realised. In contrast to other activities where we were involved in creating individual training facilities, this initiative was started on a larger scale. Sites for six Endoscopy Training Centres (ETCs), two in private hospitals and four in public hospitals, were selected from a list of almost 40 suitable candidates through meticulous application of objective criteria (see the GTZ comments below). All participating centres had to be made aware of the consequences of the agreements, and some cultural adjustment and familiarity had to be established to allow monitoring of the ETCs by GTZ to be carried out effectively.

KARL STORZ's work framed the legal networks and ensured the timely installation of equipment and proper training for potential users of the equipment. Securing the necessary permission from the administrative sections of the government hospitals and transporting the equipment into safe places in the hospitals were key tasks. Owing to the advanced technology used for MIS, additional infrastructures such as reliable power and data communication needed to be created in some environments. Because the entire project is based on self-sustainability, a vital issue was the cost of ownership in terms of the service and replacement of worn out equipment. Our experience showed early on that it is essential for the training centres to charge participants a big enough training fee in order to be able to bear the unavoidable maintenance costs incurred by a long-term project.

One of the most pressing initial challenges proved to be low physician participation. Without sufficient numbers of expert and qualified teaching doctors, training could not be provided. However, a simple mailing to potential candidates resulted in a significant increase in registration. A second problem then arose in that registration for participants from the government sector required a rather lengthy approval procedure. Despite numerous approaches to the various state-level ministries of health, progress was slow. However, we remained convinced that, where bureaucratic inertia can be overcome, the various district hospitals could contribute large numbers of physicians to the pool of trained doctors. It was particularly important that government doctors from the rural areas could be trained in MIS because only then would the potential effectiveness of endoscopic procedures for disadvantaged women be realised.

Shifting the focus of women's reproductive and maternal medical treatment towards minimally invasive techniques employing endoscopy has the capacity of reducing the country's annual medical expenses substantially due to reduced postoperative hospital stays. The individual impact on personal lives cannot be estimated, but will be drastic.

Suggestions from KARL STORZ's early experiences

KARL STORZ's experience in working to realise the WHI can provide some suggestions for how this project, or similar projects, may be adapted and developed:

- The period of monitoring project operation and patient outcomes needs to be much longer than initially planned – 5–10 years may be adequate;
- Engagement with relevant government stakeholders early in the development of the project would be useful in avoiding the delays and difficulties associated with later entry;
- Communication is vital. Regular meetings or workshops involving the coordinators of the training centres have proved to be most useful;
- Internet communication is also an essential part of the ongoing flow of information;
- More training centres need to be established following the same patterns for improved coverage of the target areas.

Reviewing our current achievements compared with the desired results, we recognise that the WHI is merely a modest beginning. The potential of endoscopic surgery for reducing recovery time and using financial resources more efficiently is truly in line with the universal human right to health as stipulated in the United Nations' Universal Declaration of Human Rights. Our experiences have led to the conviction that further improvement in health care availability in rural areas will eventually reduce the need for patients to travel to metropolitan centres or even out of the country for treatment (and thereby also reduce the outflow of funds from rural areas).We also suggest that the successful establishment of clinics offering these advanced treatment methods will further contribute to the creation of additional workplaces for the rural population and attract other related professions, such as pharmacies, to establish their operations in these vicinities.

KARL STORZ's experiences of managing the WHI have led us to conclude that the most important benefit of the availability of endoscopy at a local level is the preventive character of regular check-ups. In western countries, endoscopy has helped greatly in detecting abnormalities at an early stage, allowing for conservative treatment and preventing the need for later surgical interventions. In India, it will still be a very long time before a similar system is established. This certainly exceeds the resources of a single family-owned company such as KARL STORZ. Nevertheless, the WHI has shown the way, and the first few steps have been made in what we consider the right direction.

Management perspectives: GTZ

ANU CHOPRA

Introduction

GTZ, in coordination with KARL STORZ, had an important on-the-ground management role in realising the WHI. Following the formal launch of the initiative in April 2005, GTZ and KARL STORZ worked together to draw up initial time plans and to articulate the major project milestones. A key task was the selection of six hospitals in which the Endoscopy Training Centres (ETCs) would be established. The factors taken into account in making the assessments included:

- expertise of trainers,
- availability of infrastructure,

- geographical location,
- existing usage of endoscopic treatment in the region.

Once the sites were selected, GTZ took part in briefing the hospitals about the WHI and concluding the administrative formalities, such as the finalisation of contracts and the installation of equipment to be used in the initiative. GTZ noted that the private hospitals were quick to sign agreements and faced fewer administrative challenges in installing equipment. Although the public hospitals were also anxious to receive equipment, gaining administrative approval took much longer – two to three months. GTZ's experience here showed that support for the selected project sites through regular communications and follow-up is very important in these early stages. Despite such efforts, progress on the WHI in the public hospitals, compared with the private hospitals, was delayed by about six months owing to these administrative hurdles and then by a further two to three months while technology was upgraded to be compatible with the new equipment.

In the meantime, however, the first UN workshop as well as the first training session commenced in Chennai in October 2005, which helped maintain overall project momentum. The next centre to start the training was Belle Vue Clinic in Kolkata, with two participants.

As well as initial difficulties in attracting sufficient numbers of doctors to deliver the training, there were also low numbers of participants registered for training in the early stages. So GTZ was relieved when training commenced in the public hospitals in March 2006. However, a number of other unexpected challenges arose that required resolution before the WHI could be properly implemented. These serve as a useful reminder that effective project planning must have the flexibility to respond to unforeseen events.

For example, a country-wide strike by medical students against the reservation system brought nearly all of our activities to a halt. The public hospitals were particularly affected by it. Summer vacations of approximately one and a half months had already been taken into account when scheduling the project, but the strike caused more unplanned delays.

Further, the number of participants registered for the courses remained very low and immediate action was needed to notify medical personnel about the availability of the endoscopy training facilities. Brochures were printed and distributed to a number of medical colleges in India. It took some time initially to spread this information, but slowly the attendance at all centres started to increase.

GTZ's role in implementing the WHI training

GTZ made visits to the ETCs and briefed trainees about the WHI objectives. Interactions with trainees were interesting because of the diversity of backgrounds, age groups and level of expertise. The exchange of views and experiences with trainees was enriching both for the trainees and for GTZ staff seeking to understand and implement the project.

Outcomes were encouraging when trainees returned to their clinics/hospitals on completion of their training. Initially, their experience was limited to a few diagnostic cases and operative assistance slowly extended to their colleagues. But this is a positive development in the right direction. The treatment has been made accessible and also affordable in regions where it had not, to date, been available.

Challenges remained, however. Although the training of these providers was encouraging, the collection of patients' data from them presented a considerable challenge. The trainees were requested to provide patient data after their return to their own clinics in order to assess the impact of the WHI at a country level, particularly with a view to the project's possible further replication. There was unfortunately little cooperation, however. The trainees had no legal obligation or incentive for submitting data. However, an idea slowly emerged: sending trainees further information and updating them in the field of endoscopy might motivate them to assist by sending patient data. This proved to some extent to be the case.

Another challenge was integrating non-governmental organisations (NGOs) in the initiative to assist with the dissemination of information about this treatment to the rural population. Because doctors as well as patients were unaware of NGOs, averse to involving them, or unsure about their effectiveness, their preferred approach was mainly to spread the information by word of mouth. Unfortunately, progress in this area remained slow, which underlines the importance of GTZ's frequent monitoring visits to ETCs to ensure that realities on the ground are understood and accounted for in planning, as well as to emphasise the importance of the WHI to trainees and trainers.

Suggestions from GTZ's first experiences

GTZ's experience with this project has shown that communication about the technology involved is important. This can be accomplished most effectively if trainees and ETCs can motivate the trainer doctors to update their knowledge and share their experiences. This will have a positive impact in developing expertise in the field as well as disseminating information about the endoscopic technology for treatment to the general public and medical personnel.

GTZ found that another important issue is maintaining the quality of training being conducted by ETCs, particularly in the future as the clinics become more independent of the formal PPP initiative. In this regard, the extension of monitoring by the project's partners would help the ETCs by continuing to promote the six ETCs as centres of excellence and encouraging more hospitals to become a part of the WHI.

GTZ was pleased to discover an unexpected positive outcome of this initiative, though it remains in its nascent stage – the training of paramedics. Because endoscopy requires team work, the upgrading of skills for paramedical staff to handle the equipment is having a positive effect. In the long run it will have two beneficial impacts: quality improvement and employment opportunities for skilled professionals.

Importantly, GTZ's experience in monitoring the WHI implementation showed that a premier medical institute does not necessarily guarantee a successful ETC. The autonomy of the institutes, the leadership quality of the head of department and internal team work between the faculty members are all important. Prior to implementing the initiative, it is also necessary to check the competence level of doctors as trainers.

The objective of the WHI is to make treatment using modern technologies available to the poor and underprivileged. The most suitable institutes to fulfil this social objective are the public hospitals and medical colleges. But they must also be autonomous bodies. The administrative procedures in government colleges are already cumbersome. If, in addition, the hospitals are not autonomous, the State Health Department frequently further complicates matters.

GTZ's experience suggests that the private hospital organisations should be committed to treating a certain percentage of patients (preferably at least 20–25 per cent) free of cost or at highly subsidised prices in exchange for the state-of-the-art equipment they receive. It has been observed that, although private hospitals are in metropolitan areas and can very well afford to procure this equipment, poor patients are still charged a considerable amount. Proper monitoring of the treatment of such patients should be an integral component of future initiatives, as should a framework for regular discussion and remedial action by the project partners should one of the ETCs experience difficulties or go off track.

The academic aspect of the training was left completely to the discretion of trainers since they belong to premier institutes in India. However, feedback from trainers showed that in fact there was a preference for greater standardisation of the training modules to ensure consistency of quality and content. This may be an area for future consideration and development.

In many ways, meeting patients was the most rewarding part of the process. The poor women met by GTZ staff were given access to endoscopic treatment and, most importantly, it was also made affordable. Most of these women had not even been aware that this type of minimally invasive treatment existed. Some of them had undergone open surgery in the past, and therefore were able to compare the advantages of this treatment. They were discharged in two to three days from the hospital, and this was a relief not only to the women but also to their family members, especially since general conditions in public hospitals are overstretched.

16

The WHI: Perspectives from private and public medical doctors in the Endoscopy Training Centres

The Women's Health Initiative (WHI) is a landmark project for its capacity to self-assess, evolve and improve as a result of inbuilt assessment and reflection mechanisms. An important element of this reflection derives from the experiences and observations of those doctors in the field who have been personally involved in establishing and maintaining the project's six Endoscopy Training Centres (ETCs). Two of these doctors – Professor Dr A. Kurian Joseph of Joseph's Nursing Home, Chennai and Professor Alka Kriplani of the Department of Obstetrics and Gynaecology at AIIMS in New Delhi – comment here on their respective experiences in a private and a public ETC. As the following discussions illustrate, there were some common themes and experiences in both situations, but there were also distinct challenges relating to individual circumstances. By identifying and exploring these factors, important insights into the practical operation of the WHI can be uncovered.

Partnerships for women's health: Striving for best practice within the UN Global Compact,
Timmermann and Kruesmann (eds),
United Nations University Press, 2009, ISBN 978-92-808-1185-8

Perspectives from a private medical doctor

A. KURIAN JOSEPH

India: A paradox

India has remained a paradox of our times in several aspects. It is a densely populated country of more than 1 billion living in crowded cities and distant rustic villages, yet it also has a large number of billionaires. It is a poverty-stricken nation where many go to bed with out a decent meal, yet food grains are exported. There are large numbers of illiterate people, yet also the largest computer workforce in the world. India has a maternal mortality rate among the highest in the world, yet its high-tech hospitals are on a par with the best in the world. India is the largest democracy in the world with a large proportion of women involved in all kinds of work. When the problem of women's health in India is discussed, it immediately assumes very complex dimensions. Blame it on the politicians, the rich, the elite or the educated, but the truth of unequal distribution becomes starkly evident.

Health is wealth both in the developed world and in the developing world. With improving technology, improvements in health care developed in the west gradually percolate down and reach the developing world. However, whenever any new technique or process is introduced, high costs serve as a deterrent to its widespread use. As time passes, however, costs come down and simpler alternatives become available. Then these methods are introduced into the poorest of places as their advantages are well known. This has been the story of endoscopy in women's health in India.

The role of women in India

The role of women in Indian society has been significant for a very long time. From Sita in the *Ramayana* (an Indian epic) to Indira Gandhi (the late Prime Minister), there have always been dominant women in India. Girls outshine boys in universities, and women are employed in all walks of life, from airline pilots to judges. Even Indian-born women are astronauts in spacecraft circling the globe. Yet, strangely, the average woman, though apparently emancipated, is firmly shackled to the hearth. This remains a paradox of our times and serves to retard progress in the field of women's health. Women experience more episodes of illness than men and are less likely to receive medical treatment before the illness is well advanced, especially in rural areas. Indices of maternal health such as the maternal mortality rate and the peri-natal mortality rate are poor. From childhood, women are constantly reminded that they are the weaker sex and born to look after the "lord" of the house. This results in a negative outlook that women accept as part of their fate.

However, the winds of change are blowing and, with better education, the modern woman is no longer willing to stay quiet and accept her fate. Even the poor demand and get better facilities and better health care.

Health care in India

Health care in India is run primarily by the large government-supported public hospitals alongside the smaller private hospitals. The larger hospitals have adequate funds but they are poorly utilised, whereas the private hospitals, with fewer funds, are run more aggressively and efficiently. This picture holds good for the cities, but in the smaller towns and villages, where a majority of people live, the government set-up is mediocre, staffing is inadequate and funding is insufficient. The private health sector in the smaller towns is also inadequate and dominated by unethical methods of earning quick money. The smallest village-based primary health centres often have a shortage of doctors because the jobs are difficult but poorly rewarded. Moreover, staying in a small remote village is not attractive to the doctor's family.

Another problem facing the improvement of health care is the poor transport system coupled with poor roads. Instances of mothers with life-threatening conditions waiting for a public transport bus to come are many. Doctors in the smaller rural hospitals are barely qualified and have little scope for expanding their knowledge and skills. In the bigger cities, the presence of the large pharmaceutical companies and instrument makers results in more academic activity, and conferences and continuing medical education programmes are commonly available. Yet there are no incentives to upgrade skills to maintain the validity of one's licence. Several professional bodies and organisations are trying to step in and improve that situation. The Federation of Obstetricians and Gynaecologists of India, with over 22,000 members, is at the forefront of improving maternal health care.

In this context it may be justified to ask why endoscopy should be a priority. To answer that let me first highlight what endoscopy is.

What is endoscopy?

Endoscopy is a field of medicine where a small "scope" is passed into a body cavity. This enables a detailed study of the cavity to determine treatment. Endoscopy was introduced in the western world in the late 1940s. Today, endoscopy has made inroads into most areas of medical and surgical practice, and it has become a surgical system where procedures that required major operations are now done as simple "keyhole" surgery. The initial scope popularised in the field of women's health was the laparoscope, which was used to inspect the abdominal cavity. Then came the hysteroscope, used to inspect the uterine cavity. Several other scopes are now used in gynaecology, such as the salpingoscope and the falloposcope. The father figures of the early development were doctors/inventors from Europe such as Raul Palmer, Hans Frangenheim and Kurt Semm. Endoscopes became more effective with the development of accessories such as light sources, cameras and many surgical instruments to be used together with the endoscope. Initially, the scopes were used only for diagnosis – being of great use in finding the cause of abnormal bleeding and abdominal pain or infertility – but gradually more and more operative procedures were carried out with their aid. The advent of the small video camera converted an endoscopic procedure where the surgeon had to bend down to peer through a laparoscope into comfortable surgery where the surgeon could stand erect, view a monitor and operate.

Endoscopy came to India in the early 1970s as a method of tubal ligation (tubal sterilisation). This was very popular in towns all across the country, and large numbers of people underwent the operation as part of the National Family Welfare Programme. This resulted in several hundred surgeons becoming familiar with the laparoscope. However, owing to inadequate monitoring, these arrangements for laparoscopic sterilisation became unpopular after a couple of years. The surgeons, however, went on to more advanced procedures. The Indian Association of Gynaecological Endoscopists (1976) was one of the early associations formed to promote endoscopy. We at Joseph's Nursing Home, Chennai, started laparoscopy in 1978, and by 1992 we were doing advanced procedures. Our first endoscopy training programme started in 1994, and the centre has been recognised by the All India Federation of Obstetricians and Gynaecologists as a training centre since 1995.

What does it do in women's health?

Consider a young woman developing sudden abdominal pain. She is taken to a nearby hospital where an examination reveals that she has a tubal (ectopic) pregnancy. This is a life-threatening condition if not handled quickly. She is taken to a facility with endoscopic surgery facilities, a laparoscope is introduced and the tubal pregnancy is verified. Other instruments are introduced and the tubal pregnancy removed. The procedure is completed in an hour; the patient can go home the next day and is usually back at work in a couple of days. The same scenario, if done in a facility without endoscopy available, would need an operation to open the abdomen (laparotomy), following which the same steps of removing the tube would be carried out. A minimum postoperative stay of four or five days in hospital is needed. This is followed by a recovery phase that may take 10–14 days. During this stage, rest is essential to permit healing of the abdominal wound, and the incidence of wound infection is high. Effectively there is a difference between a two-day and a two-week period of incapacitation. This picture is further complicated by the situation at home when the women is convalescing because the routine domestic chores come to a halt, and the feeding and maintenance of the family suffers. The same situation applies if the problem is a twisted ovarian cyst or a non-malignant tumour in the abdomen. Women should not really undergo major surgery for a simple ovarian cyst or for assessing her cause of infertility because an attempt to treat her may do greater harm.

The hysteroscope is a very useful instrument in addressing abnormal uterine bleeding and growths within the uterus and in assessing fertility-related problems. Many instances of a major organ such as the uterus being removed because of such bleeding could be prevented by doing a hysteroscopy, diagnosing the cause and treating it immediately. Today, several other endoscopic procedures are increasingly in demand, for example laparoscopic hysterectomy (removal of the uterus using the laparoscope) or the removal of tumours or fibroids. These procedures, however, require surgeons to develop a greater level of competence and expertise.

This in a nutshell shows that endoscopic surgery helps in the diagnosis and the effective treatment of women's problems and also helps them to get back to work quickly. These concepts are the same wherever endoscopic surgery is practised. In addition, there are other benefits such as the low incidence of infection, minimal scarring and the ability to diagnose and handle associated problems. All these procedures are accepted as standard in hospitals in the developed world.

Problems of endoscopy

Effective treatment methods do still have their drawbacks and problems. The three main drawbacks of endoscopic surgery are the need for a hospital and special equipment, the training needed to perform the surgery and the cost.

Endoscopy needs a basic hospital where the equipment can be set up. The hospital need not be high-tech because only simple laboratory tests need to be carried out; a small efficient operating room is adequate. At present this can be done in most district hospitals and in the smaller hospitals in the small towns. Many of these centres have had prior exposure to endoscopy as part of the National Family Welfare Programme. The endoscopy equipment is expensive, but costs can be kept reasonable if the inventory is kept to a minimum and all instruments are sterilized and reused, since the use of disposable instruments is a major factor in cost escalation. Well-maintained equipment lasts longer and hence the operating room personnel need to be trained in this area.

It is here that the experience we had gained at Joseph's Nursing Home, Chennai helped. We had started endoscopic surgery in 1980 with basic instruments as part of a tubal sterilisation programme. We slowly developed the technique, taking care to keep the procedures and set-up simple and cost effective. The entire staff in the operating rooms was locally trained. As our experience improved we started doing more and more procedures laparoscopically. Today, we do most gynaecological procedures through the laparoscope. Our efforts at cost containment have succeeded to the extent that nowadays we do not charge extra for doing a procedure with the laparoscope. In other words, we charge the same for a procedure done by open surgery and by laparoscopy. Hence, we believe that, with proper training and careful control of costs, we can make endoscopy procedures practical and economical.

Quantifying the cost effectiveness of endoscopy has been the biggest problem when assessing the success of the techniques. The initial cost of the set-up, the equipment and the training of the doctors is high. The added expense of maintenance and replacements is also an issue. On the other hand, we have a quick procedure with a shorter stay in hospital, more speedy wound healing and a rapid return to work. If these advantages are measured against the costs of hospitalisation, then the procedure is very cost effective. If, however, only a basic primary set-up is sought, then investments in setting up and maintaining such technical facilities are redundant.

Given this, is it fair to decide that poor/rural women should not get more effective treatment? The answer seems to lie in the effective and proper management of funds.

Endoscopy training

The training of an endoscopic surgeon is quite specific. The surgeon has to develop hand/eye coordination so that they can look at a monitor screen and operate at the same time. Further, endoscopic instruments are small and quite different from the ones the doctors are used to. This means that surgeons have to enrol in dedicated endoscopy training courses where these skills are taught. In our initial experiences, these courses were hard to find and expensive. Furthermore, they were based on the personal ability of the tutor, with no prepared curriculum. In fact, most were weekend courses where the dinners appeared more important than the training.

This led us to develop a two-week course in 1994 in which we incorporated the guidelines provided by several endoscopy associations. To this we added demonstrations on equipment maintenance and trouble-shooting. The lack of trained, competent support personnel was a problem, and at times the surgeon had to double up as the electrician, the theatre technician, the photographer and the plumber. The first groups of trainees were more socialites in nature trying to add to their qualifications with another certificate, but then there were also dedicated learners who would diligently go through the entire course. Some of these surgeons have today become competent endoscopic surgeons.

The initial training consisted of simple exercises on a "Pelvi-trainer", picking up peanuts or mints and putting them on a marked spot. This helped with hand/eye coordination. The exercises then became more complex, with skills such as cutting, coagulating and suturing. This was practised on both inanimate and animate tissue. Over the two-week period, most trainees became quite adept at handling the instruments. In a period of 10 years we trained more than 700 doctors from India and abroad, and when we followed up on our trainees we found that about a third of them regularly carry out endoscopy; another third carry out endoscopy infrequently; and the rest do not carry out the procedure at all. On further analysing the situation of those who did not carry out endoscopy, we became aware that there was a lack of formal credentialing, which made many hesitant to venture out and perform surgery. It was at this point that we received the offer of support as part of the Women's Health Initiative through KARL STORZ. We accepted the offer to train 40 doctors every year from smaller towns in the country so that they could go and use this knowledge in the service of the poor patients in their towns. At the end of the training and after a post-course test, the doctors were awarded certificates.

What the WHI aims to achieve

The aim of the WHI is to spread the concept and practice of endoscopy to benefit the poor. The major metropolitan areas in India are quite well served by endoscopy centres, and the aim was therefore to train doctors from smaller towns and cities. This would update their management principles from the ones they learnt at medical school, and in turn they would be able to use the new skills to the benefit of their patients. The demand–supply cycle will lead to the creation of more endoscopy centres in smaller towns. More endoscopy would mean more patients recovering quickly, with fewer infections and lower morbidity.

We started the training course in October 2005 and completed the full quota of training for that year. By 2007, we had trained nearly 70 doctors. Our trainees have come from all over the country; the majority of them are women and all are postgraduate doctors. Approval of the courses by the doctors has been uniformly good. However, not many of them have started work with the endoscope in their own health centres yet. The major difficulties are the time and the funds needed to set up endoscopy facilities at their home locations. We are trying to remedy the situation by organising a "basic set" of instruments that will be sufficient to start endoscopic work in otherwise unsuitable centres. The KARL STORZ Company has offered to provide the instruments at a subsidised cost.

Where do we go from here?

A good beginning has been made in organising structured training in the field of gynaecological endoscopy to benefit the poor in smaller Indian towns. We are thankful for the private public partnership that has enabled this. However, this is only a small step. For the attempt to improve the lot of women in smaller towns and villages to be effective, we must persist with the programme in the longer term. Training around 200 doctors at all the training centres each year is just a drop in the ocean of need. Further steps to support and update the skills and expertise of doctors already trained will be needed, and monitoring their work and helping them to solve the problems they encounter will encourage them to do more.

We believe in the words of a great Indian spiritual leader, Swami Vivekananda: "All the powers in the universe are already ours. It is we who have put our hands before our eyes and cry that it is dark." So let us raise our hands and stand counted in the effort to improve the health of Indian women.

Perspectives from a public medical doctor

ALKA KRIPLANI

Introduction

In medical terms, the majority of gynaecological surgeries previously requiring a laparotomy can now be performed using laparoscopy or hysteroscopy. In comparison with traditional techniques, laparoscopy and hysteroscopy have minimal surgical impact on the patient. This includes a shortened postoperative hospital stay and recovery period, reduced postoperative discomfort (less need for analgesia), better cosmetic outcomes and generally lower overall costs. Hysteroscopic surgery for intra-uterine deformities such as uterine septa or submucosal fibroids eliminates the need for laparotomy and incisions in the uterine wall. Where tubal sterilisation is sought as a permanent method of contraception (as it may be in India), laparoscopic methods of tubal ligation again offer advantages over the traditional minilaparotomy approach.

In the developed world, incorporation of laparoscopic and hysteroscopic surgery into daily gynaecologic practice is widespread, imparting a distinct advantage in the health care of those women. For the women of developing countries, in contrast, the availability of endoscopic surgery is very restricted, owing to the lack of accessibility of sophisticated equipment and the necessary skills and training facilities.

At present the health system in India is run by both government and private sectors. The government health care systems deliver health care at primary, secondary and tertiary health centres. Treatment in government hospitals is free of cost, but most minimally invasive surgery (MIS) is available only in expensive private hospitals, which are not accessible to the majority of the population. Very few gynaecologists in India currently practise endoscopic surgery and, of those, most are located in urban areas.

Common gynaecological problems in women include infertility, adnexal pathology including endometriosis, pelvic inflammatory disease, ectopic pregnancy and dysfunctional uterine bleeding. The majority of these problems can be successfully managed endoscopically. However, owing to the lack of infrastructure in government hospitals and high costs in private hospitals, the majority of Indian women are unable to benefit from MIS.

If endoscopic surgery facilities with trained physicians were made available to more women, it would help improve the health care of those young women who are in the most productive years of their lives and whose health is largely neglected in developing countries for various reasons, including gender bias.

Proper training and certification are important to ensure the highest quality of health care, to maximise success and to minimise morbidity. Training is also essential for the medicolegal protection of the doctor. Proper training also minimises the risk of complications during and after surgical procedures. Addressing some of these issues is a key objective of the Women's Health Initiative.

Goals of the programme

The WHI is a programme committed to improving women's health care in India, particularly in small towns and rural communities. The programme aims to provide equipment and training facilities to increase the use of gynaecological endoscopic surgery (including laparoscopic and hysteroscopic surgery). The main objective of the Endoscopy Training Centres established under the WHI endeavour is to train practising gynaecologists from various locales in India, with a special emphasis on training those from smaller cities and rural areas. In addition to surgical education, gynaecologists receive basic training in diagnosing and treating infertility cases and in reducing surgical complications; they are also taught the basic functioning and maintenance of endoscopic equipment. This training will help provide the increasing numbers of poor girls and women who require surgery with all the benefits of this MIS approach.

Expectations regarding results of the programme

After completing their training, practitioners are expected to gradually incorporate more advanced minimally invasive gynaecological surgery into subsequent work at their usual health facilities, including performing laparoscopic sterilisation operations rather than open laparotomy procedures. During the training sessions, trainees are taught how to implement laparoscopic training in their own health facilities. Routine procedures benefiting from endoscopic techniques include infertility diagnosis and management, ectopic pregnancy and common gynaecological diseases such as endometriosis and adnexal pathology. With increasing experience it is also expected that practitioners will become adept at managing fibroids and removing the uterus endoscopically. The gynaecologists should also be able to perform laparoscopic ligation operations, select patients for appropriate endoscopic procedures, select the necessary instrumentation, minimise intraoperative/postoperative complications and manage a postoperative course.

The set-up of the programme

The WHI programme for endoscopic training for doctors was started in 2006 and is presently running in six centres in India, of which four are government institutes and two are private hospitals owned by individual doctors. Four times a year, 10 gynaecologists who have submitted their curriculum vitae are selected from health care centres in various parts of the country to participate in a 10-day training programme, including practical interaction between the trainee doctors and the trainers. The course details are advertised through various news bulletins and KARL STORZ stalls. Circulars are sent to major teaching institutions and announcements are made at all academic conferences and on teaching programmes.

The programme plans to train 40 doctors every year. Trainees are charged a nominal fee of Rs 15,000, which is to be used for the maintenance and upgrading of existing equipment in the training centres. Selected trainees are practising gynaecologists with a postgraduate diploma or degree and who have, in their current positions, limited facilities and exposure to minimally invasive surgery. Four training courses had been successfully completed by February 2007. The trainers are department faculty currently practising in various government and private hospitals.

At the beginning of each session, an evaluation is done to assess the basic knowledge of the trainees; the trainers can then demonstrate the surgeries and deliver lectures with Q&A sessions accordingly. At the end of a training session, a second assessment is undertaken to evaluate the effectiveness of the programme. At the end of each session, trainees are also able to give their feedback and suggestions to improve or modify the training.

Pelvi-trainers are supplied during the training session for practical training purposes. During live demonstrations, basic principles and practical aspects are also explained: for example, the insertion of a verres needle, the creation of a pneumoperitoneum, the umbilical port, accessory ports, explanations about the working principles of monopolar and bipolar electrocoagulation, the handling of hand instruments and laparoscopic suturing (intracorporeal and extracorporeal). Among the various surgical procedures demonstrated are laparoscopic tubal ligation, diagnostic laparoscopy and chromotubation, ovarian cystectomy, myomectomy, tuboplasty, tubal recanalisation, adhesiolysis, laparoscopic assisted vaginal hysterectomy, total laparoscopic hysterectomy, laparoscopic radical hysterectomy, diagnostic hysteroscopy, hysteroscopic adhesiolysis and hysteroscopic septal resection.

There have been several challenges in setting up the programme. Prior to starting the programme, obtaining the necessary government permission, installing the equipment, acquiring training facilities and setting up ISDN lines were all early challenges, but once these were overcome there have been no serious issues in this area. One ongoing challenge, however, has been an increased demand for training availability because only 10 trainees are accepted per session. This is a very popular programme with a long waiting list of trainees. It has also been a challenge for trainers to make time in their busy schedules to conduct Pelvi-trainer sessions and deliver lectures over a 10-day training period.

Set-up of the training

Surgeries are conducted in the major operating theatre in the Endoscopy Training Centre and a live telecast is broadcast to the conference hall. The trainees usually watch and are able to discuss the procedure through a two-way audiovisual system. ISDN line access allows surgical procedures to be transmitted anywhere in India. With this access, trainees performing surgeries in their individual facilities can continue to contact trainers for expert advice. Pelvi-trainers are kept in the conference hall for trainees' practice. At the end of each day, a detailed discussion is held regarding the surgeries performed that day and on any particular surgical procedure.

At the end of the session, participants are provided with CDs of the procedures performed throughout the course. The KARL STORZ Company, which supplies the endoscopic equipment for the entire programme, also provides CDs containing video clips of operative procedures and correct use of the equipment, in addition to course materials and books. After returning to their own health care facilities, the trainees' subsequent progress is monitored by GTZ, which keeps a record of procedures subsequently performed by these doctors and which continues to support them by providing the latest CDs with video recordings of procedures performed by experts.

Conclusions and future prospects

The majority of trainers' expectations of the programme concerning the provision of state-of-the-art equipment have been fulfilled. The WHI is expected to provide maintenance for the basic units (for example, camera, cautery and monitors) in the case of malfunction. Smaller units such as hand instruments can be maintained with money raised from the course fees. Further provision of the latest equipment as and when it is introduced on the market is also anticipated. To ensure continued education and skill upgrading, the WHI should go on providing course materials, including CDs containing video clips of the latest surgical procedures and techniques.

Experience with the programme so far allows some perspectives and ideas on its possible future development to be suggested.

Structure of the training

From the perspective of medical doctors involved in the WHI, it is recommended that some changes to the structure of the training be considered. In particular, it is suggested that, apart from doctors, there should be separate training programmes/modules for nurses and occupational therapy (OT) technicians. Nurses should be trained with more emphasis on the maintenance and care of equipment and hand instruments. OT technicians should be trained in the basics of equipment, troubleshooting in case of minor malfunctioning, and the care of equipment and energy sources. A formal examination at the end of the training would also help increase the involvement of trainees, encouraging a more serious approach to training.

It could be considered whether the programme might be extended outside India to neighbouring countries in the future. For example, one session has already included four trainee doctors and two nurses from Nepal, and there have been more requests.

A separate programme could be started for training in laparoscopic sterilisation procedures. Other state government authorities have requested this. Because India has problems of overpopulation, female sterilisation is a popular method of contraception. At present, the facilities for laparoscopic sterilisation are limited, owing to the lack of widespread availability of laparoscopic equipment and trained doctors who could perform these procedures.

Participation of government agencies

Greater government participation could enhance the programme and its aims in several ways. Endoscopic training should be incorporated in the basic postgraduate degree training curricula. Because endoscopy is a permanent fixture in our society, the younger generations, if exposed to it from the beginning of their careers, would adopt minimal access surgery without encountering the difficulties that the present generation of practising gynaecologists faces.

Government agencies could also play a stronger role in maintaining and enhancing doctors' surgical skills after the initial endoscopic training. Doctors embarking on a new endoscopic programme face many problems at first, and they often need help. For example, trainers could be supported to conduct workshops at a trainee's workplace and to help set up a new endoscopic facility at peripheral hospitals.

Mobile vans with endoscopic equipment could also be taken to peripheral/rural areas to provide practical training.

More practical experience

There is an increasing demand for hands-on training in medical procedures, which becomes difficult in projects such as the WHI for medicolegal reasons and where there is a commitment to train postgraduate trainees. If virtual reality Pelvi-trainers could be provided, like computer training programmes, or Pelvi-trainers simulating human bodies, basic skills such as inserting a verres needle or a primary trocar insertion could be taught. This would increase a trainee's self-confidence in performing these procedures independently. In general, more Pelvi-trainers should be made available. In the feedback given at the end of training, all trainees request more time to work on Pelvi-trainers.

More live minimal access gynaecological surgery workshops should be arranged after finishing the 10-day course. This would allow the frequent exchange of knowledge and skills between trainees and trainers and ensure regular improvements of both trainees' and trainers' skills.

17

The economic logic of the Women's Health Initiative as a business model for poverty alleviation

Christina Gradl

Introduction

"Endoscopy for the poor in developing countries" – the proposition of the Women's Health Initiative (WHI) – sounds almost cynical. Surely, such high-tech treatment would be unaffordable for anybody qualifying as "poor" in a low economic development context? In fact, endoscopy reduces the cost of treatment, compared with alternative methods, by raising productivity. The technology enables both doctors and patients to save time and other resources, and it is thus appropriate to include it in a "business model for poverty alleviation". Such models describe ways in which companies can sell profitably to the poor while simultaneously improving the latters' well-being. This chapter looks at the WHI as such a business model. It shows how social and business goals are combined, describes the special challenges of the "market of the poor", and suggests lessons that can be learned from the project.

Partnerships for women's health: Striving for best practice within the UN Global Compact,
Timmermann and Kruesmann (eds),
United Nations University Press, 2009, ISBN 978-92-808-1185-8

My focus is on the economic logic of the WHI and, to this end, the chapter portrays all actors as rational agents seeking their own benefit. This assumption should not be misinterpreted as a descriptive ("all actors are exclusively self-interested") or even a normative statement ("all actors should act in a self-interested manner"). Rather, this standard economic assumption helps to reveal the incentive structures that actors face when making decisions. Understanding these structures allows statements about what actors are likely to do, which in turn explains why a business model works as it does and what challenges to its success may remain.

The following discussion has three main components. After a brief outline of the project set-up, I introduce the concept of business models for poverty alleviation as one of mutual benefit, and I describe the gains to both KARL STORZ and the patients from the WHI. I then show how business models for poverty alleviation are different from standard business development by highlighting the special challenges of the "market of the poor". It becomes clear that, in order to achieve its social and business goals, such a model must be integrated into the existing "ecosystem" by creating the right framework conditions and aligning the interests of the relevant actors.

The discussion of the WHI from an economic perspective suggests four key lessons on how to approach the market of the poor: businesses must (1) think systemically; (2) invest in market framework conditions; (3) involve local actors; and (4) plan long term.

The WHI at a glance

The WHI seeks to improve access to endoscopic treatment for women in India. In essence, it is a training programme in endoscopic treatment methods for gynaecologists. Endoscopy refers to the examination of a cavity or organ inside the body by means of an optical device, the endoscope. The technology allows for precise diagnosis of intracorporal problems and a minimally invasive approach where surgery is required. The programme was initiated by KARL STORZ, a German medical technology company that develops, manufactures

Figure 17.1   Set-up of the WHI

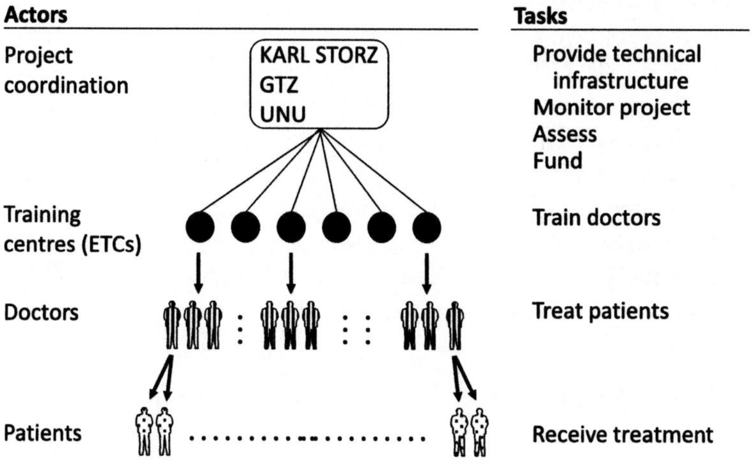

Actors		Tasks

Source: the author.

and sells endoscopy equipment, mainly for medical applications. The basic set-up of the project is illustrated in Figure 17.1.

The initiative is a partnership between KARL STORZ, the German Society for Technical Cooperation (Deutsche Gesellschaft für Technische Zusammenarbeit, GTZ) and the United Nations University (UNU). All three partners share responsibility for coordinating the project.[1] KARL STORZ provides the equipment and ensures its technical implementation. GTZ monitors the implementation and social impact of the programme. UNU assesses the project from a broader policy perspective, discussing its relevance for poverty alleviation, the protection of human rights and the governance of cross-sectoral partnerships. KARL STORZ and GTZ share the project costs. The project commenced in December 2004 and concluded in June 2007.

Six Endoscopy Training Centres (ETCs) were set up within the gynaecology departments of renowned hospitals in India. Two of the ETCs are in private hospitals in Chennai and Kolkata, the other four are in public hospitals in Chandigarh, Cuttack, Delhi and Lucknow, and all are medical teaching institutions. ETCs have been provided with state-of-the-art endoscopy equipment, and in the future they will also form a virtual network linked by an Internet platform that can be used to observe and advise on surgical procedures in other hospitals. ETCs offer regular two-week training courses where doctors learn how to use endoscopic equipment for both the diagnosis and treatment of gynaecological problems. The availability of endoscopic equipment is a prerequisite for participation, and doctors pay a fee for the course.[2] After training, it is intended that doctors will apply their new skills in their own medical practice. A particular goal of the WHI is to reach out to doctors from rural areas in India, and all doctors must also commit to treating patients from poor backgrounds.

Patients who do receive endoscopic treatment benefit mainly from better diagnosis and the reduced invasiveness of treatment. Endoscopy provides exact information from inside the body, thus allowing for a precise identification of irregularities, and it requires no or only small incisions to access the body. Compared with the standard procedures of open surgery, the approach reduces both the length of stay in hospital and the postoperative recovery period. Moreover, the risks of infection, as well as the need for medication after the operation, are reduced.

The concept of business models for poverty alleviation

A concept of mutual benefit

Today, responsible business is no longer only about reducing a company's negative impact, but is also about having a positive impact by solving social and environmental problems. In recent years, calls for a more "responsible" way of doing business have increased. Companies have come under greater scrutiny from civil society actors and, as a result, have started to examine their business practices with a view not only to economic but also to ecological and social impacts.[3] The initial activities of companies to comply with their "corporate responsibilities" have focused on limiting the damage particular business practices do to "people and the planet", a focus that could largely be described as risk control – avoiding the risk of bad publicity, disloyal employees or the loss of the licence to operate. More recently, an alternative conception of corporate responsibility has been adopted by business executives: that of developing solutions to social and environmental problems. Solving problems through innovation is indeed the core competency and *raison d'être* of some companies. This type of responsible business is driven by a call not to limit activities but to extend them.[4] The challenges people living in poverty face have been identified as an opportunity for responsible business development.[5]

The concept of "business for poverty alleviation" refers to business models that can profitably provide products and services to the poor in developing countries while simultaneously improving their well-being. "Poverty" is best understood here as the absence of opportunity resulting from a lack of material, physical, intellectual and social resources.[6] Translated into economic terms, poverty can be described as a lack of productivity owing to the absence of capital.[7] Access to products and services can improve the situation of the poor because they can then increase their productivity and gain new opportunities. Providing products to the poor can benefit a company because it creates new customers and thus increases its revenues. Moreover, these engagements can also improve a company's reputation and lead to transferable innovation.

Supplying goods and services to the poor via the market has (at least) three advantages over philanthropic donations. First, these businesses are compatible with people's own incentives. There is no need for continuous extensive monitoring and enforcement systems, since people benefit from complying with the system. Second, sustainability is already built into any functional business model for poverty alleviation. A successful business model is, above all, a profitable one. If the company supplying the product or service benefits from it, the model will simply become part of its mainstream business after the implementation phase. There is no previously defined "project end", as with typical aid projects that have no refunding mechanism. Third, a functional business model can also be scaled up and transferred to other places. Once the mechanisms for the business model are well understood, it can be implemented elsewhere, as long as the new circumstances correspond to it. There is no inherent limit to scale, since the business model ensures a sufficient return on investment.

The WHI follows the basic logic of "business for poverty alleviation". It seeks to provide a service to the poor that is rarely available to them, namely endoscopic diagnosis and treatment of women's gynaecological problems. It seeks to increase the number of doctors who offer this treatment by providing training. If more doctors use endoscopy, women gain better access to quality health care and KARL STORZ gains new potential customers. In this context, the benefits both to KARL STORZ and to women in rural India will be described in more detail below.

Business benefits

The WHI corresponds well with KARL STORZ's market position and strategy in India: the company has been actively selling endoscopic equipment in that country for more than 40 years. It has established a strong brand, which is associated with best-in-class quality. Even though the price of the equipment is comparatively high, it holds a major share of the market for endoscopic equipment in India.[8] However, competition is increasing steadily in the Indian market. Today, there is a multitude of local manufacturers offering their products at a fraction of the price of KARL STORZ equipment. Moreover, they frequently copy the technology and design developed by KARL STORZ and, despite evident differences in quality, customers often choose these much cheaper copies.

The WHI responds to this challenge in two ways:

(a) The publicity associated with the WHI reinforces the perception of KARL STORZ as a cutting-edge technology provider and as a company investing in education. Collaboration with renowned medical institutions supports this claim of high brand quality.

(b) The WHI also expands the overall market for endoscopy technology in India. At an individual level, the training enables doctors to practise endoscopic treatment in their own practices, and thus the doctors become potential customers. By using the KARL STORZ instruments during the training, doctors become familiar and comfortable with their handling and quality, and this creates customer loyalty and increases willingness to pay the price premium of KARL STORZ products. At an institutional level, the WHI encourages policy changes. Although endoscopy is already used in other areas, such as urology, it has not been as popular in gynaecology. Formal public policy does not actively support endoscopy in gynaecological practice, and it is barely taught in either undergraduate or postgraduate medical studies. The WHI can highlight the benefits of endoscopic treatment in gynaecology from both a medical and a financial point of view. This may lead to changes in medical curriculums and in public policy, which would make endoscopy a standard practice in gynaecology.

With these benefits, KARL STORZ can expect a positive return on investment in the WHI. Even though competitors will reap some of the benefit, KARL STORZ is likely to capture the majority of the newly created market, thanks to its strong market positioning.

Consumer benefits

For patients, endoscopic treatment has a number of advantages. It allows precise and early diagnosis of abdominal problems and minimally invasive therapy. It thus reduces the cost and risk of treatment and minimises the need for hospitalisation. This prevents families from falling into poverty and increases their willingness to seek medical care.

In gynaecology, endoscopy is used for three major indications: abnormal bleeding and abdominal pain, infertility and sterilisation.[9] Only endoscopic sterilisation is already widely available (including in rural areas), owing to public policy efforts to control population

Figure 17.2   Change in the burden of disease in India:
Estimates and projections, 1990 and 2020

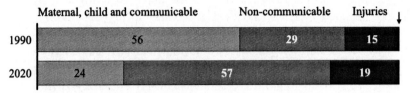

Source: World Health Organization, *Investing in Health Research and Development*, Geneva: WHO, 1996, p. 57.

growth. Endoscopic treatment of pain and bleeding problems and of infertility is available only in cities and mostly in private hospitals. In public policy terms these are subordinate problems, because they constitute only a minor part of women's burden of disease in India. The most important causes of female morbidity and mortality today are related to pregnancy and birth as well as communicable diseases.

However, the burden of disease is changing, with non-communicable diseases such as cancer and cardiovascular problems becoming more important. And, even today, the number of women affected by the above-mentioned problems is significant. It is estimated that more than 1 million hysterectomies are performed each year and that more than 20 million women suffer from infertility.[10]

Endoscopy improves both the diagnosis and treatment of gynaecological problems. Endoscopic diagnosis allows for a precise identification of the cause of the problem, which is essential for targeted therapy. With a clear diagnosis, surgery can often be avoided and, if required, can be concentrated closely on the identified problem area. Surgery can be performed without or with only small incisions since doctors access the body through the vagina or through "keyholes" in the abdomen.

This minimally invasive surgery has a number of advantages for the patient compared with the alternative of open surgery. Most importantly, recovery times are reduced significantly. Even major surgery such as hysterectomy can be ambulatory or with one overnight

Figure 17.3   Hospitalised Indians falling into poverty as a
result of medical costs, 1995/96 (per cent)

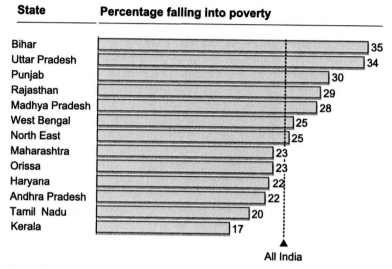

State   **Percentage falling into poverty**

Source: World Bank, *India: Raising the Sights – Better Health Systems for India's Poor, Overview*, Washington, DC: World Bank, 2001, p. 3.
Note: Selection of states based on location of ETCs.

stay in hospital, and women can fully resume their normal activities after one week. After open surgery, women stay in hospital for at least one week and have to wait four to six weeks before they can go back to normal life. Moreover, endoscopic surgery reduces postoperative problems. The risk of infections and complications after surgery is less, and women experience less pain because of the minor incisions. Consequently, less medication such as painkillers and antibiotics is needed and for a shorter period of time. Finally, body aesthetics are improved because scars are small or absent.

Minimising hospitalisation helps to prevent people from falling into poverty. Statistics show that, on average, one-fifth of patients fall below the poverty line after a stay in hospital, as shown in Figure 17.3.[11] In Uttar Pradesh, one of the poorest states in India and the location of one ETC, the percentage of inpatients falling into poverty is as high as 34 per cent.

The reason for this economic decline is threefold. First, a stay in hospital is expensive. In public hospitals, treatment is free but patients have to pay for medication and catering for themselves and their family members, who always accompany the patient. In private hospitals, patients also need to pay for the treatment, and charges can easily exceed a poor person's annual income.[12] Second, there are no risk-sharing mechanisms in place that would protect families from unexpected high expenses owing to illness and injury. Health insurance covers less than 10 per cent of the population, mostly upper-income governmental or industrial employees.[13] Most payments for health care are made out-of-pocket, and the poor finance more than 40 per cent of their medical expenses through debt.[14] Third, patients and their families forgo earnings during their time in hospital. They cannot attend to their housework and fieldwork or to paid employment. Avoiding or minimising hospitalisation is thus a direct contribution to the economic stability of a family.

Reducing the duration of incapacitation also increases acceptance of women seeking medical care. Women in the village have many responsibilities and work very hard from early morning to the evening hours. Hence, they find it difficult to take time off for a stay in hospital. Women also depend on other family members to make decisions for them; they cannot simply go to see a doctor but must ask their husband or in-laws for permission. Therefore, women often delay necessary medical examinations, especially when they expect surgery. As a result, problems are often detected only when they are acute. The reduced cost of treatment can make it more acceptable, and thus women may be less reluctant to seek medical care.

The market of the poor

Clearly, both KARL STORZ and poor women benefit from more doctors offering the treatment. But what is so special about this concept of business models for poverty alleviation? After all, exchange for mutual benefit is the basis for any business model; it is indeed the very essence of market logic. The specialness lies in the particular "ecosystem" prevalent in the market of the poor. In this section, the notion of a "business ecosystem" is introduced to explain the challenges that companies face in the market of the poor and how to respond to them.

The WHI ecosystem

Looking at a market as a "business ecosystem" helps to understand the difference between developed and developing markets. In biology, the term "ecosystem" refers to "a system formed by the interaction of a community of organisms with their physical environment".[15] Here, this idea is translated from an ecological to an economic interpretation. An economic ecosystem can be defined as a system formed by the interaction of a community of actors with their market framework conditions, as illustrated Figure 17.4. A market is often described simply as a set of sellers and buyers but, in reality, markets are complex systems with a variety of actors and based on varying conditions. The framework conditions describe the environment of a business ecosystem. They include all the factors required to establish a market, such as contract enforcement systems and infrastructure. The actors in a business ecosystem are all parties that affect or are affected by the business activity – the stakeholders.[16]

In a business ecosystem, framework conditions and actors influence each other. Actors respond to the existing framework conditions, but they can also change them. In fact, the framework conditions are largely (except for the natural physical environment) designed by the members of a society. The difference between framework conditions and actors thus corresponds closely to the difference between the social and the individual: as a society, we define a certain set of rules and provide certain common goods; as individuals, we respond to these conditions based on our own interest in achieving private goods.

A business model describes how a new product or service offer fits into an existing ecosystem. A successful business model will ensure that the right framework conditions are in place and that the

Figure 17.4   The WHI ecosystem

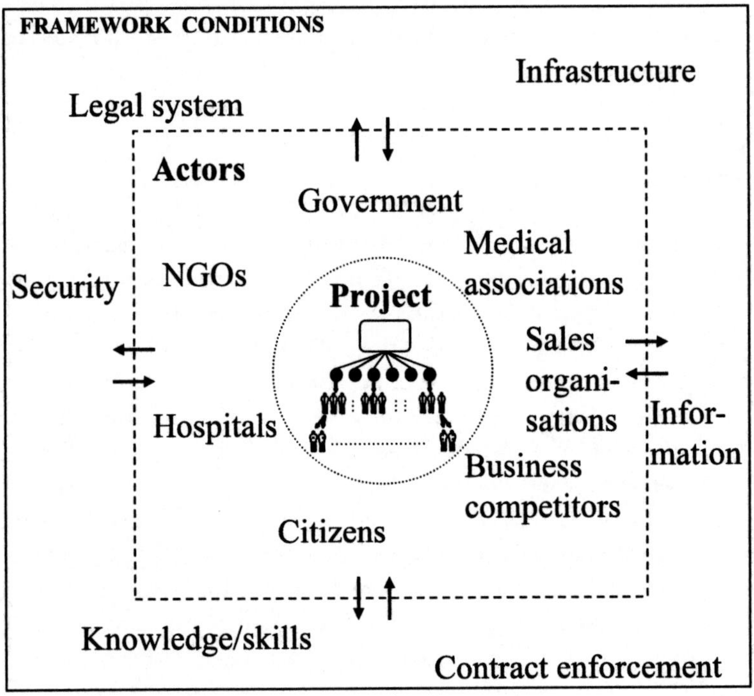

Source: the author.

interests of the relevant actors are aligned with the business interest. The development of a new business model must thus start with a careful analysis of the business ecosystem.

Framework conditions

Any functioning market requires certain enabling framework conditions. These include a legal system to ensure contract enforcement and individual security; a certain level of education and skill amongst the agents; the availability of information about sellers, buyers and goods sold; and the existence of physical infrastructure. These framework conditions are to the benefit of all actors within the system.

Without them, exchanges would simply not take place because actors would not be able to trust each other, to understand a product offer or even to meet. Usually, however, no single actor has a strong enough incentive to take responsibility for establishing these framework conditions. Since these goods are accessible to everybody, there is no way to charge people for using them, recover costs and make a profit. These types of goods are called "public goods" in economic theory because they are by nature to the benefit of a whole community of people.[17]

When everybody wants to use a good, but nobody wants to put it in place, a coordination problem arises. Take the example of training. Two companies need skilled doctors who would be able to use their instruments. Both would benefit if each of them trained some doctors. However, each benefits even more if it leaves the investment of education to the other company and only reaps the benefit of new potential customers. As a result, both will rely on the other for training. If no coordination mechanisms are in place, no training will be provided and the market for both remains at the status quo. In other words, by trying to improve their individual situation, actors make themselves worse off collectively.[18]

In developing countries, this coordination problem often leads to the absence of crucial market-enabling framework conditions. In developed markets, such factors are normally provided by the state, and companies typically do not need to worry about law enforcement or about the availability of basic skills among their customers and employees. The government implements the common interest of its citizens. In this way, the ecosystem of developed markets enables individual actors to contribute to social goals while achieving their personal goals. In developing markets, in the urban slums and rural villages where the poor live and where framework conditions are often not in place, lack of effective governance structures prevents the implementation of a flourishing business environment.

If companies want to operate in the market of the poor, they must therefore contribute to building the required framework conditions. Business models in these markets are special because companies must first put certain public goods into place in order to be able to sell their private goods. Obviously, the expected returns from the business must be sufficient to justify such an investment, even though competitors may reap some of the benefit. This is what makes the development of these models a challenging task.

In India, there is a lack of endoscopy education for gynaecologists; it is not a component of the general medical education provided as part of a four-year undergraduate degree in India. After graduation, many students leave university to start work, but even those who continue on to a three-year postgraduate qualification in obstetrics and gynaecology get little exposure to endoscopy because few medical colleges use the technology. For those who wish to acquire the relevant skills, there are a number of private training centres in place that offer training (some of which are also supported by KARL STORZ), but none of these programmes aims specifically to improve the situation in rural markets.

Training provided through the WHI is an investment in market framework conditions, and WHI trainees acquire generic endoscopy skills that can be used with any endoscopic equipment. Hence, a gynaecologist becomes a potential buyer of endoscopic equipment from any company offering such equipment, and KARL STORZ is thus building a market of endoscopy buyers that is free for anybody to use. The strong brand and market position of the company allows KARL STORZ as an individual player to put this public good into place and still expect a positive return on its investment.

Actors and interests

The WHI involves a variety of actors. Directly, it includes all the members of the project: the three coordinating partners, the ETCs, the trained doctors and the patients. Indirectly, it involves a much broader range of actors, including national and state governments, universities, medical associations, non-governmental organisations (NGOs) working on women's health, and business partners and competitors, as well as citizens generally, especially women in rural areas. All these actors can affect the achievements of the WHI and are affected by them.

The framework conditions of an ecosystem influence actions by defining the incentives people have to engage in or avoid an activity. Actors may have a *prima facie* interest in an activity and still not engage in it because the cost is too high or the benefit too low. For example, without easy access to education, it may be too costly for doctors to acquire the skills for endoscopic treatment, even though they have an interest in the practice. Adverse incentives can also discourage actors from entering into exchanges of mutual benefit. This problem often arises where one party has to provide a part of the deal first, trusting that the other party will comply with the agreement. For example, a hospital may have an interest in training a doctor in order to improve its capacity for treating poor patients. The doctor may promise (and even genuinely intend) to treat poor patients, but, if there is no real incentive to comply with this promise, the hospital has no reason to trust the doctor and may offer the training to somebody else. Because the doctor cannot ensure that he or she will comply, the opportunity for beneficial cooperation between the two is lost.[19]

By understanding incentives, the barriers to the successful implementation of a business model can be identified. Changing framework conditions can change actors' incentives and align them with the business interest. The benefits to KARL STORZ and to patients from the WHI have already been described. In what follows, the incentives of the other actors within the project – the ETCs and doctors – are analysed.

An overview of the basic situation of India's health care landscape will facilitate this analysis. India has a mixed system of public and private medical care. Although, according to the constitution, everybody in India has the right to free public health care, in reality 80 per cent of all health spending is private.[20] Whereas outpatient care is mostly provided by private practitioners, the public sector is still an important provider of inpatient care: public hospitals receive 40 per cent of all patients above and 60 per cent of patients below the poverty line, as shown in Figure 17.5.

The two sectors pose different problems of access for poor people. Generally, poor people rely more on the services of the public health system because treatment there is free. By contrast, charges in the

Figure 17.5   **Public and private sector shares in service delivery for those above and below the poverty line: All India, 1995/96**

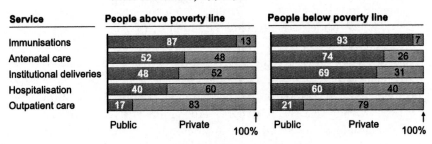

Source: World Bank, *India: Raising the Sights – Better Health Systems for India's Poor, Overview*, Washington, DC: World Bank, 2001, p. 3.

private sector, especially with regard to inpatient care, are high. However, the motivation of doctors in the public sector is often poor owing to low pay and lack of performance incentives. As a result, service is often inadequate, doctors are absent and specialists are not available. In a nutshell, services in the private sector are available but not affordable to the poor, whereas services in the public sector are affordable but not available. Because of diverging incentives in both sectors, doctors in the public sector and in the private sector are discussed separately in the following analysis.

Public doctors

Most poor patients rely on public hospitals for inpatient care because this is what they can afford. Costs are lower than in the private sector because patients and their families have to pay only for medication and catering, not for the treatment itself. Therefore, because one of the objectives of the WHI is to improve access to treatment for poor women, there is a preference to focus on training doctors from the public sector.

In principle, using endoscopy is attractive for public hospitals because it increases efficiency. Though the operation itself takes about the same time and may require even more staff than open surgery, the recovery time for the patient is much shorter and less medication is required. This increases overall hospital capacity: more patients can be treated with the limited resources of beds, nurses and drugs available. Even though endoscopic treatment requires a considerable investment, the increased productivity reduces the cost of treatment per patient as long as the number of patients treated is high enough. However, in India, public hospital management is driven not so much by productivity as by public policy, and governmental support to establish endoscopy practice is widely lacking.

Participating in the training is attractive because doctors can learn and take time off from the hospital. Practising endoscopy is also interesting in itself because doctors can improve their skills and offer a better service to their patients – both of which make work more rewarding. In their home hospitals, however, doctors face a number of challenges that can frustrate their intentions to transfer and continue the practice: a busy schedule in the operating theatre; lengthy administrative and organisational hurdles to setting up the equipment; the need to train other staff to assist; and so forth. The amount of effort required to continue practising may not seem worthwhile given the lack of economic reward for better work, as well as possible negative reactions from staff and superiors and the possibility of being transferred to a different hospital at any time.[21] In fact, at the time of writing no more than half of the doctors from the public sector had taken up the practice after the WHI training.

In order for endoscopy to be practised more widely in public hospitals, it needs the support of public policy. Policy support would reduce the cost of starting the practice by removing the existing financial and organisational hurdles, and it could also increase the return on effort by improving career prospects. Such an encouraging environment would lead more doctors to practise endoscopy in public hospitals after the training.

Why does public policy not support the application of endoscopy in gynaecology? Productivity increases in hospitals and the reduced recovery times of patients seem to be compelling reasons to extend the practice. The biggest hurdle is the lack of information. Although the patient benefits of endoscopy have been clearly proven in many medical studies, these insights have not been translated into a cost-effectiveness analysis that relates the cost of the treatment to the gains in "disability adjusted life years" (DALYs), which would make it comparable with other medical interventions.[22] Moreover, no cost–benefit analysis has been undertaken that would articulate the economic rationale of a hospital investing in endoscopic equipment in terms of potential savings. Cost-effectiveness and cost–benefit analyses are necessary to provide public policy with a basis for decision-making on whether, where and when to implement endoscopy technology.

Private doctors

Doctors in the private sector have long recognised the benefits of endoscopic treatment – for their own interests. Endoscopy improves the quality of their service, with all the patient benefits described above; and a private practitioner who offers the treatment can attract more patients and charge higher prices. For example, the price premium for a hysterectomy by most of the private practitioners interviewed is around Rs 5,000 (approximately US$100), which is a 25–50 per cent premium over the cost of open surgery. In other words, investing in the training and equipment really pays off for private doctors. Indeed, the interest of private gynaecologists in endoscopy is growing and more and more doctors offer the treatment.

However, private doctors rarely offer their services in rural areas. Demand and the ability to pay are simply much higher in big cities. Within the WHI, doctors commit themselves to provide access to treatment to poor women. Yet there is no way to enforce this commitment, and doctors have incentives not to comply with it. In fact, even for doctors who are now practising in rural areas, the training can increase the tendency to offer their service to a more profitable clientele. Nevertheless, the role of the private sector in hospital care can hardly be neglected. The percentage of inpatients treated in private institutions is increasing steadily, growing from 40 to 56 per cent from 1985 to 1995.[23]

If the payoffs from treating the poor could be increased, this would benefit both the poor and private doctors.[24] Payoffs will increase if demand for treatment increases. At the moment, the poor cannot really articulate their need for endoscopic treatment because they do not have information about it and they lack financial backing.

Women in rural areas simply do not know about endoscopy technology and its benefits. Although they have been widely exposed to endoscopic sterilisation and thus are familiar with the concept of "keyhole surgery", they have no knowledge of other applications of the technology. In their medical decisions, people in rural India rely to a great extent on the consultation in the primary health care centre or the community health centre, their first point of contact.[25] Practitioners working in these health centres have usually left university after graduation, are not aware of endoscopic applications in gynaecology and cannot provide guidance in this direction.

Even if they had adequate knowledge, women in rural areas may not be able to articulate their demand properly for financial reasons.[26] In India, there are hardly any risk-sharing mechanisms such as health insurance in place to cover people's health risks. In these circumstances, hospitalisation becomes a major source of indebtedness and poverty, as shown above.

Consequently, demand for endoscopy among poor women in India is latent. Improving awareness and creating ways for women to afford the treatment could promote this demand and create income opportunities for doctors in rural areas. If there were enough patients who requested and could afford the treatment, doctors would surely offer endoscopy also in rural areas.

Endoscopy Training Centres

The incentives for ETCs to enable doctors to practise endoscopy are mixed. Certainly, it is attractive for ETCs to accept KARL STORZ's offer to install high-tech equipment in their hospitals. But is it really in their interests to increase the number of gynaecologists offering endoscopic treatment to the poor? First of all, all training centres receive additional income from providing the training through the course fee. However, this income is mostly used to run the training and maintain the equipment. Public ETCs have an interest in more doctors providing the treatment because this would reduce some of the patient load on their own hospital. Private ETCs benefit from trainees who refer patients for advanced surgery. At the same time, doctors providing the training have less time to attend to their patients while they are teaching, and additional effort is required to publicise and organise the programmes. Overall, the benefits may or may not outweigh the additional effort required, depending on the individual situation, and ETCs may reduce their efforts after the intense monitoring phase of the WHI is over.

The benefits for ETCs increase if the WHI manages to implement a really innovative model of medical care in the market of the poor. So far, the WHI is little more than another offer of medical training in India. But part of the vision of the WHI is the implementation of a data network that will allow all members of the WHI to observe and advise on surgical procedures from a distance. With this network, doctors can support trainees in their home hospitals, making it easier for them to start practising and allowing relatively complicated problems to be solved at the local hospital. For the ETCs, such a tele-medical system would offer various benefits. For private hospitals, distance counselling can provide a new source of income. For public hospitals, it can increase the number of doctors practising endoscopy by de-specialising its use. Moreover, ETCs could reduce the cost of training per patient by providing distance teaching and leveraging each other's resources. Being part of such an innovative model provides international recognition and new career opportunities. Building the WHI into this innovative model could thus compel ETCs to fully support its success.

Achieving ecosystem integration

The WHI will achieve its objectives only if the interests of the project members are aligned. To ensure sustainable success for the WHI, the identified issues need to be addressed in a targeted approach. The WHI has already achieved its first goal of providing better training opportunities for gynaecologists. It has brought together a good set of players, installed the required technical infrastructure and started the training courses. However, my analysis has revealed a number of challenges.

The interests of trainees and trainers are not fully aligned with the WHI owing to deficiencies in four areas: (a) the tele-medical network; (b) public policy information; (c) patient awareness; (d) risk-sharing mechanisms in health care. All of these goods form part of the framework conditions of the WHI: they are public goods that require the cooperation of actors. In order to make the WHI self-sustainable, these framework conditions also need to be addressed. Here, KARL STORZ can exercise only a partial influence since some of these goods can be supplied only by other actors. The following suggestions represent one possible way to overcome the hurdles and provide the missing framework conditions.

(a) KARL STORZ can help to implement the tele-medical network. In fact, it is already in the process of putting the six training centres onto a common digital platform. The company benefits from building this network because it can showcase the applications of its tele-medical equipment and furthermore set technical standards in this up-and-coming area. The WHI could thus become the cornerstone of a new tele-medical network for endoscopy in India. I have argued that using this network to create a really innovative model of health care provision would increase the commitment of ETCs to the goals of the WHI.

(b) If ETCs really see a benefit in increasing the number of gynaecologists using endoscopy, they will also be motivated to encourage the necessary policy changes. This kind of advocacy work, which involves informing politicians about the rationale for using endoscopy in gynaecology, can only be taken on convincingly by medical experts. The information required to supply the necessary basis for public decision-making – that is, the cost-benefit and cost-effectiveness analysis – must also be provided by doctors and scientists. ETCs could either generate such studies themselves or collaborate with other universities to do so.

(c) The task of raising awareness among the poor can be accomplished only by a party that reaches out to rural doctors and patients. Again, if doctors fully accept and adopt the goal of the WHI, they can leverage their resources to spread the use of gynaecology in endoscopy. Increasing patient awareness first requires education for doctors in the rural areas about the benefits of the practice. Since all the public ETCs are in teaching institutions, they already train their students in the technology; by attracting doctors from other medical colleges and postgraduate institutions for training, a wider cohort of medical students could quickly be exposed to endoscopy. A second step would be to educate doctors from the district hospitals, who regularly undertake outreach work to their colleagues in the smaller hospitals. If the treatment were offered by all medical colleges, postgraduate institutes and district hospitals, of which there are a maximum of 800 in all of India, coverage would improve enormously because most people live less than 100 km from one such hospital. Targeted dissemination would facilitate information exchange with doctors at the primary and community health centres and translate into increased patient awareness.[27]

(d) The lack of risk-sharing mechanisms in health care is a general problem in the Indian health care system. Implementing health insurance systems is not within the scope of the WHI; it is a formidable task that currently makes even large donor agencies struggle. The WHI can, however, react to women's financial constraints by reducing the price of endoscopic treatment. In fact, if the treatment could be offered at a lower price but with the same profit margin, this would certainly be in the interests of private doctors, who could then capture a new market of middle-class and even poor patients. There are two ways to reduce the cost of treatment per patient. One is to increase the number of patients treated, thus reducing the cost of equipment and human resources per patient. In order to increase the volume of patients, hospital capacity can be improved through efficiency measures and more patients can be attracted through awareness-raising programmes.[28] The second way is to reduce the cost of equipment. Here, KARL STORZ could offer a special product range for the market of the poor. These products would offer basic functionality and high quality at a low cost.[29] Both strategies would increase KARL STORZ's market penetration and revenues while improving access to treatment.

No matter which strategies are pursued, it is essential to take the WHI to the next level of system integration. Although the first phase of the WHI concluded in June 2007, it would be a mistake to end the project right after the introduction and set-up of the technical equipment. If no coordination among ETCs is maintained and there is no follow-up on the outcome of the training, there is a risk that trainers and trainees will simply return to "business as usual" without driving the goals of the WHI forward. The next phase of the WHI must build a system that encourages doctors to practise endoscopy in rural areas and ETCs to train these doctors. This will create new users of endoscopic equipment and improve women's access to the treatment. In other words, only if a systemic integration of the WHI is achieved will the investment by KARL STORZ pay off for all parties.

Conclusion

Business for poverty alleviation is a promising way to address the unmet needs of the poor. The advantage of supplying needed goods and services via the market rather than through philanthropic donations is that these systems of mutual benefit can be sustained and scaled up over time without any inherent resource constraint. On the contrary, the supplier has a strong interest in extending the activities in order to increase the benefits from the model.

The challenge is to identify a business model that integrates seamlessly into the existing ecosystem. The WHI case study provides some suggestions on success factors for building business models for poverty alleviation:

(1) **Think systemically:** To ensure that the model reaches its target group and delivers a return, it must be integrated into the existing ecosystem. It is therefore crucial to analyse the existing ecosystem carefully, identify the relevant actors and their interests and understand the framework conditions.

(2) **Invest in market framework conditions:** The ecosystem of poor markets is particularly challenging because the framework conditions of the market are often wanting. Market-enabling goods such as education, security, legal enforcement and so on are frequently absent. Consequently, a need arises for private actors to invest in these market conditions. In other words, businesses need to provide public goods first in order to deliver their private good.

(3) **Align the interests of the relevant actors:** It is essential to understand the incentives of all the actors who affect or are affected by the achievements of the business. Actors may often be discouraged from entering a collaborative venture owing to the lack of necessary framework conditions. It is, again, crucial to put the right framework conditions into place to ensure that actors contribute to the success of the business.

(4) **Plan long term:** Building business in the market of the poor requires a long-term perspective. It certainly takes some time to understand the dynamics of the system and even longer to scale up such a model to achieve real business impact. A two-year project, the time-frame of the WHI, is hardly enough to establish the basic infrastructure, not to mention the system integration of the model. Concluding the project too early risks wasted resources and lost social and business impact.

Thanks to its capacity to increase productivity for both hospitals and patients, endoscopy technology is appropriate for a business model that improves the situation of the poor while making a profit. However, health care systems are complex constructs that vary widely among countries. To replicate the model in another country, it will be vital to analyse the ecosystem in that country and adapt the model to those conditions. With this approach, KARL STORZ will certainly find its engagement in the market of the poor a rewarding venture – and so will the poor.

Sources of information

This article is based on a case study of the WHI conducted between November 2006 and January 2007. It involved a visit to the KARL STORZ headquarters in Tuttlingen, participation in the second UNU evaluation workshop in Bonn and a five-week visit to India. During the case study, I spoke to many people both within and outside the WHI: doctors, trainers, trainees, patients, scientists, NGO representatives, diplomats and business representatives. I wish to thank all of them for sharing their insights and ideas with me and for always offering a cup of tea. All those who were formally interviewed are listed below, in alphabetical order:

Mrs Aarti, Dr Anjoo Agarwal, Dr Arun K. Aggarwal, Dr Namita Agrawal, Stefan Ahlhaus, Vikas Ahuja, Dr Arun, Dr Seema Asthana, Amit Awasthi, Dr Richu Baharani, Dr Peter Berman, Ms Chanili, Anu Chopra, Dr Neelam Choudhary, Dr Manti Chowdry, Dr Vinita Das, Mrs Dawender, Dr Achim Deja, Dr Lakhbir K. Dhaliwal, Eric Dourver, Dr Geetika, Dr Rabiswar Ghosh, Dr P. K. Goswami, Christian J. Grünwald, Dr Gurprut, Dr A. K. Gupta, Dr Dinesh Gupta, Mrs Hardjidkur, Dr Rupa Jahudar, Dr Jatander, Dr Kurian Joseph, Mr Junker, Basal Kaul, Dr Gautam Khastgir, Dr Anju Huria Khosla, Diana Kraft, Dr Trivendra Krishnan, Dr Christian Kühnl, Peter Laser, Dr S. Mahapatra, Dr Arvind Mathur, Dr N. K. Mishra, Suneeta Mittal, Dr Rajesh Modi, Dr Rajat Mohanty, S. Nanduakumar, Dr Mahendra Narwaria, Dr Neelu, Dr Nirlep, Dr Nirmilla, Dr Andreas Pfeil, Dr Hubertus Pleister, Dr Pradheema, Shishu Raksijk, Ramanathan, Dr Ramesh, Dr Ravindran, Dr Pradip K. Saha, Dr Ratna Sanyal, Dr Tejaswini Sasnur, C. S. Sathyamurthy, Susanne Schmidt, Dr Shanti, Mrs Sharda, Dr Sargeeta Shrivastava, Dr Nirujsama Singh, Dr Sankalp Singh, Dr Vikesh Srivastava, Sven Steckeler, Dr Peter Steinmann, Regina Stern, Ruchi Taxani, Dr Tevari, Dr Shradda Thakur, Dr Martina Timmermann.

Notes

1. Overall coordination among the three partners was done by Dr Achim Deja (TIMA GmbH) in his role as GC coordinator and representative of KARL STORZ until the end of December 2006.
2. The course fee within the WHI is currently Rs 15,000 (approximately US$300).
3. On the concept of sustainable business management, see, for example, J. Elkington, *Cannibals with Forks*, Gabriola Island, B.C.: New Society Publishing, 1998.
4. On the business opportunities arising from social and environmental problems, see, for example, S. L. Hart, *Capitalism at the Crossroads: The Unlimited Business Opportunities in Solving the World's Most Difficult Problems*, Upper Saddle River, NJ: Wharton School Publishing, 2005.
5. On the idea of alleviating poverty by selling to the poor, see, for example, C. K. Prahalad, *The Fortune at the Bottom of the Pyramid: Eradicating Poverty through Profits*, Upper Saddle River, NJ: Wharton School Publishing, 2005.
6. On the conception of poverty as a lack of opportunity, refer to the work of Amartya Sen – for example, A. K. Sen, *Development as Freedom*, New York: Knopf, 1999.
7. This conception of poverty is based upon the idea that people produce, as it were, their own well-being. They use goods, human capital and time to produce the things they want, such as health or enjoyment. The term "capital" is also used in a broad sense here, including material, financial, human and social capital. On the theory of household production, see the work of Gary S. Becker – for example, G. S. Becker, *Human Capital: A Theoretical and Empirical Analysis, with Special Reference to Education*, New York: Columbia University Press, 1964.
8. This information relies on observations and interviews with business competitors. Exact market size and shares are not obtainable.
9. These three indications highlight the most common areas of application for endoscopy in gynaecology. The technology is also used for a broad range of other diagnostic and therapeutic procedures. For more information on the application of endoscopy in gynaecology, please refer to Chapters 7 and 9 in this volume.
10. Estimate for hysterectomy: 600,000 hysterectomies are performed in the United States annually; the female population aged 40–69 years (the typical age group for hysterectomy) was 55 million in the United States and 120 million in India in 2000; the incidence of hysterectomy in this age group is assumed to be similar in both countries. Estimate for infertility: 10 per cent of all women of reproductive age suffer from infertility; the female population aged 15–39 years in India was 225 million in 2005. (*Sources*: US Department of Health and Human Services, <http://www.cdc.gov/reproductivehealth/WomensRH/Hysterectomy.htm>, accessed 15 June 2009; American Society for Reproductive Medicine, <http://www.

asrm.org/Patients/faqs.html>, accessed 15 June 2009; US Census Bureau International Data Base, <http://www.census.gov/ipc/www/idb/>, accessed 15 June 2009)

11. The figure also shows the enormous discrepancies between states. Throughout the chapter, I abstract from this complex landscape by referring to the predominant structures and tendencies. It should be kept in mind, however, that the differences between states in terms of economic attainment and governance can be much larger than those between different European countries.

12. In India, average income is Rs 3,000 per month (US$60). The national poverty line is defined by the amount it takes to buy 2,400 calories a day. In 2000, this amount was set at Rs 327 per month (approximately US$6.50) in rural areas and Rs 454 per month (approximately US$9) in urban areas. Based on this definition, the number of people living below this line was estimated to be 260 million, or 26 per cent of the population (data available from the Indian Ministry of Statistics and Programme Implementation, <http://www.mospi.nic.in/mospi_social_pr.htm>, accessed 15 June 2009). A hysterectomy in a private practice costs at least Rs 10,000 (US$200), about three times the annual income of a poor person.

13. National Development Council, *Tenth Five Year Plan – 2002–2007. Volume II: Sectoral Policies and Programmes*, 2002, p. 137.

14. Ibid.

15. Definition from Princeton WordNet, <http://wordnet.princeton.edu/perl/webwn>, accessed 15 June 2009.

16. This description of a relevant actor corresponds closely to Ed Freeman's definition of a "stakeholder" as "anybody who can affect or is affected by the achievement of the firm's objectives" (R. Edward Freeman, *Strategic Management – A Stakeholder Approach*, Boston: Pitman, 1984, p. 25).

17. A public good is "a good that must be provided in the same amount to all the affected consumers" (Hal R. Varian, *Intermediate Microeconomics: A Modern Approach*, London: Norton, 2003, p. 644). On the private provision of public goods, see R. Cornes and T. Sandler, *The Theory of Externalities, Public Goods, and Club Goods*, Cambridge: Cambridge University Press, 1996.

18. This coordination is known as the "prisoners' dilemma" in the game-theoretic literature. For an introduction to the prisoners' dilemma and game-theoretic reasoning generally, see, for example, R. Duncan Luce and Howard Raiffa, *Games and Decisions: Introduction and Critical Survey*, New York and London: Wiley, 1957.

19. This problem is typically described as the "one-sided prisoners' dilemma". For a discussion of the ethical relevance of both the one-sided and the two-sided prisoners' dilemma, see Ingo Pies and Markus Sardison, "Wirtschaftsethik", Discussion Paper No. 05-2, Wittenberg-Zentrum für Globale Ethik, Lehrstuhl für Wirtschaftsethik, Martin-Luther-Universität Halle-Wittenberg, 2005, <http://www.wcge.org/downloads/DP_05-2_Pies__Sardison_-_Wirtschaftsethik.pdf> (accessed 15 June 2009).

20. World Bank, *India: Raising the Sights – Better Health Systems for India's Poor. Overview*, Washington, DC: World Bank, 2001, p. 3.
21. In India, doctors working in the public sector are transferred at least every five years. They cannot choose the destination of their transfer. The possibility of being transferred to a hospital without endoscopic equipment can discourage doctors from making the effort to exercise their newly acquired skills.
22. Cost-effectiveness analysis is the standard management tool for public health investment decisions. In order to compare the effectiveness of different medical interventions, the "disability adjusted life years" (DALYs) gained through an intervention are related to the cost of the intervention. Without any detailed analysis, it can be said that the DALYs gained through endoscopic surgery as compared with conventional open surgery will not be very high, since the main benefit to patients is the time saved through faster recovery. A much more compelling reason for investing in endoscopic equipment is the financial saving to both patients and hospitals that can be achieved through reduced recovery times. The relation of these savings to the cost of the treatment would be stated in a cost–benefit analysis.
23. National Development Council, *Tenth Five Year Plan*, p. 94.
24. The governments of many states already try to encourage private doctors to treat poor people by providing financial incentives. For example, doctors who treat 10–20 per cent of their patients for free receive tax benefits and can purchase land for a hospital on preferential conditions. As a result, many private hospitals provide (limited) access to poor patients.
25. In India, alternative medicine, subsumed under the label of AYUSH, also plays a major role. People in villages often prefer alternative practitioners because they are more accessible and enjoy greater trust and their services are more affordable than those of allopathic practitioners.
26. For a discussion of the difficulty of the poor in articulating their demand for health care owing to a lack of risk-sharing mechanisms, see Ingo Pies and Stefan Hielscher, "Das Problem weltmarktlicher Arzneimittelversorgung: Ein Vergleich alternativer Argumentationsstrategien für eine globale Ethik", Discussion Paper No. 2007-5, Lehrstuhls für Wirtschaftsethik, Martin-Luther-Universität Halle-Wittenberg, 2007, <http://wcms.uzi. uni-halle.de/download.php?down=1114&elem=1016129> (accessed 15 June 2009).
27. NGOs working in the area of women's health can also make an important contribution to raising patient and doctor awareness in rural areas through their interactions with doctors and villagers. Furthermore, collaborating with a women's health NGO can bring more information into the WHI on the situation of women and their problems of access to health care.
28. An example of this approach is the Aravind Eye Hospitals in Tamil Nadu, India. These hospitals use the best equipment from Germany and the United States. They treat 60 per cent of inpatients for free, but still achieve a 40 per cent margin of income over expenses (information from <http://www. aravind.org/, accessed 15 June 2009).

29. An example of this approach is General Electric (GE). GE has decreased the price of its ultrasound equipment in India tenfold. To do this, it has reduced the product to the basic components, adapted it to the special conditions of the rural markets and reorganised production processes to produce locally. Today, ultrasound diagnostics is widely used in rural areas – to the benefit of both GE and patients.

18

A PPP for women's health and human rights in India: Striving for best practice within the framework of the UN Global Compact

MARTINA TIMMERMANN AND MONIKA KRUESMANN

Looking back to the first meeting on the project in October 2004, the shared goal of all three project partners was to contribute to improving women's reproductive and maternal health (care) in India. The approach was to form a public private partnership (PPP) between a corporate partner specialising in endoscopy and the Deutsche Gesellschaft für Technische Zusammenarbeit (GTZ) as the monitoring partner in India. The idea was to equip six hospitals (public and private) with endoscopy equipment and to initiate and run endoscopy training sessions based on the train-the-trainer principle. The trainees were preselected according to their background and motivation to accept the project requirements to treat economically disadvantaged women and girls for free after having been accepted on the training course at considerably reduced rates. The hospitals were to raise money from the training to enable them to acquire and maintain new hospital technology and to be able to provide state-of-the-art or best attainable

Partnerships for women's health: Striving for best practice within the UN Global Compact,
Timmermann and Kruesmann (eds),
United Nations University Press, 2009, ISBN 978-92-808-1185-8

health care. In addition, the PPP project was deliberately placed within the framework of the United Nations Global Compact (UN GC) by requiring particular attention to the demand for business ethics, transparency, accountability and compliance with the ten UN GC Principles in order to achieve effectiveness, sustainability and a quality that would allow this rather small pilot project to be up-scaled within India and transferred to other countries and regions in the world.

To ensure an impartial assessment, the United Nations University (UNU) joined the project as the third partner. It is UNU's mission to contribute to thinking on issues of global concern, that is, to function as a think tank of the United Nations and for the people of its member states. Capacity-building projects in developing countries are of particular interest to the UNU. Joining this PPP as external academic assessment agency gave UNU the opportunity to do genuine valuable research and to contribute to the many vital debates on the Millennium Development Goals (MDGs), women's reproductive and maternal health care in India and beyond, PPPs as opportunities for (or impediments to) creating viable health care systems, the opportunities offered by the UN Global Compact for such PPPs and the role that small and medium-sized companies (SMEs) can play in such processes and future projects.

In retrospect (i.e. about a year after finishing the pilot project with the final monitoring report by the GTZ (2008)), we can now do a stock-take and discuss whether the project has met its UN GC embedded goals. In order for the project to be up-scaled or transferred to other countries and regions and to contribute to global approaches to improving women's reproductive and maternal health, our central question is: Can this pilot project for "Improving women's reproductive and maternal health in India through a PPP within the UN Global Compact" serve as a "blueprint for best practice"?

Defining the criteria for a "blueprint for best practice"

What criteria would need to be met to qualify this project as "best practice"? And what would be the particular requirements of a "UN GC PPP model of best practice"?

Defining "best practice"

Here, we will proclaim best practice if the goals of the project are achieved and continuous self-learning is demonstrated: from design to implementation to results, the project avoids the typical weaknesses and challenges found in other global health PPPs and therefore demonstrates that it is effective, transparent (ensured through continuous independent monitoring), sustainable and up-scalable/transferable.

We will affirm **good practice** if the project has met its major goals but there are some weaknesses in design and implementation and results in terms of its effectiveness, transparency, sustainability and up-scalability/transferability; progress can nevertheless clearly be noted and there has been encouraging potential for learning and positive development in the future.

We would certainly need to speak of a **failure** if the project goals have not been achieved, the typical weaknesses and challenges of previous health PPPs have been repeated and no learning process and potential for future improvements, up-scaling and transfer have been detected.

If we finally add to this understanding the requirements of an evaluation of the project's outcome by an independent partner (as suggested in the Introduction), our acceptance of a best practice PPP within the framework of the UN GC would rest on the structural potential for self-learning, a sustainable impact, effectiveness, up-scalability and independent monitoring to ensure transparency (see Figure 18.1).

Figure 18.1   Blueprint for a best practice PPP within the UN Global Compact

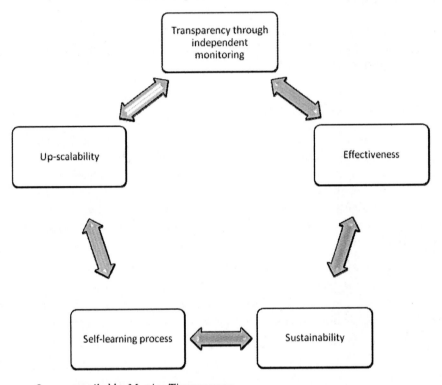

Source: compiled by Martina Timmermann

The Women's Health Initiative (WHI) – effective, transparent, sustainable?

Has the project qualified as a role model for best practice? Based on our preceding definition of best practice within the framework of the UN Global Compact, it is useful to break down our main over-arching question into several sub-questions:

1. Has the project been effective?

    a. Have the project shareholders (i.e. the partners) met their joint goal?

  b. Have the project shareholders achieved their individual
     goals?
2. Has the project become sustainable?
3. Has the project been transparent?
4. Has the project gone beyond previous health PPPs?
5. What would be needed for the project to be up-scaled or transferred?
6. Has the WHI made contributions beyond the immediate
   project?

Has the PPP been effective?

Effectiveness is a measure of quality and goodness. Effectiveness says ... that getting it right is more important than cost or time (in contrast to efficiency, which is a measure of speed and cost).

Neil Kendrick[1]

A major joint goal of the shareholders of this PPP was to improve women's reproductive and maternal health in India and to help economically disadvantaged women (with an annual income of less than Rs 25,000) to have better access to the best attainable health care. A second major shared goal was to make this initiative sustainable by being transparent and avoiding the mistakes of other health PPPs. So, have they "got it right"?

Have the project shareholders met their joint goal?

The joint goal to contribute to improving women's reproductive and maternal health in India and to efforts to provide economically disadvantaged women with better access to the best attainable health care has been achieved in absolute numbers. The final monitoring report by GTZ notes that, by the end of the first project period (the end of June 2007), a total of 2,023 women had been treated (see Table 18.1); 702, or 36 per cent, of them fell into the category of economically disadvantaged women.[2]

GTZ concluded in its report that: "The project has achieved its objective to a great extent in terms of the direct benefits of

Table 18.1 Number of doctors trained and patients treated at each
           ETC

No. of study	Endoscopy Training Centre	No. of doctors trained	No. of patients diagnosed and treated	No. of states covered
1	Joseph Nursing Home, Chennai	70	579	12
2	Belle Vue Clinic, Kolkata	35	385	5
3	All India Institute of Medical Sciences, New Delhi	41	399	10
4	SCB, Medical College, Cuttack	40	83	3
5	Queen Mary's Hospital, KGMC, Lucknow	20	380	1
6	Postgraduate Institute of Medical Education & Research, Chandigarh	37	197	9
	Total	243	2,023	

Source: "Reaching beyond Boundaries – Women's Health Initiative: A Public–Private Partnership", GTZ Monitoring Report by Dr Nisha Lal and Dr J. Peter Steinmann, New Delhi, May 2008, Table 1.

establishing the ETCs [Endoscopy Training Centres], training doctors in minimally invasive surgery at a lower cost, and increasing access of endoscopic diagnostic and treatment services to women." The endoscopy trainees were also required to treat economically disadvantaged women after their training. With regard to this outcome, however, the GTZ final report critically notes that "there are some missing links in the activities implemented under WHI, which if taken care would certainly give the direct benefits a significant leap. Results do not depict a positive correlation between the number trained ... and number treated."[3] Further, the desired number of at least 40 doctors trained in each hospital was not achieved across the board.

What might be the reasons? Has the project really been effective?

To answer this, it is necessary briefly to discuss some questions that ran all the way through this project: (1) the relevance of high technology for improving women's reproductive and maternal health, (2) the contribution of economic and social incentives to the effectiveness of this PPP, (3) the dissemination of information necessary for reaching the patients and achieving a wider impact, (4) the involvement of the Indian government and (5) the relevance of monitoring to ensure transparency and accountability.

Improving women's reproductive health via high-tech + primary health care

The fundamental question of whether or not high technology such as laparoscopy is actually the right approach for improving economically disadvantaged women's reproductive and maternal health on a grand scale has been controversial since the beginning of the project. At UNU's first workshop, critics argued that endoscopy serves only the economic interests of the medical doctors and the company delivering these high-end products (KARL STORZ). Some project participants considered the focus of this project on endoscopy to be too technology oriented and therefore not fully meeting the basic needs of poor women. For instance, Lynn Freedman from Columbia University and director of the part of the Millennium Development Project related to MDG5 on women's maternal health, argued that there was a much greater need to change conditions outside the hospitals if the maternal mortality rate was to be reduced by 2015. Whereas endoscopy was likely to assist doctors in their personal careers and hospitals in making money, the real poor, who have to pay for the technical equipment such as simple gloves, scissors or needles that the doctors need for surgery, would be left out. She also referred to Staffan Bergström from the Division of International Health (IHCAR), Department of Public Health Sciences, Karolinska Institute, Stockholm, Sweden, who had voiced the criticism in one of his articles that "[o]bstetricians show a disproportionately small or even insignificant interest in alarming maternal mortality and maternal ill health in underserved and impoverished countries".[4]

Freedman suggested that the aim should be the fundamental improvement of primary care by the Indian public health system.

Bergström, too, emphasised the need for awareness-raising among obstetricians and gynaecologists about the external causes of maternal mortality (calling it "ectoscopy") and also stressed the need to focus on specialised training and an audit of various aspects of quality care.[5]

KARL STORZ and several medical doctors, however, underlined the advantages of high technology. They suggested that it provides several important benefits to consumers that are as vital for better off patients as for economically underprivileged patients. Such technological advantages include:

- better and earlier diagnosis and less invasive therapy;
- shorter stays in hospital (1–2 days instead of 7–10 days) and a speedier recovery, enabling patients (and partners) to resume work quickly;
- cost reduction as a result of shorter hospital stays and less medication;
- risk reduction through fewer infections and complications after minimally invasive surgery;
- more aesthetic (smaller) scars and less psychological strain.

Freedman's and Bergström's positions result from practical experiences in the field, which may have caused them to question the willingness of medical doctors to continue being involved in interventions that do not meet their economic interests. And in fact, albeit that they were not the sole factors, economic incentives have proven vital to the effectiveness of this project.

The economic incentive – engine for and impediment to improvement

In interviews conducted by GTZ, medical doctors criticised the fact that in reality it was possible that doctors with little training might decide to treat poor people in exchange for the training and then – having gained experience – exclusively cater for better off patients in private hospitals and move to the cities where incomes are higher.[6]

The message was therefore – and in synergy with Bergström's suggestion – that the medical doctors needed a frame of reference for accountability, a code of conduct with standardised quality rules and procedures, and a certification process. Efforts to reach these goals were made by some of the doctors participating in this initiative. Their approach seemed promising in 2007 because they were then in leading positions in the Federation of Obstetric & Gynaecological Societies of India (FOGSI). According to those participants, the debate at FOGSI reached the point where they suggested certain rules and standards. In 2008, however, upon enquiry from UNU on the situation, then-FOGSI president, Prof. Malhotra, replied that she did not know about any such initiative, but would appreciate support for progress in this area. The original drivers of the process reported that the discussion at FOGSI had ended in deadlock over the level of fees FOGSI would charge endoscopy trainees for certification. It was, therefore, also economic interest that hindered such important progress.

In addition to the economic interests of the doctors, there has also been some pressure from better off patients. One director of a private clinic participating in this initiative admitted that he had faced trouble with private patients who had paid substantially more money for their treatment and therefore (understandably) expected visibly more privileged treatment. They did not feel fairly treated when they realised that less economically fortunate people were in effect receiving the same treatment. To avoid further friction, the director of the hospital therefore decided to treat the less well-off patients at a different location. This example illustrates that, beyond the benefits to mere medical doctors, other stakeholders' economic and social incentives can substantially influence the effectiveness of a PPP because, outside such a pilot scheme, it can be assumed that private hospitals would be unlikely to provide another location for treatment unless there was a convincing economic incentive.

Another lesson was that medical doctors need to have an incentive to stay in rural hospitals when more lucrative options are available to them in the cities – not only but especially after the training measures. One idea of the project stakeholders had been to set up video-conferencing for expert counselling and also to reduce possible feelings of professional isolation in rural environments.

In addition, there were plans for creating a WHI stakeholder platform for e-communication to attract new interested project participants and thus build a community of highly skilled practitioners. In 2008, however, UNU was informed by KARL STORZ that this goal could not be realised because of a lack of installations and problems in installing ISD lines at each ETC for medical video-conferencing. KARL STORZ was confident in May 2008, however, that it would "revert to it once the technical conditions improve[d]".[7]

At this point it became obvious that earlier and closer cooperation with the Indian government would have been helpful to such efforts through support in administration, infrastructure and logistics.

Spreading the news – reaching the poor

Another challenge was to reach people in the rural areas and inform them about their options. Here again the perspectives of the private and public protagonists varied in approach.

From a business point of view, Gradl suggests in Chapter 17 of this volume that information about the advantages of endoscopy for women in rural areas should be distributed through medical doctors:

> If doctors fully accept and adopt the goal of the WHI, they can leverage their resources to spread the use of gynaecology in endoscopy. Increasing patient awareness first requires education for doctors in the rural areas about the benefits of the practice. Since all the public ETCs are in teaching institutions, they already train their students in the technology; by attracting doctors from other medical colleges and postgraduate institutions for training, a wider cohort of medical students could quickly be introduced to endoscopy. A second step would be to educate doctors from the district hospitals who regularly communicate on training or other medical matters with their colleagues in the smaller hospitals. If the treatment were offered by all medical colleges, postgraduate institutes and district hospitals, of which there are a maximum of 800 in all of India, coverage would improve enormously because most people live less than 100 km from one such hospital. Tar-

geted dissemination would facilitate information exchange with doctors at the primary and community health centres and translate into increased patient awareness (see Chapter 17 in this volume).

From a corporate point of view, this approach might make sense at first glance but, looking at the overall picture, doctors would certainly be hard-pressed to be the sole providers of information to far-flung rural villages. It seems to be more effective to pursue a joint approach with the Indian government, which is already in the process of implementing comprehensive and nationwide strategies – such as within the Reproductive and Child Health Programme (RCH-I & RCH-II) – for improving access to the best attainable health care (see also Chapter 19).

The authors of Chapters 1, 2, 7, 8, 9 and 10 in this volume all mention the importance of taking into account the particular national challenges affecting women's awareness of and access to the best attainable health care. The overall lack of infrastructure, which limits access to health care facilities, institutional challenges within the health care system and socio-cultural constraints pose challenges that undoubtedly need to be tackled comprehensively by the local and national governments. Ghosh (Chapter 10 in this volume) further emphasises the importance of literacy and education for girls and women so that they can assess the information on the best and the best available health care opportunities.

All these suggestions point to the urgent need to involve the Indian government in any initiative for improving women's reproductive and maternal health in order to make it sustainable. Despite initial approaches at the beginning of the WHI project by the GTZ team in India, the GTZ final report states that there is still a need for greater cooperation with the Indian government, which is responsible for the administration of the public hospitals (among the many other issues outlined above). Effectiveness could therefore have been higher if the Indian government had been more strongly involved from the very beginning or at least during the project implementation period.

Have the project shareholders achieved their individual goals?

Beyond the joint goal of improving women's reproductive and maternal health in India, each partner had additional objectives that were not always made explicit but that nevertheless influenced their perception of their roles and tasks and consequently also their perception of success.

Reflecting the perspectives of the private partner

KARL STORZ's first objective was not only to contribute to the women's reproductive and maternal health situation in India, but also, having joined the UN Global Compact in November 2004, to celebrate the company's 60th anniversary with a UN GC showcase project. If the project also helped to increase the brand's reputation by presenting a positive image when competing against companies offering less expensive copies of its products, this was considered a positive side-effect. It would also help increase its range of customers (see Chapters 12 and 17 in this volume).

Looking at a letter to UNU from the director of business development, Peter Laser, who was KARL STORZ's WHI project director in India during the time of the project pilot, it seems that KARL STORZ perceived the project as a success:

> After this preliminary conclusion of the initiative the project can be attributed a positive resonance ... we are pleased to report that we have increased our sales market through the trained doctors and as a result of catering to this group we have also achieved economic success. In conclusion it can be said that because of these positive experiences KARL STORZ would be willing to repeat such a project any time or, alternatively, extend the initiative.[8]

Reflecting the perspectives of the public partner

For GTZ, as the technical branch of the German Ministry for Economic Cooperation and Development (BMZ), there were several BMZ-related targets to be met because BMZ benchmarking for success poses several challenges.[9] BMZ wanted to see:

- efforts that boosted private sector interest in becoming involved in health PPPs;

- PPP partners undertaking a harmonised approach to ensure that both partners are able to achieve their objectives better, faster and at lower cost;

- the project going clearly beyond usual business activities to avoid any impression of subsidisation;

- a measurable contribution by the PPP to improving the gynaecological health situation for underprivileged women and girls in India;

- the PPP complying with the BMZ development policy guidelines, which included that the main target group of development cooperation are the poor and health PPPs are designed according to their needs;

- the development cooperation project being implemented according to the policy priorities of the partner country. Since the German contribution in India is marginal compared with the dedication of the Indian government's own resources, the Indian government itself determines whether or not health PPPs are promoted. Consequently, it would be vital for success to include the Indian government in this project.

According to Kraft and Hartmann from GTZ (see Chapter 14 in this volume), the WHI by its very design fulfilled these requirements. Kraft and Hartmann consider the WHI PPP project as contributing to two focus areas of impact in German development policy: promoting women's and girls' health in a development policy context and closely involving the private sector.

The close involvement of a private partner also aims at transforming the private partner's commitment at the project level into a longer-term business case for entrepreneurial engagement in the partner country's markets – based on mutual advantages for all project partners. In this way it would be possible to develop a model for a sustainable improvement in health services for disadvantaged parts of the population that can be transferred to projects in other regions.[10]

Since the beginning of the twenty-first century, public private partnerships have been an international and national trend – including at BMZ. Consequently, a special section for PPP has been established at GTZ. It was therefore important for GTZ to participate in PPPs such as this one and thereby stimulate its PPP programme. Moreover, health-related PPP projects on women had been rare, so the WHI offered a good opportunity to fill this gap and thereby support BMZ's other policies and pledges to contribute to achieving the MDGs.

A second-tier goal may have been the fact that GTZ also serves as the focal point for the UN Global Compact network in Germany. It was very convenient to cooperate closely on a project with a medium-sized German company that had just joined the UN Global Compact and the German GC network. Thus, the WHI could also serve as an example for projects with other SMEs in the future.

With reference to the letter from Peter Laser of KARL STORZ, GTZ could assume that the business-related goals had been achieved. This implied the accomplishment of another GTZ goal, that of contributing to fostering German business involvement in India through a PPP.

Nevertheless, the question needs to be addressed of whether this approach can indeed serve as a model for sustainable improvement in health services for disadvantaged parts of the population, and whether it can be up-scaled and transferred to other regions. Within this context, in order to be able to conclude that the project has contributed to reaching the MDGs – as for instance stipulated in the BMZ development policy guidelines – we need to take a closer look at the sustainability of the initiative.

Has the project become sustainable?

The sustainability of this initiative was a major concern of the partners and the stakeholders,[11] but the very term "sustainability" seemed to convey a different meaning to the partners.

The private perspective on sustainability

For corporate business, sustainability plainly means that the business model must have paid off, that is, the return on investment must have been continuously satisfactory and thus proven "sustainable". Gradl, for instance, who discussed the economic perspectives of the business model with a strong leaning towards the company, writes in Chapter 17:

> [S]ustainability is already built into any functional business model for poverty alleviation. A successful business model is, above all, a profitable one. If the company supplying the product or service benefits from it, the model will simply become part of its mainstream business after the implementation phase. There is no previously defined "project end", as with typical aid projects that have no refunding mechanism.

From the perspective of the business sector there were several economic incentives to ensure the sustainability of this initiative also for the poor.

For instance, Gradl particularly alluded in Chapter 17 to the economic need to find compelling reasons for the participating ETCs to cooperate beyond the initial period of the project. She recommended continuous monitoring and tele-medicine, arguing that this approach would contribute to new career opportunities, create more potential for income generation and enhance the international reputation of the doctors and also of KARL STORZ. Her view of the need for monitoring was in line with the original business model, preferring to stress incentives rather than governmental control. Any extension of the project would therefore indicate the corporate perception of the initiative as economically sustainable.

With reference to the letter from KARL STORZ in August 2007, we might conclude that economic sustainability has been achieved. In the process of updating our information in May 2008, we also asked for any up-scalings or plans for up-scaling the project in India and/or for transferring the initiative to other countries. Such a move would also indicate perceived sustainability by the company. We received the following response from KARL STORZ:

> We maintain a close relationship with all ETCs as per the general policy of KARL STORZ. We are partners in the effort to further train doctors in MIS [minimally invasive surgery] in order to further improve the reach into the rural areas. This relation will continue to exist even beyond the official end of the project. In a very concrete way the contact between KARL STORZ and the six ETC could be described as follows: KARL STORZ is still involved in the continuous reprint and sending out of ETC's promotion flyer. This flyer explains and promotes the WHI training courses towards potential participants in order to win new surgeons to participate in this initiative. In co-operation with the ETC KARL STORZ still supports the ETCs in handling the registrations of new participants. KARL STORZ is still providing adequate training brochures on a regular base to the ETCs for distributing them to the trainees. To handle all these mentioned aspects we have one employee at our subsidiary KARL STORZ India who is working full-time on these aspects in order to continue an optimal and further co-operation with and support of the six ETCs.[12]

Thus, from a business point of view, sustainability is said to have been achieved. Still, by May 2008 no up-scaling or transfer seemed to have taken place. Our question about any plans to transfer this project to other countries elicited the following response: "We will certainly be interested to do similar projects wherever it makes sense. Details can be made available as and when such opportunities arise."[13]

Whereas in Peter Laser's letter an extension (up-scaling or transfer) seemed in reach, the email reply indicated that (until September 2008) no such activities were yet being undertaken. Moreover, there was no reference to maintaining the particular quality of this GC-embedded PPP project structure, that is, the continuous monitoring designed to ensure accountability, compliance and transparency.

The public perspective on sustainability

To ensure full-fledged sustainability, however, monitoring to ensure transparency and compliance has been considered absolutely vital and was therefore demanded by the GTZ implementing staff, by the medical doctors in the six ETCs, by UNU in its mission report of April 2007 and later on also by KARL STORZ (see Chapter 15).

Monitoring needs to be financed and staffed. Since this PPP was seen as a start-up PPP by the shareholders from BMZ/GTZ and KARL STORZ, long-term monitoring was not originally planned for, which was in accordance with BMZ and GTZ rules. And because there was no strong involvement by the Indian government, there was also nobody on that side to take on this important role.

GTZ's idea of sustainability was that the initiative had to run independently after the initial start-up period. This included the hospitals that had participated in the WHI initiative being able to raise enough money through their endoscopy training to fund new instruments and to pay for their maintenance. In short, the project would move on from its charity-supported infant step to become a clear-cut independent business. (Note that the training participants were not obliged to buy KARL STORZ equipment after the training sessions ended.)

In interviews in April 2007 with the All India Institute of Medical Sciences (AIIMS) – the largest public hospital and one with a high reputation – it was mentioned that this goal had been achieved. The fees were permitting an independent business to operate, creating a win–win situation for AIIMS and the doctors, and more women had been treated simply because of more sessions with trainee doctors. We can therefore assume that this approach is contributing to a sustainable improvement in the public health care sector.

There was nonetheless a clear request for advice in terms of the development of a business plan, which the doctors (rightly) felt was beyond their tasks and capabilities. They also asked for support for coordination between the partners and their hospital administration in order to be able to spend more time on the training and on their patients. Finally, they insisted on continuous monitoring by a third party to make sure that comparable and reliable standards would be applied and standards and rules would be complied with.

Has the project been transparent?

Transparency is a vital component of PPPs but especially so for a UN GC PPP. Transparency ensures accountability and compliance, therefore contributing to anti-corruption.

The tool for achieving transparency is skilled, reliable and continuous monitoring. As Kent Buse (a member of the first WHI workshop) and many others have found in their analyses of PPPs, monitoring often produces substantial challenges to the partners involved. Differing loyalties, business rationale, the personal motives and interests of the participating shareholders and stakeholders, unexpected administrative problems and many other causes may make monitoring and assessment a difficult task.[14] In particular, PPP partners' performance is often insufficiently assessed or not assessed at all.[15] For that reason, this project was deliberately designed to include not only field monitoring but also a final assessment of the project's activities. This final assessment was to depend strongly on the viewpoints of the invited experts.

From the start of the project the corporate partner, KARL STORZ, in cooperation with GTZ India provided detailed quarterly "plans of operations" where each partner's tasks and progress as well as the remaining stages were presented. Communication at the steering committee level took place at four meetings (in Geneva, October 2004; in New Delhi, February 2005; in Chennai, October 2005; and in Bonn, December 2006). In addition, exchanges between all shareholders and stakeholders took place during the two workshops (October 2005 and December 2006). Monitoring still turned out to be an issue of concern for several reasons.

Unexpected medical strikes in India and administrative problems in some public hospitals led to delays of up to six months in setting up the training programmes. Because the period of monitoring had to be the same at each site, the full project had to be extended for a year. The extension caused different challenges for each partner. From a corporate point of view, the design and success of the project rested on a precise business plan. GTZ had to pay attention to the timely and proper spending of BMZ money and this entailed meeting German budgetary planning deadlines at the ministry. These deadlines had to be extended. GTZ also needed to take into account the parameters for success at the ministry (see Chapter 13 by von der Goltz in this volume). From its perspective, the project was understood to be a start-up initiative and therefore should not last too long (i.e. monitoring for a longer period was not in its original plan). It also turned out that the personnel for the monitoring function in India needed methodology training, which required additional time and funding that was originally unplanned for.

The monitoring challenge was further exacerbated by several personnel changes within the GTZ monitoring team. This personnel turnover in the field delayed production of the final report for about a year in addition to causing communication problems with the other partners.

UNU, as last actor in line, equally had to reorganise and adjust its personnel resources according to the changing timing. This also included the planning of the workshops with experts, who might be available only at certain times. The chain of impact was felt right to the end, when the publication process was delayed and contracts needed to be readjusted.

In sum, each partner organisation suffered from the changes in personnel, because valuable project memory/wisdom was lost. This also impaired the efforts for transparency and effectiveness.

Interim conclusions: Has the project gone beyond previous global health PPPs?

The WHI project falls within the parameters of a number of contemporary global debates: debates about the MDGs, about human rights, about business and ethics and the Global Compact, about accountability and transparency, about health financing, about public private partnerships and about the role of SMEs. As such, it was a complex project and there were challenges assessing its overall effect and sustainability.

Based on our definitions of good and best practice, and guided by the input of the project stakeholders and invited project experts, we can conclude that the WHI constituted an example of 'best practice', within the purposes and parameters that shaped its establishment. Partners were engaged and remained connected and committed, ETCs were established, equipment was supplied, training was undertaken, and procedures were carried out while striving for transparent, open and accountable processes. Notably during the course of the WHI's implementation, a number of new principles for successful partnerships came to light. Thus, a continuous learning process can be identified that allows us to conclude that there is room for further improvements and reaching all goals in a process of up-scaling and/ or transfer.

The project was deliberately set up as a self-learning process with two workshops and outside expert participants. During the two workshops – at the beginning and near the end of the implementation period – weaknesses were openly discussed and awareness was raised about issues that had not been considered persuasively enough before.

So has this project been like other health PPPs? Or has it broken new ground in striving for best practice? The seven opportunities of global health PPPs as suggested by Kent Buse[16] also apply to this PPP: (1) the PPP was rapidly established; (2) funds for this project as well as the profiles of the partners were raised; (3) R&D was enhanced on the social scientific/business planning side; (4) access to products was improved for hospitals and patients; (5) service delivery capacity was enhanced on the business side, one lesson was noted that not only the business but also the quality of the governmental and non-governmental service would need to be raised and ensured; (6) policy and planning processes were strengthened during the initial project period (further conclusions are difficult because the project ended just as it was taking off and gaining in momentum, but there are several important lessons that could and would need to be applied if the project were to be up-scaled or transferred to other countries); and (7) standards were applied during the monitoring process in the later stage in line with demands for monitoring in, for instance, the 2006 *Global Corruption Report* by Transparency International (TI).[17]

At the beginning of the project, the relevance of monitoring in the field and of a third party (or "supra") assessment by an independent source was not equally recognised. This changed during the project process. The importance of monitoring for providing the overall transparency, compliance and accountability of the participating shareholders was finally realised by all the public parties. It was for this reason that the medical doctors, GTZ India and UNU (in its mission report of April 2007) strongly encouraged ongoing monitoring far beyond the initial phase of the project.[18] With the end of the implementation period, the monitoring stopped – but the business activities carried on. This illustrates the special driving role business has in such PPPs, and the great need to involve the relevant governments to ensure continuous monitoring beyond start-up projects funded by foreign donor countries.

The results and experiences of the WHI project therefore coincide to quite some degree with the findings of Kent Buse, who concluded in 2007 that beneficial actions for best performance should attempt:

- to embrace the agenda of the Paris Declaration on Aid Effectiveness (i.e. national harmonisation),
- to strive for balanced representation,
- to address problems of participants' divided loyalties and accountabilities,
- to apply the PPP approach to non-communicable diseases and lifestyle challenges,
- to enhance business practices to improve efficiency and accountability, and
- to assess the cost-effectiveness of public versus public private versus private approaches.[19]

In this project, the lessons were: to cooperate with the Indian government; to raise awareness of the relevance of gynaecological endoscopy in general and among medical doctors in particular; to develop certification guidelines for a rigorous check on the quality of the training in gynaecological surgery and the appropriate staff; and to find convincing ways of spreading information about the available options to patients via medical doctors and by making use of existing governmental health care policies and instruments.

Beyond that, it was learned in the process of reporting and analysis that, because of the UN GC ethical framework chosen by the partners, the project had achieved a new and higher level of quality. Transparency through independent monitoring was now considered a key tool to ensure accountability and, ultimately, the success – i.e. the effectiveness and sustainability – of this (and any) UN GC PPP.

Finally, the complexity of the issues and actors underlines that it is not a question of improving women's reproductive and maternal health through *either* high technology *or* primary health care but rather one of *combining both* approaches in a complementary fashion. In Indian health care programmes, laparoscopy plays an important role in population planning. For women, minimally invasive surgery is definitely a better, less painful and quicker way to be treated. They and their families can get back to work earlier, which helps to avoid the poverty trap that can develop during a longer period of ill health and hospitalisation.

It is therefore of great importance to develop combined health care programmes that unite the political health care goals of the Indian government with the high-tech health care opportunities and to ensure the utmost transparency and accountability by bringing all stakeholders to the table. If this happens in the process of up-scaling or transferring this PPP, the WHI will develop into a best practice PPP within the framework of the UN Global Compact .

Towards a blueprint for best practice

Being a think tank of the United Nations, the United Nations University joined this project with several visions. Besides ensuring the transparency of the PPP it was important to UNU to study this project with respect to several important debates related to maternal mortality. These debates concern women's maternal and reproductive health in India and beyond (as manifested in the Millennium Development Goals); women's health needs and human rights, especially their human right to the best attainable health care; the role of PPPs in health care provision; the UN Global Compact, with a particular focus on the opportunities and challenges for small and medium-sized enterprises in public private partnerships and the search for incentives to join the UN GC; and the development of fair compliance mechanisms for companies that are committed to the UN Global Compact. Thus, for UNU, the project has had a much wider scope than "just" assessing the partners' activities in relation to transparency. In line with UNU's mission, there was the academic goal to explore and develop a PPP approach for improving women's and girls' reproductive and maternal health that could be used on a wider and maybe even a global scale – in the same way that women's health and human rights challenges extend to women all over the world even though a large majority of current problems are found in Asia and Africa.

Such ambitious goals were fully in accordance with the important requirement of the UN Global Compact that PPPs should bear the potential for up-scaling to achieve a wider impact and thereby contribute to reaching the MDGs:

> The most significant contribution of the private sector to the MDGs is to invest and to be successful and to do so in a socially and environmentally responsible manner – thereby creating enormous social benefits including employment and income generation. The challenge for governments, business, NGOs and other societal actors is to find ways to scale-up collaborative efforts in order to achieve wider impact.[20]

Consequently, any effort towards developing a blueprint for best practice within the UN Global Compact would need to include the potential for up-scaling. What are the prospects and potential for up-scaling the WHI?

Coordinating the WHI with existing governmental health policies

One important lesson learned during the WHI pilot was the crucial need for deep cooperation with the Indian government and Indian civil society in order to increase transparency, accountability, effectiveness and sustainability. Any up-scaling measures of the WHI

would therefore need to include joint efforts towards stronger cooperation between project stakeholders, government and civil society.[21]

Efficiency would be further increased by identifying and building
on synergies between the project and existing governmental health
policies and by inviting all major stakeholders to the planning table.
For best results from planning to implementation these stakeholders should include representatives from the Indian government, the
public health sector, the non-governmental health research sector
and quasi-non-governmental and non-governmental organisations
that are active in the health care sector for distributing information
and monitoring compliance. The potential for synergies between the
WHI and recent governmental initiatives can, for instance, be found
in the National Rural Health Mission (NRHM 2005–2012), the Reproductive and Child Health Plan, Phase II (RCH-II) and the Vande
Mataram health scheme.[22]

Options for aligning the WHI with the
National Rural Health Mission

The National Rural Health Mission (NRHM) is a combination of
national programmes, including the Reproductive and Child Health
Plan, Phase II (RCH-II), the National Disease Control Programmes
(NDCP) and the Integrated Disease Surveillance Project (IDSP). It functions like an umbrella for the various existing national government
policies, such as the National Health Policy 2002, National Population Policy 2000 and the UN Millennium Development Goals.

Sharing several goals and targeting the same groups, the WHI
and the NRHM offer several opportunities for cooperation. First, the
NRHM – like the WHI on a much smaller scale – aims to provide
quality health care that is accessible, affordable, accountable, equitable and effective, especially to the vulnerable rural population, with
women and children constituting the specific target groups. The
Mission focuses on 18 selected states with particularly poor demographic and health indicators.[23]

Second, in order to achieve its public health goals, the NRHM
specifically argues in favour of public private partnerships. In order
to own, keep control of and manage public health services in those

partnerships, the NRHM has adopted strategies for training and enhancing the capacity of local bodies (Panchayati Raj Institutions, PRI) to participate in PPPs.

Third, the NRHM and the WHI jointly contribute to tackling the overall shortage of gynaecologists in India, and especially of doctors with expert knowledge of gynaecological surgery. Here, the WHI, with its particular focus on minimally invasive surgery by gynaecologists, could – in a strategically planned PPP on capacity-building – contribute to strengthening the Indian government's efforts towards high-quality training of doctors, especially in the public sector.

Fourth, the challenges experienced by the WHI when trying to implement the initiative effectively in rural areas underline the need for joint initiatives with actors beyond the medical sector. In fact, it might be interesting to think about cross-sector PPPs combining health care, construction and logistics, as well as IT project planning. It could be an option, for instance, to form an overarching PPP with the particular task of installing broadband technology in public hospitals at the national level and thereby create the technical pre-conditions necessary for Internet-based video-counselling. This would support the Indian government's cross-sector health approach as well as NRHM's intentions to strengthen the community health centres and rural hospitals accredited under Indian Public Health Standards for curative care. Finally, this would further support WHI efforts by generating new incentives for medical experts to stay in rural areas instead of moving to the big cities with more attractive working conditions and professional challenges.

Fifth, informing the poor about their options was a major challenge in the WHI project. The NRHM has been facing the same challenge. Being much bigger in size and scale than the WHI, the NRHM has started to establish "accredited social health activists" (ASHA) at the village level (with a target of 1 per 1,000 inhabitants). ASHAs inform underprivileged women and girls about their primary health care options. Cooperation with the WHI could, for instance, involve ASHAs not only promoting access to primary health care but also the options for the best attainable health care, including technically more advanced options such as minimally invasive surgery.

Options for aligning the WHI with the
Reproductive and Child Health initiatives

Under the broad auspices of the NRHM, Phase II of the Reproductive and Child Health Plan (RCH-II) aims to deliver high-quality health services. This is an extremely complex area involving a host of public and private, local and international players. Within the UN GC framework, the WHI places particular emphasis on accountability and transparency, and this points to useful synergies with the RGH-II initiatives.

The RCH-II plan articulates the specific roles and responsibilities of public, private and civil society institutions engaged in the health sector to ensure the timely supply of quality pharmaceuticals and health sector goods and services at competitive prices. In order to address weaknesses in procurement processes and pharmaceutical quality, the Indian government aims at improvement through five specific measures:

1. increasing competition and lessening collusion;
2. strengthening procurement implementation and contract monitoring;
3. handling procurement complaints;
4. disclosing information and promoting oversight by civil society;
5. improving certification of the quality of pharmaceuticals.

The Ministry of Health and Family Welfare has established an Empowered Procurement Wing (EPW) to professionalise the procurement of health sector goods and services. In support of such new policies and actions, the EPW aims at ensuring fairer competition and more transparency in the procurement of health sector goods, pharmaceuticals and services in India. The WHI, with its particular focus on providing the best attainable health care and fair competition in high-tech procurement, as well as helping in the development of a business model at the hospitals, could make substantial contributions to such efforts.

Options for aligning the WHI with the Vande Mataram health scheme

More options for synergies in a potential process of up-scaling the WHI can be found in the Vande Mataram health scheme. The Vande Mataram health scheme envisages increased involvement of the private sector in achieving national maternal health goals. The specific objectives of the scheme are to bring about change in health-seeking behaviour by and for expectant and new mothers and to create awareness in the family and community of the need for safe motherhood. It proposes to involve practising obstetricians and gynaecologists from the government sector, the private sector and NGOs to provide free outpatient services and antenatal check-ups to all pregnant women at their clinics or the nearest community health centre (CHC) on a fixed date once a month. It is expected that public private and civil society partnerships will be strengthened, and that there will be greater acceptance of spacing and family planning methods, leading to a reduction in unwanted pregnancy. Finally, it is also hoped to reduce maternal and neo-natal deaths and to raise recognition that safe motherhood requires medical care and antenatal checks.

This voluntary scheme – which will be assessed every three months for progress – is run under the auspices of the Federation of Obstetric & Gynaecological Societies of India (FOGSI), one of the biggest medical associations in India. This is also a step towards better public private and civil society partnerships. Ultimately, the scheme aims also to involve those gynaecologists who are not members of FOGSI.

In terms of awareness-raising in the communities, the WHI could additionally profit from the Vande Mataram approach, which envisages placing advertisements every month in local papers to highlight the details of the scheme and provide a list of participating medical doctors. If the WHI were included in this scheme, its doctors practising gynaecological surgery via laparoscopy could be included in such a list. In this way, the doctors in the initiative could be given more incentives and more patients could be reached. As a result, one of the bigger challenges of the WHI, namely disseminating information, could be overcome.

Moreover, efforts have been made in the Vande Mataram scheme to develop a communication package for awareness-raising among people in the rural communities. If there were cooperation between the WHI and the scheme, this package might also include information on the advantages of minimally invasive surgery.

FOGSI for its part is to involve all 192 local societies and identify in each one at least two volunteer specialists.[24] These volunteers will offer free services on the ninth of every month to all antenatal cases. Initially the free services were to comprise only antenatal and postnatal examination and counselling and advice regarding contraceptives, diet, immunisation, delivery and so on. More complicated cases were to be counselled separately. Basic or advanced counselling could also cover minimally invasive surgery options.

As in the WHI, the goal of the scheme is to give the participating doctors a logo and certificate from the Indian government indicating their provision of free voluntary services as part of the RCH programme. Such logos can be prominently displayed at their clinics. This suggests the easy potential for combining these two approaches.

Moreover, the Vande Mataram enrolment card for patients could be used for the additional data collection and monitoring necessary for measuring the sustainability of the WHI (which would then turn into a sub-initiative) and other future (sub-)initiatives culminating in a comprehensive data set for further health care planning by the government (as, for instance, demanded by Moazzam Ali in Chapter 1 of this volume). Such an approach would also provide a new basis for initiatives and cooperation with the private sector.

Finally, the WHI could additionally profit from the scheme's example of the government taking steps to provide some kind of insurance or indemnity protection for the volunteer Vande Mataram specialists against any problem that might arise with regard to the Consumer Protection Act. This approach would also meet the demands of critics such as Freedman and Bergström and support the Indian government's efforts to strengthen the health and human rights of women.[25]

Ensuring compliance, accountability and transparency

In order to meet UN GC's demand that up-scaling measures should ensure a wider impact and a real contribution to the MDGs, the WHI would need to become a German–Indian PPP. This shift would also be in accordance with the international development principles of the Paris Declaration, which the German Ministry for Economic Co-operation and Development (BMZ) has signed and which have been milestones of success for BMZ[26] and the international experts of this project. The shift to national ownership of this project would, in fact, be an indication of the overall success of the project.

Compliance and transparency through Indian monitoring

In order to respond to Baru and Nundy's request in Chapter 9 of this volume for stronger monitoring of all PPP partners' activities and the quality of their contributions, a monitoring third partner is needed to assess the socio-economic and institutional prerequisites for the partnership and to ensure that equity is not compromised. Self-monitoring by foreign implementing organisations may raise external doubts about the credibility of the results and create internal problems because of institutional dependencies, loyalties and result-ing restrictions.[27]

In any up-scaling processes of the WHI, a local monitoring partner needs to be involved that will strengthen harmonisation with na-tional health policies (thereby meeting another demand of the Paris Declaration). Here again, the involvement of civil society as well as medical expert associations in peer-reviewing would be essential. The monitoring should be guaranteed by an Indian scientific organisa-tion and in accordance with such new health policies. This would be a PPP according to the Paris principles (i.e. a PPP with national ownership).

GTZ rules for PPP did not foresee continuous monitoring in a project that was essentially intended to serve as a start-up PPP and then carry on by itself. Since this poses substantial challenges for projects that depend on compliance structures – which often need to be created from scratch – and where people need to be trained to be aware of their responsibilities and accountability, short-term PPP measures do not really serve the purpose of creating a sustainable UN GC PPP with lasting success.

In the case of up-scaling the PPP in India, one approach could be the involvement of the Indian Council of Medical Research (ICMR), which on 5th October 2007 was integrated into the new Department of Health Research (DHR) of the Ministry of Health and Family Welfare, Government of India, and which has an active network of 26 disease- or discipline-specific institutes (for example, leprosy, tuberculosis, malaria, pathology, cytology and preventive oncology, desert medicine, reproductive health, nutrition and occupational health) and over 70 field stations in various parts of the country.[28] The ICMR could improve the efficiency and effectiveness of monitoring throughout the country and ensure national ownership. Monitoring by a government-related agency would also be necessary to raise the standards of treatment itself because the use of endoscopy is a challenge also in terms of training – it coincides with the Indian government's health care plans but also with the very ethics of the medical doctors involved.

In accordance with GC principles, both the Indian stakeholders and the private partner would therefore be well advised to keep the PPP fully transparent. In terms of the accountability and transparency of Indian monitoring, the involvement of Indian nongovernmental institutions would be advisable. This would also help improve transactions in the process of reaching the economically disadvantaged women in India who need to know about their options in relation to the best attainable health care at affordable costs. This comprehensive approach would contribute to achieving sustainable improvement in the overall situation of women's maternal and reproductive health and thereby also substantially contribute to reaching the MDGs by 2015.

Strengthening women's reproductive health and human rights: Creating a code of conduct for gynaecological endoscopy surgery

In the search for a blueprint for best practice PPPs within the UN GC, the issue of human rights is fundamental and hotly debated.

The focus of the debate has been on compliance and potential mechanisms for ensuring compliance. Some argue in favour of state control; others prefer self-regulation. This project, however, illustrates that there is more to be taken into consideration than the mere question of how to control partners' immediate commitment.

One important lesson has been learned during this project: the importance of training in gynaecological endoscopy and the need for certification of training standards beyond this project. What is required is a code of conduct for endoscopy surgery that would be in line with medical ethics and with the UN Global Compact's Ten Principles.

Our suggestion is in line with the demands of Transparency International (TI), which considers a code of conduct "a must for regulators, medical practitioners, pharmacists and health administrators. These codes ought to make explicit reference to preventing corruption and conflicts of interest that can lead to corruption, detail sanctions for breaches and be enforced by an independent body."[29]

In this regard it is extremely important that FOGSI decides on general rules for content and certification in order to deal with unwelcome developments that are in clear contrast to the existing human rights and medico-ethical understanding of providing the best attainable health care for all. In fact, it is the medical doctors who are to protect poor people from being exploited by unskilled personnel for dangerous personal endoscopy training. It will be necessary to increase:

- awareness-raising about the need for gynaecological endoscopy;
- awareness-raising about the need for common curriculums and uniform standards of quality;
- awareness-raising about the need for continuous training.

Such awareness, in addition to strong government-led monitoring, will ultimately also contribute to strengthening the Indian health research system, a request discussed by Ganguly and Roy in Chapter 8 in this volume.

In order to create and maintain the utmost transparency and to create further room for progress, it will also – as mentioned before – be advisable to invite women's health NGOs to the stakeholders' table. The voluntary sector, with an estimated 7,000 voluntary health agencies, has a high presence in the rural areas (see Chapter 9 in this volume). The majority of these agencies safeguard and complement government work by providing guidance, criticism and expertise to explore ways and means of doing things differently. They participate in supplementing health education, undertake demonstration projects and mobilise public opinion on health legislation.

In order to contribute to the strengthening of women's health and human rights, the WHI stakeholders are requested to support efforts to develop a code of conduct for gynaecological endoscopy surgery. Any kind of assistance with such efforts will contribute to accountability, transparency and ultimately an improvement in the human rights and health situation of women in India – and beyond.

Notes

1. Neil Kendrick, "Effectiveness vs. Efficiency", in *The Reporting Skills and Professional Writing Handbook*, 2nd edn, 2008, available at <http://www.reportingskills.org/secure/5_moreaboutreporting.htm> (accessed 22 June 2009)
2. "Reaching beyond Boundaries – Women's Health Initiative: A Public–Private Partnership", GTZ Monitoring Report by Dr Nisha Lal and Dr J. Peter Steinmann, New Delhi, May 2008.
3. Ibid., p. 8.
4. Staffan Bergström, "Obstetric Ectoscopy: An Eye-Opener for Hospital-Based Clinicians", *Acta Obstetricia et Gynecologica Scandinavica*, 84, 2005, pp. 105–107.
5. Ibid.
6. "Reaching beyond Boundaries", p. 13.
7. Email from KARL STORZ, Tuttlingen, 23 May 2008.
8. Letter from Peter Laser, KARL STORZ GmbH, to UNU, 21 August 2007.
9. On this and the following, see Chapter 13 in this volume.
10. Chapter 14, p. X.
11. See Monika Kruesmann, "Report of the Women's Health Initiative Workshop, Bonn, Germany, 3–5 December 2006", unpublished manuscript.
12. Email from *KARL STORZ, Tuttlingen, 23 May 2008.*
13. Ibid.

14. Kent Buse and Andrew Harper, "Global Health: Making Partnerships Work: Seven Recommendations for Building Effective Global Public–Private Health Partnerships", Overseas Development Institute (ODI), Briefing Paper 15, January 2007, p. 3.

15. See especially Baru and Nundy in Chapter 9 of this volume.

16. See Buse and Harper, "Global Health: Making Partnerships Work".

17. Transparency International, *Global Corruption Report 2006*, Ann Arbor, MI: Pluto Press, 2006.

18. Martina Timmermann, "Findings and Recommendations Resulting from Communications with Project Stakeholders and Outside Observers in Delhi, Chandigarh and Chennai 8–15 and 23 April 2007", UNU Mission Report, 25 April 2007, unpublished internal document.

19. Buse and Harper, "Global Health: Making Partnerships Work".

20. See the United Nations Global Compact website "Partnerships for Development", <http://www.unglobalcompact.org/Issues/partnerships/business_development.html> (accessed 20 June 2009).

21. The most valuable advice was provided by the participants at UNU Workshop II; for details, see Kruesmann, "Report of the Women's Health Initiative Workshop Bonn, Germany, 3–5 December 2006".

22. Such programmes are discussed and quoted by Mittal and Mathur in Chapter 7 and by Ganguly and Roy in Chapter 8 of this volume.

23. Uttar Pradesh, Uttaranchal, Madhya Pradesh, Chhattisgarh, Bihar, Jharkhand, Orissa, Rajasthan, Himachal Pradesh, Jammu and Kashmir, Assam, Arunachal Pradesh, Manipur, Meghalaya, Nagaland, Mizoram, Sikkim and Tripura.

24. For more information on FOGSI, see <http://www.fogsi.org/about_us.html> (accessed 20 June 2009).

25. Lynn Freedman, Director, Averting Maternal Death and Disability Program, Columbia University, was a participant in UNU Workshop I in Chennai and was critical about the approach of using high technology. Her arguments basically concurred with those of Staffan Bergström in his paper "Obstetric Ectoscopy: An Eye-Opener for Hospital-Based Clinicians", which she kindly provided for this report.

26. See Chapter 13 in this volume.

27. S. Garg and A. Nath, "Current Status of National Rural Health Mission", *Indian Journal of Community Medicine*, 32(3), 2007, pp. 171–172, available at <http://www.ijcm.org.in/text.asp?2007/32/3/171/36818> (accessed 23 June 2009).

28. See Ganguly and Roy in Chapter 8 of this volume; more information is available at <http://icmr.nic.in/abouticmr.htm> (accessed 20 June 2009).

29. Increased transparency is one pertinent way to combat corruption, which TI discussed as particularly widespread in the health care sector (Transparency International, *Global Corruption Report 2006*).

PART C

CONCLUSION

19

PPPs for women's health and human rights beyond India: Probing new standards and methodologies

Martina Timmermann and Monika Kruesmann

The Women's Health Initiative (WHI) aimed at contributing to strengthening women's and girls' health and rights not only in, but also beyond India. An aspiration for the WHI was that, following the original project's successful completion, the model might be further developed, extended and translated to different contexts.

Talking about this public private partnership (PPP) in terms of "beyond India", therefore, refers not only to the transfer of this project to other countries and regions of the world but also to its contribution to current international debates related to women's re-productive health and their right to the best available health care. It also refers to debates on financing health care via PPPs with ethical guidelines as provided by the United Nations Global Compact (UN GC).

Thus, if we wish to discuss the WHI "beyond India" we will need to refer to both territorial and issue dimensions.

Partnerships for women's health: Striving for best practice within the UN Global Compact, Timmermann and Kruesmann (eds),
United Nations University Press, 2009, ISBN 978-92-808-1185-8

Transferring the PPP beyond India

In terms of transfer to other countries and regions, the WHI illus-trated that improving women's reproductive and maternal health is a challenge that needs to be met at different social levels and through a multi-sector approach.

The first step would be awareness-raising about the magnitude of the problem. This would include recognising that the complexity of the issues and actors in the challenging process of improving ma-ternal and reproductive health care calls for a combined approach involving primary health care and high technology. What is needed is a "both/and" instead of an "either/or" solution.

Another vital step would be to ensure accountability, as was, for instance, demanded by Dr Francisco Songane, Director of the Panel on Maternal Mortality and Human Rights (PMNCH), in his speech at the Human Rights Council in Geneva in 2008:

> The challenge is not technological, but strategic, organizational and, above all, political. Women rights are being violated on a grand scale. We all have a role in fostering political accountability – of UN agencies, of donors, and of national leaders in countries. We have now a unique opportunity for building accountability for mothers and children.[1]

With regard to the alarming situation of women's maternal and reproductive health in South Asia and Africa, Moazzam Ali (Chapter 1 in this volume) advised first identifying the key factors inhibiting improvements in health outcomes, which would require strengthen-ing gender-related human indices in South Asian and African coun-tries. Only once the distribution of the causes of maternal deaths is understood can there be reliable information on which to base overall reproductive health policies and programmes. In line with Arabinda Ghosh (Chapter 10 in this volume), who stressed the importance of including literacy in any governmental policy for improving women's health in order to be able to inform the poor properly, Moazzam demanded that due attention be paid to cultural, educational and economic barriers.

Based on such recommendations for multi-sector cooperation, as well as the findings of Baru and Nundy in Chapter 9 in this volume, transfer of this project as a PPP would require several concrete steps:

- Because in most developing countries there are no overarching regulatory frameworks for the private sector or for PPPs, there needs to be an assessment of the socio-economic and institutional prerequisites for the partnership.

- The PPP should be deliberately embedded in the UN GC to meet the requirement of developing criteria for the registration and regulation of private and voluntary players.

- Awareness needs to be raised among medical institutions and doctors about the value of laparoscopic gynaecological surgery.

- Closely related is the need to raise awareness about the importance of training guidelines, monitoring and certification of training and accountability. There should be a clear milestone plan for developing a shared level of quality in terms of teaching and training modules.

- The monitoring should be done by one or more independent partners. To meet the request for national ownership, monitoring could be done by a third party in the particular country. This could for instance be a quasi-non-governmental organisation (quango). For the utmost transparency and credibility, however, it would be more effective to additionally invite local NGOs into the process at any time during the project when needed. In order to allow for such flexibility, the PPP should stay open to a deliberate self-learning process.

- It will be essential to provide support to the hospitals and medical doctors for business plan development and capacity development. Such a process could be supported by consultant experts from the health care sector who have specialised in health care economics (see, for instance, Chapter 4 by Neubauer and Driessle in this volume) and can draw on their experiences in other countries.

- As Buse has already suggested, it is necessary to bring all stakeholders to the table.[2] To ensure the smooth implementation of a project within hospitals, it will be very important from the very beginning of the project to invite participation by representatives of the hospital administration and finance department, who also need to accept being monitored in the name of transparency and accountability – and to avoid incentives for corruption.

- With particular regard to the relationship between corporate business and the public sector, it is important that there are the same or at least comparable business conditions for all partners, which can be ensured through transparent procedures. All hospitals that cater for the poor should receive the same contractual treatment by the company in terms of maintenance and warranties.

- In relation to the monitoring of the project, this implies that the same time-frame and services are applied to all the project's Endoscopy Training Centres (ETCs). To get the project successfully off the ground, implementation in the field should start at the same time and realistic goals and timelines need to be developed between the project designer, the funders and the implementers in the field. In this regard it is essential that the rationale and goals of the project are comprehensively and continuously *explained* to all shareholders and *repeated* at different stages of the project. Personnel can change and valuable knowledge can be lost, which has a negative impact on the effectiveness and efficiency of the project.

- As the WHI project showed, it is highly desirable to have a project coordinator who ensures overall communication among the partners.

- In addition, clear and transparent communication within the partner organisations themselves is vital to make sure that the plans developed in the head office are transmitted and accepted by the implementers in the field. Partners thus need to ensure sound communication within their own organisations. They need to create – in Buse's words – internal loyalty in implementation.[3]

- For the measure to be sustainable, an e-platform for communication and advice should be set up that allows medical doctors in rural areas to seek expert guidance when needed. In addition, this e-platform will enhance the overall transparency of the measure and communication among all shareholders and stakeholders.

Contributing to relevant debates on issues beyond India

United Nations University, with its mission goal to serve as a think tank for the United Nations on issues of global concern, aspired to provide new inputs to the debate on health-related MDGs, women's maternal and reproductive health needs and human rights, corporate business, ethics and the demand – especially by human rights representatives – for accountability.

Contributing to UN GC debates on assessment and strengthening UN inter-agency cooperation

One major UNU goal was to develop a methodological approach for voluntary assessment through an international UN platform that, if accepted by a company, would clearly indicate that company's GC commitment to transparency and accountability. Because of this project's very structured approach (i.e. its self-learning structure and dual monitoring approach at the field level and above), it has contributed to the UN GC debates on how to undertake voluntary and fair assessments of UN GC company activities.

The WHI was designed in 2004. It was deliberately embedded in the UN GC framework, with two of its partners being members of the Compact; it was based on a regular business model; and the partners agreed to have their work assessed by an international agency, the United Nations University. This already makes this project a role model within the UN GC framework. Within the design process in 2004, UNU developed a particular GC assessment model, which was first presented to the public at the International Conference on Human Rights and Development at the City University of Hong Kong in May 2005.[4]

The business model, which had been essential for the company's business case and which had been designed by a consultant representative (TIMA) from the corporate sector, was discussed from an academic viewpoint in Chapter 17 in this volume by Christina Gradl, the first Kofi Annan UN Global Compact fellow.[5] Ms Gradl had the opportunity to look at relevant materials, conduct in-depth interviews with all stakeholders and thus study and discuss the business design of the project from an economic perspective. Her fellowship included three months at KARL STORZ company, three months in the UN GC office and three months at Harvard University, which ensured a widespread exchange of ideas on this project and its perspectives beyond the group of project participants. Other eminent participants in this project, such as Paul Hunt (the Special Rapporteur on the right of everyone to the enjoyment of the highest attainable standard of physical and mental health, until June 2008), and Klaus Leisinger (Special Advisor to the UN Secretary-General on the Global Compact, until December 2006), have also contributed chapters, but in addition have increased awareness of this approach in their work with the UN Global Compact and the human rights community in Geneva. The Foreword in this volume by Mary Robinson is another indication of UNU's successful efforts at serving as a think tank for the United Nations and at providing fresh intellectual input on issues of global concern.

Finally, through this multi-player approach, UNU has strengthened its cooperation with other UN agencies and civil society. The result of this fruitful interaction was reflected when the UN Global Compact Office put its "Business Case Studies: Guidelines" online.[6] Thus, the UN Global Compact Office recognises the UNU's contributions and those of its experts to a new framework for analysis – what could be better success for UNU, its mission and its goals in this project?

Contributing to the debates on SMEs and the Global Compact: Profit, protection and human rights progress

Another important question, but one that has not yet been fully discussed here, is why small and medium-sized enterprises (SMEs) should join the UN Global Compact. SMEs are responsible for the majority of economic activity worldwide. In industrialised countries such as Germany, SMEs – not the multinational corporations, as public opinion tends to assume – make up over 90 per cent of all companies that are decisive carriers of the economic performance and economic leverage. In order to meet the MDGs and to make the UN Global Compact, and with it human rights, a reality worldwide, it is therefore of the utmost importance to involve SMEs, even if it may look easier to focus on multinational corporations (see Chapter 6 by Bethke and Bösendorfer in this volume). Similarly, the UN Global Compact, with its requests for transparency, accountability and compliance, could be an extremely significant platform for SMEs in our globalising world.

Yet many SMEs are hesitant to join the global scene and the GC initiative for various reasons. In Europe, for instance, SMEs do not consider the UN GC important. They clearly remain focused on their national markets. "Only 8% of EU27 SMEs export and only 12% of the imports of an average SME are purchased abroad. The main reason is usually lack of financial resources, but most of all the lack of skills or skilled human capital to tackle the demands of globalization."[7]

Another reason for the lack of interest is the UN GC demand for transparency, which provokes the fear among SMEs that they would have to reveal too much internal information, which might create a backlash against the company. So what would be the actual benefits for SMEs if they joined the UN Global Compact? Here, there is a lot to learn from the WHI project, in which KARL STORZ GmbH was considered a medium-sized company– admittedly, with more than 3,300 employees worldwide when the project started, at the very upper level of the category.

Copyright protection

Many SMEs in medical technology, such as KARL STORZ, focus on innovation in close cooperation with medical doctors. Indeed, their products are often developed as a result of demand from medical doctors. The outcome of such cooperation is therefore unique and creates development costs. By up-scaling the product and its distribution, such SMEs thereby also contribute substantially to progress in the development of new health care options. But, because of their small size, they are also more vulnerable with regard to copyright protection. SMEs do not usually retain permanent legal staff. And even if they did and were able to use the law to retaliate, their actual competitive advantage − the first-mover effect triggered by quick and creative innovation − would be lost, but the costs of development would remain. For SMEs in such an environment, both the Global Compact and civil society's demand for business transparency are therefore often perceived as dangerous for the company.

Moreover, the demand for greater transparency raises fears that their competitors might profit from additional inside information. Any kind of difficulty that might occur could negatively influence public opinion, to the benefit of a competitor. In harsh global competition, any bad news can easily have an impact on and endanger the very survival of a small or medium-sized company.

Transparency, therefore, is seen as a double-edged sword, and trust is even regarded as a naive ivory tower concept. What is overlooked is the fact that, through participation in the Global Compact and cooperation on projects with other UN GC participants of all sizes and within the framework of the UN GC rules, transparency and compliance with the rules will increase trust, reliability and opportunities for cooperation. UN GC cooperation can thus lead to enhanced copyright protection and consequently allow for more freedom and resources for development because the companies that are part of such undertakings can reduce their transaction costs and increase their profits. Moreover, patients will benefit from more easily available and up-to-date technological treatment and hospitals will gain from more transparent cost structures.

There is obviously a close causal relationship between copyright protection for SMEs and health care development that – if compliance and accountability are ensured – benefits the patients. Unfortunately, however, this relationship based on trust and reliability is often overlooked.

With regard to property rights, the Global Compact could also cooperate with the World Intellectual Property Organization, which already has a special eye on SMEs.[8] Through such cooperation there would be a support platform for the SMEs. This platform could be further strengthened in size, coverage and quality by the United Nations Industrial Development Organization, which has also been running programmes on PPP with SMEs (as mentioned in Chapter 6 in this volume).

The highest level of legitimacy would be achieved if this challenge of creating and ensuring trust and accountability were tackled at both global and local levels, with the UN GC providing an ethical framework that allows for more trust to develop and local entities taking care of the monitoring in order to ensure compliance. Based on our experiences in the WHI, national monitoring (governmental and non-governmental) together with international overview assessment seems to be the most useful way to ensure a credible and comprehensive sustainable approach. The lesson here is that transparency increases trust and reliability among UN GC participants and offers protection.

Protection from corruption: Strengthening SMEs' performance and patients' rights

Transparency and compliance are also vital issues for SMEs with regard to the problem of corruption, especially for those in the health care business.

Transparency International defines corruption as "the abuse of entrusted power for private gain",[9] and the health business has a definite tendency towards such abuse of power. Owing to the number of public and private shareholders and stakeholders in health projects, there are many circumstances in which temptations to behave corruptly can arise. There might be opportunities for bribing regulators and medical professionals, for corruption in procurement and for overbilling. When hospital administrators or physicians (public or private), company executives or employees of international institutions strive to enrich themselves through such a project, they are not formally abusing a public office, but they are abusing the power and resources with which they were entrusted in order to improve the overall health situation.

Especially with regard to gynaecological endoscopy, it has become apparent that corruption prevents equal access by patients to the best available health care, and can even lead to inexpert and life-threatening treatments, with poor people suffering the most. The poor are disproportionately affected by corruption, because they are less able to afford bribes for health services that are supposed to be free. And they certainly cannot pay for private alternatives.

In addition to legitimate demands for transparency in order to ensure access to the best available health care for all, there is also an important lesson for the SMEs. If they are faced with corruption and act in compliance with their GC commitments – a clear reference to being a GC member with the obligation to report its business transactions publicly – this ultimately protects the company, and thereby also the patients. Transparency and compliance thus contribute to the strengthening of the business position and also enforce the patients' positions and rights.

This underlines (again) the necessity and importance of monitoring by governmental and non-governmental society in order to improve accountability and transparency in such processes.

Conclusion

The WHI illustrates that PPPs must not substitute the fundamental responsibility of governments to provide services and infrastructure, and develop and implement standards and operating regulations.

Rather, public private partnership organisations must work *together* with governments to ensure activities are mutually beneficial, rather than obstructive or duplicative. The WHI demonstrated considerable success as a public private partnership within the ethical framework of the Global Compact. It thereby constitutes a concrete example of the potential of the GC for accommodating diversity and buffering and meeting the challenges of globalisation. In particular, the PPP initiative demonstrates the difficulties of engaging effectively with state actors; but it also demonstrates the value of the GC model in opening the way for actors with different foci, expectations and practices to come together on a common ethical platform to pursue a shared goal. Although this project has been small in size, we hope that the results and options for up-scaling and transfer will encourage the project stakeholders (former and future) to continue or to start afresh and go even further – with the vision to reach out on a much greater scale – and thereby contribute to achieving the MDGs and strengthening the human rights of women and girls.

The WHI in India showed the importance of cooperating with the government to raise awareness of the relevance of gynaecological endoscopy in general and among medical doctors specifically, to develop certification guidelines for a reliable quality check of the training of gynaecological surgeons and corresponding staff and to find convincing ways of spreading the news of available options to patients via medical doctors and by making use of existing governmental health care policies and instruments.

Beyond that, it was learned in the process of reporting and analysis that, because of the UN GC ethical framework chosen by the partners, the project was able to reach a new and higher level of quality. Transparency through independent monitoring was considered a key tool to ensure accountability and, finally, success.

SMEs, which account for more than 90 per cent of world economic power, are vital for increasing the strength and viability of the UN Global Compact and its many initiatives in the health, environmental and technology sectors – which all interlink with human rights issues. SMEs therefore need to be attracted to join the UN Global

Compact. There are several advantage to SMES from joining the UN Global Compact: they would, for instance, find new options for entering markets together with bigger UN GC partner enterprises. Such GC enterprises can, in fact, act as door openers for small and medium-sized firms.

The transparency required by the UN GC increases trust and reliability among UN GC participants and offers protection. In the short and medium terms, SMEs profit from greater respect for, and therefore protection of, copyright, resulting in less corruption. The long-term effect of SMEs joining the UN GC would be their vital contribution to improving the human rights situation, with more people having access to the best attainable health care and with a safer environment for people and more options for lucrative business.

In conclusion, a best practice UN GC PPP needs to be transparent, effective, efficient and sustainable in order to be successful and contribute to the advancement of women's health and human rights. If the lessons learned in this UN GC PPP are applied in any process of up-scaling and transfer, if follow-up PPPs were set up with particular consideration of the socio-cultural and economic circumstances of the host country, and if there were continuous impartial third-party monitoring throughout the project, there would be a good chance of seeing such UN GC PPPs turn into vital carriers of improvements in women's reproductive and maternal health care not only at a global scale but also at a more comprehensive local scale.

In sum, a successful sustainable UN GC PPP requires a *glocal* design as well as implementation involving all major stakeholders and requiring particularly close cooperation between the public and private partners. The need for transparency must be accepted by the partners and provided by engaging with civil society. It is also important to maintain a loyal and (as much as possible) permanent project staff with a joint project mediator/coordinator in order to ensure continuous and smooth inter-partner communication. Thus, the overall project know-how and knowledge that are essential for the efficiency of transactions, for progress and for the success of the project will be guaranteed throughout the partnership. The winners will be the partners but also – most of all – the women, their health and their human rights.

Notes

1. Human Rights Council, Panel on Maternal Mortality and Human Rights, Thursday, June 5, 2008, Palais des Nations, Geneva, Speech by Dr Francisco Songane, <http://www.who.int/pmnch/media/news/2008/20080606_unhumanrights_songanespeech.pdf> (accessed 15 June 2009).
2. Kent Buse and Andrew Harper, "Global Health: Making Partnerships Work – Seven Recommendations for Building Effective Global Public–Private Health Partnerships", Overseas Development Institute (ODI), Briefing Paper 15, January 2007.
3. Ibid., p. 3.
4. The article was published as Martina Timmermann, "Meeting the MDG Challenges of Women's Health, Human Rights and Health Care Politics: The Women's Health Initiative (WHI) for Improving Women's and Girls' Reproductive and Maternal Health in India", in C. Raj Kumar and D. K. Srivastava (eds), *Human Rights and Development: Law, Policy and Governance*, Hong Kong: Lexis Nexis, 2006, pp. 475–493.
5. The fellowship was additionally funded by KARL STORZ.
6. See "Business Case Studies: Guidelines", at <http://www.unglobalcompact.org/docs/issues_doc/human_rights/Resources/Business_Case_Studies_Guidelines_17_Jun_08.pdf> (accessed 26 June 2009). We are grateful that our project had the opportunity to provide input to the process of developing these guidelines through in-depth exchanges with the UN GC Office, other UN bodies and universities (most notably Harvard University). The UN GC Office and its partners have further detailed this first approach with particular regard to the human rights dimension. Their template for UN GC human rights case studies is available at <http://www.unglobalcompact.org/HowToParticipate/guidance_documents/index.html> (accessed 16 June 2009).
7. *Supporting the Internationalisation of SMEs. Final Report of the Expert Group*, European Commission, Enterprise and Industry Directorate-General, Brussels, December 2007, p. 4.
8. See <http://www.wipo.int/activities/en/> (accessed 16 June 2009).
9. See <http://www.transparency.org.uk/> (accessed 16 June 2009).

APPENDICES

Appendix A

UNU Workshop I, 1–4 October 2005, Chennai, India: "'Improving Women's Health in India' – Public Private Partnership of KARL STORZ and GTZ. Background, Method, Potential"

Programme and participants

Welcome	**Ramesh Thakur** Senior Vice Rector, Assistant Secretary General, UNU
Introduction to the Project and the Workshop Structure	**Martina Timmermann** Director of Studies on Human Rights and Ethics, UNU
I: Women's Health	**Chair: Lynn Freedman**
Keynote Speech: Women's Health, MDGs and Human Rights	**Lynn Freedman** Director of the Averting Maternal Death and Disability (AMDD) Program, Mailman School of Public Health, Columbia University
Improving the Health of Poor Women in Asia	**Meera Chatterjee** Senior Social Development Specialist, World Bank India
The Situation of Women's Reproductive/Maternal Health in India	**Arvind Mathur/Antigoni Koumpounis** Cluster Coordinator for 'Family and Community Health' WHO-India
II: India's Health Politics	**Chair: Ramesh Thakur**
India's Medical System	**N. K. Ganguly** Director, Indian Council for Medical Research (ICMR)
India's Health Policy	**V. R. Muraleedharan** Head of Department of Humanities & Social Sciences, IIT-Madras
Women's Health and the Role of Insurance	**Alka Narang** Head HIV/AIDS Unit, UNDP India

III: PPP, Health and Governance	**Chair: Peter Berman** Harvard School of Public Health / Lead Economist, World Bank India
PPP, Health and Governance	**Guenter Neubauer** Director of the Institute of Health Economics, Munich
Seven Deadly Sins of Global Public Private Health Partnerships	**Kent Buse** Research Fellow, Overseas Development Institute (ODI), London
World Bank and Health PPPs – Examples from Tamil Nadu	**Preeti Kudesia** Senior Public Health Specialist, World Bank India
IV: Government Experiences with PPPs in the Field of Women's Health	**Chair: V. R. Muraleedharan**
Indian Women's Health Policy: The Value of PPPs as Seen from the Point of View of the Indian Government	**Rajesh Bhushan** Director, Department of Health, Ministry of Health & Family Welfare (represented by Arvind Mathur, WHO)
The BMZ Approach towards Improving Women's Health in India: The Promise of PPPs	**Nicolaus von der Goltz** Division for Cooperation with the Business Sector, German Federal Ministry for Economic Cooperation and Development (BMZ), Berlin
Visit of the Hospital and ETC	
V: The Project from Within	**Chair: R. Thakur / M. Timmermann**
KARL STORZ's WHI-Goals and Expectations	**Achim G. Deja** KARL STORZ WHI Project Coordinator / CEO TIMA GmbH
KARL STORZ's WHI-Experiences "On the Ground"	**Peter Laser** KARL STORZ, Managing Director India

GTZ's WHI-Goals and Expectations	**Johann P. Steinmann** Director of Indo-German Health Programme, GTZ India
GTZ's WHI-Experiences "On the Ground"	**Ellen Soennichsen** GTZ India
Joseph's Nursing Home's WHI-Expectations	**Vasant Kumar, M.D.**, Joseph's Nursing Home, with **Diethelm Wallwiener**, University of Tübingen (via Video)
Medical doctors' expectations and goals	Two MDs – participants in the upcoming training session
Summary Discussion Impressions/suggestions regarding: • Approach • Method • Perspectives	
VI: Conclusions and recommendations for WS II: The WHI within the framework of the Global Compact	**Chair: Martina Timmermann**
Discussion of the potential and replicability in other countries Recommendations for the project	
Workshop Closing	
Steering Committee	**Chair: Achim G. Deja**

Additional distinguished participants who supported us in our programme included:

• **Dr. hc. Sybill Storz, CEO, KARL STORZ GmbH & Co.KG,** Tuttlingen

- **Karl-Christian Storz**, Senior Management, KARL STORZ GmbH & Co.KG, Tuttlingen
- **Helmut Wehrstein**, Senior Management, KARL STORZ GmbH & Co.KG, Tuttlingen
- **Regina Stern**, Assistant to CEO, KARL STORZ GmbH & Co.KG, Tuttlingen
- **Prof. Gundapuneni Koteswara Prasad**, Director of the Mahatma Gandhi Centre for Peace and Conflict Resolution, University of Madras, India
- **S. Chidambaranathan (Nathan)**, Special Advisor to the rector of the United Nations University, New York
- **Prof. Tehemton Udwadia**, President of the International Federation of Societies of Endoscopic Surgeons (IFSES), Head, Department of M.A.S. Hinduja Hospital

Appendix B

UNU Workshop II, 3–5 December 2006, Bonn, Germany: "The WHI: Aspirations, Actions and Achievements"

Programme and participants

Official Opening	**Hans van Ginkel** Rector, UN Undersecretary, UNU Tokyo **Janos Bogardi** Director UNU-EHS, Bonn **Baschar Al-Frangi** Center for Cooperation with the Private Sector – GTZ, Berlin
Introduction to the Project and the Workshop	**Martina Timmermann** Director of Studies on Human Rights and Ethics/UNU WHI Project Director
Keynote: The Role of Endoscopy and Laparoscopy for Women's Health	**Kurian Joseph** Chairman Endoscopy Committee, Asia Oceania Federation of Obstetrics & Gynaecology
I: PPP Project Reports: Partner Perspectives	**Chair: Hans van Ginkel**
Experiences and Perspectives from KARL STORZ India	**Peter Laser** Director KARL STORZ India
Experiences and Perspectives from GTZ India	**Anu Chopra** GTZ-India
Experiences and Perspectives from Public Medical Doctors Involved in the Project	**Suneeta Mittal** Dean of Department of Gynaecology, AIIMS **Alka Kriplani** WHI-Co-Chairperson, AIIMS
Experiences and Perspectives from the Project-Coordinator	**Achim Deja** KARL STORZ/TIMA GmbH
What Were the Challenges in the Planning and Implementation Process?	Q&A/DISCUSSION

II: Improving women's health care in India?	**Chair: Moazzam Ali** Assistant Professor, Tokyo University
India's Women's Health Situation: Programmes and Policies	**Arvind Mathur**
Health PPPs in India: Stepping Stones for Improving Women's Health Care?	**Rama Baru** Associate Professor, Jawaharal Nehru University
Pro-poor Capacity Building in India's Women's Health Sector	**Arabinda Ghosh** Joint Director, State Government, West Bengal
What Has Been, Could or Should Be the WHI Contribution in India?	DISCUSSION
III: Contributing to Sustainable Development? Role Model for PPPs within the GC framework?	**Chair: Günter Neubauer**
Economic Rationality and Human Rights – Can CSR Work as a Tool for Sustainable Development?	**Minna Gillberg** Senior Advisor to EU Vice-President M. Wallström **Pamela Bell** Research Fellow, Louvain University
Winning SMEs for PPPs within the GC Framework: In Need of Role Models?	**Manuela Bösendorfer** UNIDO
Interviews with Indian WHI participants	GTZ – Video
IV: The WHI: Going beyond India?	**Chair: Martina Timmermann**
Improving Maternal and Reproductive Health beyond India	**Moazzam Ali**

What are the Major Achievements? Can and Should the WHI be Replicated beyond India? What Would Be the Challenges?	FINAL DISCUSSION (internal)
Public Debate – Business, Ethics and the Right to Health (with a Focus on the WHI's Future Perspectives)	**Chair: Janos Bogardi**
Welcome	**Janos Bogardi** Director UNU-EHS **Ulrike Haupt** Head of Department, Federal Ministry of Economic Cooperation and Development (BMZ)
Health Care Ethics from a European Perspective	**Stefan F. Winter** State Secretary, Ministry of Labour, Health and Social Affairs, North Rhine-Westphalia
Keynote I: Corporate Social Responsibility and the Right to Health	**Klaus Leisinger** Special Advisor to the UN SG on the UN Global Compact President & CEO, Novartis Foundation
Doing Business within the UN Global Compact: The "Women's Health Initiative" in India	**Martina Timmermann**
Keynote II: Improving Women's Health: What Are the Needs and Challenges in Africa?	**Peter H. Katjavivi** Ambassador of the Republic of Namibia to Germany, Chair of the UNU Council
Final Discussion	
Closing	**Janos Bogardi**

Independent Rapporteur in WS II:

- **Monika Kruesmann**, Assistant Director, Department of Education, Employment and Workplace Relations (DEEWR), Australian Government. For a copy of Monika Kruesmann's "External Report on the Women's Health Initiative: Evaluation and Progress", updated in June 2008, kindly contact the author (e-mail: Monika.Kruesmann@gmail.com).

Additional participants in our programme included:

- **Dr. hc. Sybill Storz**, CEO, KARL STORZ GmbH & Co.KG, Tuttlingen
- **Helmut Wehrstein**, Senior Management, KARL STORZ GmbH & Co.KG, Tuttlingen
- **Regina Stern**, Assistant to CEO, KARL STORZ GmbH & Co.KG, Tuttlingen
- **Jörg Hartmann**, Head Public Private Partnership, GTZ, Berlin
- **Diana Kraft**, PPP Manager, GTZ, Eschborn
- **Dr. Johann P. Steinmann**, GTZ India
- **Jasja van der Zijde**, Director of SAMA Advies, Netherlands
- **Christina Gradl**, Martin-Luther Universität Halle-Wittenberg, Germany

Appendix C

Paul Hunt's 2008 Preliminary Mission
Report on India

**UNITED
NATIONS**

A

General Assembly

Distr.
GENERAL

A/HRC/7/11/Add.4
29 February 2008

ENGLISH ONLY

HUMAN RIGHTS COUNCIL
Seventh session
Agenda Item 3

**PROMOTION AND PROTECTION OF ALL HUMAN RIGHTS,
CIVIL, POLITICAL, ECONOMIC, SOCIAL AND CULTURAL
RIGHTS, INCLUDING THE RIGHT TO DEVELOPMENT**

**Report of the Special Rapporteur on the right of everyone to the enjoyment of
the highest attainable standard of physical and mental health**

Preliminary note on the mission to India

Addendum[*]

---

[*] The present note was submitted later than the indicated deadline, in order to incorporate the latest available information on the subject matter. Due to late submission, it is circulated as received.

GE.08-11270

A/HRC/7/11/Add.4
Page 2

Introduction

1.   At the invitation of the Government, the Special Rapporteur on the right of everyone to the enjoyment of the highest attainable standard of physical and mental health ('right to the highest attainable standard of health' or 'right to health') visited India from 22 November to 3 December 2007.

2.   The mission focused on the issue of maternal mortality with a view to understanding, in the context of the right to the highest attainable standard of health, the steps taken by India to reduce this phenomenon, and to make constructive recommendations. The Special Rapporteur visited the states of Rajasthan and Maharashtra to engage with the authorities on their approaches to the issue. The Special Rapporteur also discussed maternal mortality with India's central Government in Delhi.

3.   During the mission, the Special Rapporteur met with the Minister of Health, Dr Anbunmani Ramdoss, Minister of State for Women and Child Development, Ms Renuka Chowdhury, Minister of State for External Affairs, Mr Anand Sharma, Chairperson of the National Human Rights Commission, Mr Rajendra Babu, a number of senior officials in Rajasthan and Maharashtra as well as officials from the UN County team.

4.   The Special Rapporteur is grateful to the Government of India for the invitation to undertake a mission and for the support provided before, during and after the mission.

5.   This Note provides some preliminary observations arising from the mission. The Special Rapporteur will submit his mission report to the Human Rights Council in September 2008, and will go beyond the brief observations presented in this Preliminary Note.

Maternal mortality

6.   Globally, over 500,000 women die each year in childbirth or during pregnancy, leaving over a million motherless children. Crucially, the great majority of these maternal deaths are preventable.

7.   The Special Rapporteur underlines that maternal death is not only a health issue. It is also a human rights issue, relating to - for example - women's rights to life, health, equality and non-discrimination.

8.   In India, 100,000 women die yearly in India during childbirth or pregnancy. There is an average of 300 maternal deaths for every 100,000 live births in India, which is higher than in many other middle-income and some low-income countries[1]. Furthermore, in some of the country's states, the situation is considerably worse – for

---

[1]   Brazil – 110 deaths for every 100,000 live births; Chile - 16; China – 45; Cuba-45; Egypt - 130; Namibia – 210; Sri Lanka – 58 (WHO, UNICEF, UNFPA, World Bank 2005).

instance, in Uttar Pradesh there are over 510 - and in Rajasthan 445 - maternal deaths for every 100,000 live births.

9.   Even though the Indian rate of maternal deaths is declining, at the present rate neither India, nor any of its states, will reach their maternal mortality targets for 2015 arising from the Millennium Development Goals (MDGs). Financial bottlenecks, often caused by insufficient absorptive capacity, obstruct India's progress towards achieving its MDGs. In some local authorities, over 50% of the health budget is unutilised.

10.   The Special Rapporteur commends and supports the efforts of the Government for introducing policies designed to improve maternal health and reduce maternal deaths. He commends the Government's commitment to increase funds for the public health sector, as well as for establishing the National Rural Health Mission, an ambitious initiative that represents a very significant step in the right direction.

11.   However, the Special Rapporteur was concerned about the uneven level of healthcare services in Rajasthan and Maharashtra. During the mission, the Special Rapporteur visited a number of public sector health facilities in both states, from very large hospitals to very small health posts in slums and rural areas. Regrettably, some of these facilities were clearly seriously inadequate: dilapidated, ill-equipped, under-staffed, and offering very low-quality services. However, some other public sector facilities he visited were inspirational: community-supported, well-equipped and staffed by dedicated teams of health and other workers.

12.   By adopting various measures, the central and state authorities have successfully managed to increase the number of women delivering babies in public health facilities. In other words, they have increased the demand for services in the public sector. But, in many cases, the range and quality of services offered in those facilities has been seriously neglected. In short, the supply-side has received too little attention. The focus has been on increasing institutional delivery – but institutional delivery does not always provide access to life-saving care, such as emergency obstetric care, and therefore cannot be regarded as a proxy for access to life saving care.

13.   It is imperative that the sequencing of reforms ensures a balance between the demand-side and supply-side. Getting pregnant women to go to facilities that do not have the services that they need is not a satisfactory outcome.

14.   The Special Rapporteur also found that the authorities are collecting data on the number of institutional deliveries. However, there is little or no data on the crucial issue: access to improved life-saving care which does not appear to be automatically accompanying institutional deliveries as could have been expected.

Registration system and maternal death audits

15.   The Special Rapporteur noted with concern that there is no effective, reliable and comprehensive civil registration system for accurately reporting births and deaths in India. There is evidence that women are silently dying in childbirth and during

A/HRC/7/11/Add.4
Page 4

pregnancy. As many of these deaths are not registered, they remain uncounted and unreported.

16.   The Special Rapporteur strongly recommends that all States introduce, as a matter of urgency, a comprehensive, effective registration system, as well as a system of maternal death audits, such as those already in existence in Tamil Nadu and on a pilot basis in Rajasthan. It is of the utmost importance that all the circumstances of maternal deaths are examined in order to find out why the death occurred. A maternal death audit should be a non-judicial review, one that goes beyond medical reasons to identify the social, economic and cultural reasons that led or contributed to the death.

17.   The emphasis of the maternal death audits should be on fact-finding rather than fault-finding. In this way, they can help to identify the structural and systemic failures that are leading to women's preventable deaths.

Health workers

18.   The Special Rapporteur was concerned about the massive, crippling crisis in India's health workforce. In many areas, life-saving care is unavailable to women giving birth. Rural and disadvantaged areas are those most likely to be without a provider in public facilities. This compels many women either to go without any care at all, or to go to the private sector for life-saving services that should be publicly available for free. Recourse to the private sector impoverishes many women and their families.

19.   A human rights approach will call for all health practitioners to contribute to the provision of predictable and sustainable medical care in public facilities in rural and underserved areas. For example, for the life of the present National Rural Health Mission (2005-2012), private practitioners should provide their services to the public authorities for one day a month at governmental rates of pay. In turn, the governmental authorities have a corresponding duty to ensure that such contributions are supported by the necessary facilities and equipment, so that the contributions have maximum impact.

20.   However, such arrangements do not provide a long-term solution to a complex, systemic, workforce problem. Therefore, the Special Rapporteur strongly recommends that the Government establish, as a matter of urgency, a high-level, high-profile independent committee to prepare a report on human resources in health, both the public and private sectors, with a particular focus on the needs of rural and underserved areas. The report should be wide-ranging and include the issue of posting and transfers of staff.

National and State Health Commissions

21.   The Special Rapporteur notes that, under international human rights law, governments have a binding legal obligation to ensure that third parties, including the private sector, are respectful of individuals' and communities' human rights. Especially in the absence of adequate self-regulation, this requires a State to establish an appropriate, effective, regulatory framework.

22.   There are about 1.4 million health practitioners in India. Only about 10% of them are in government service. In other words, the Indian private health sector is enormous. Crucially, it is largely unregulated. Also, to a large extent, the public health authorities act as both provider and regulator, whereas it is clear that these functions should be separated. In other words, the existing monitoring and regulation of both the private and public health sectors is inadequate.

23.   Accordingly, the Special Rapporteur recommends that autonomous Health Commissions be established, at the federal and State levels, reporting to their legislatures, to monitor and regulate the private and public health sectors, to ensure that they deliver quality health services to all.

24.   Such Commissions need not constrain the health sector but ensure that it operates in a fair and reasonable manner, thereby securing the public's confidence

-----